CASE REVIEW
Head and Neck Imaging

FOURTH EDITION

SERIES EDITOR

David M. Yousem, MD, MBA
Professor of Radiology
Director of Neuroradiology
Russell H. Morgan Department of Radiology and
  Radiological Science
The Johns Hopkins Medical Institutions
Baltimore, Maryland

David M. Yousem, MD, MBA
Professor of Radiology
Director of Neuroradiology
Russell H. Morgan Department of Radiology and
   Radiological Science
The Johns Hopkins Medical Institutions
Baltimore, Maryland

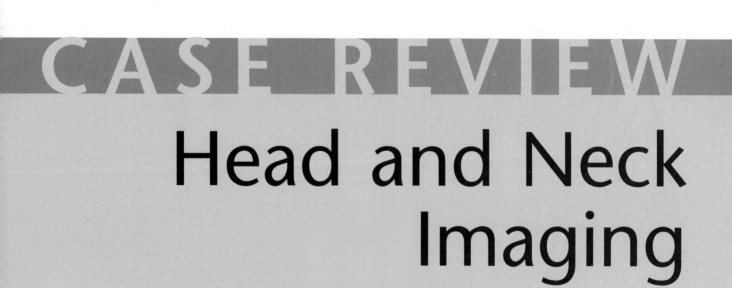

CASE REVIEW

Head and Neck Imaging

FOURTH EDITION

CASE REVIEW SERIES

ELSEVIER
SAUNDERS

ELSEVIER
SAUNDERS

1600 John F. Kennedy Blvd.
Ste 1800
Philadelphia, PA 19103-2899

HEAD AND NECK IMAGING: CASE REVIEW SERIES, FOURTH EDITION   ISBN: 978-1-4557-7629-0

International Standard Book Number: 978-1-4557-7629-0

Senior Content Strategist: Don Scholz
Content Development Specialist: Katy Meert
Publishing Services Manager: Catherine Jackson
Design Direction: Ellen Zanolle

Printed in China

Last digit is the print number: 9   8   7   6   5   4   3   2   1

To all the residents, fellows, and trainees preparing for examinations and the world to follow, and to all the practicing radiologists uncomfortable with head and neck radiology (95% of us??): Good luck. I hope this is helpful on your journey.

To Kelly, my partner now and forever:

To my kids and extended family:

You *are in every second of my life, every day and every way. Thank you for the love and support … always and all ways.*

—DMY

I have been very gratified by the popularity and positive feedback that the authors of the *Case Review* series have received on the publication of the latest editions of their volumes. Reviews in journals and online sites as well as word-of-mouth comments have been uniformly favorable. The authors have done an outstanding job in filling the niche of an affordable, easy-to-access, case-based learning tool that supplements the material in *The Requisites* series. I have been told by residents, fellows, and practicing radiologists that the *Case Review* series books are the ideal means for studying for oral board examinations and subspecialty certification tests.

Although some students learn best in a non-interactive study book mode, others need the anxiety or excitement of being quizzed. The selected format for the *Case Review* series (which consists of showing a few images needed to construct a differential diagnosis and then asking a few clinical and imaging questions) was designed to simulate the Board examination experience. The only difference is that the *Case Review* books provide the correct answer and immediate feedback. The limit and range of the reader's knowledge are tested through scaled cases ranging from relatively easy to very hard. The *Case Review* series also offers feedback on the answers, a brief discussion of each case, a link back to the pertinent *Requisites* volume, and up-to-date references from the literature. In addition, we have recently included labeled figures, figure legends, and supplemental figures in a new section at the end of the book to provide the reader more information about the case and diagnosis.

Because of the popularity of online learning, we have been rolling out new editions with electronic content as well. We also have adjusted to the new (non-oral) Boards format, which will be electronic and largely case-based. The *Case Reviews* are now hosted online at www.expertconsult.com, powered by Inkling. The interactive test-taking format allows users to get real-time feedback, "pinch-and-zoom" figures for easier viewing, and links to supplemental figures and online references. Personally, I am very excited about the future. Join us.

David M. Yousem, MD, MBA

This is the fourth edition of 200 head and neck cases that I have prepared for the *Case Review Series (CRS)*. I wrote this edition with the kind and considerate help of Katy Meert, Content Development Specialist at Elsevier, who worked hard to format and review my cases so that they met the specifications of the new CRS electronic format. This new electronic offering through www.expertconsult.com is a hybrid of the textbook and the fully interactive CRS product we had previously offered. It is now more light and nimble but still very effective in teaching you head and neck radiology.

As I look at my career in neuroradiology (now that I am in my mid-50s), the most gratifying moments have been twofold: (1) having someone come up to me and say "I read your book (*Neuroradiology: The Requisites* or *Head and Neck Imaging: Case Review*) and it helped me get through the Boards. I really enjoyed it," or (2) having someone who I have employed/trained/written letters for get his or her green card and/or become a U.S. citizen. Those two events, passing the Boards and getting a green card, are very special moments.

I hope that this contribution to the literature will allow more people to feel comfortable with head and neck imaging. This is a neat area of radiology, and if you know it well, you add significant value to your imaging team *and* the clinicians. The skull base surgeons, plastic surgeons, dermatologists, oral surgeons, endocrinologists, and otorhinolaryngologists will gravitate to you if you show interest and expertise. You can become the "go to" person for a finite field of radiology in your group. That is special.

I want to thank all my residents and fellows who have inspired me to continue to write textbooks and casebooks that they find valuable. The worth of *Case Review* books is unquestioned. They apply the knowledge base to the interpretation of images that can benefit patient care. *Case Review* books reinforce the didactic teachings of other literature. They allow the development of pattern recognition that is so critical to "knowing" a diagnosis at a glance.

Thank you to Nafi Aygun for the help on the third edition and for his expertise in head and neck imaging. Thanks to the Neuroradiology Division at Johns Hopkins Medical Institutions.

I am proud to submit, for your perusal, *Head and Neck Imaging: Case Review*, Fourth Edition.

David M. Yousem, MD, MBA

CONTENTS

Opening Round

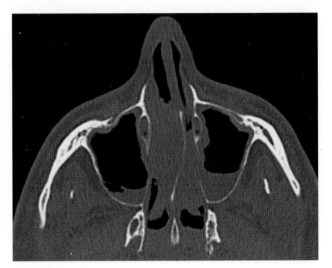

Figure 1-1

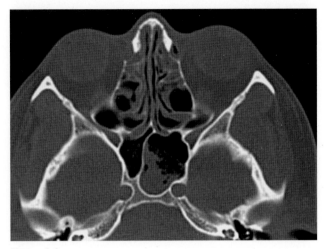

Figure 1-2

HISTORY: A young adult complains of nasal congestion and a runny nose.

1. Which of the following would be included in the differential diagnosis for the imaging findings presented? (Choose all that apply.)
   A. Sinonasal polyposis
   B. Mucocele
   C. Acute sinusitis
   D. Acute on chronic sinusitis

2. Which of the following is *true* about sinusitis?
   A. Acute sinusitis in a patient who is receiving a bone marrow transplant is associated with increased mortality.
   B. Acute sinusitis in a patient who is receiving a bone marrow transplant is associated with transplant rejection.
   C. Chronic sinusitis in a patient who is receiving a bone marrow transplant is associated with decreased mortality.
   D. Screening for sinusitis in a patient receiving a bone marrow transplant has little value.

3. The routes of paranasal sinus drainage include which of the following?
   A. Frontal sinuses to nasolacrimal duct
   B. Maxillary sinus to inferior meatus
   C. Posterior ethmoid to sphenoethmoidal recess
   D. Anterior ethmoid to agger nasi

4. What finding is not indicative of chronic sinusitis?
   A. Air-fluid levels
   B. Mucosal thickening
   C. Osteitis
   D. Polyps
   E. Mucous retention cysts

See Supplemental Figures section for additional figures and legends for this case.

CASE 1

Acute Sinusitis

1. **C and D.** The presence of an air-fluid level implies acute sinusitis. Mucosal thickening may occur with acute or chronic sinusitis. Polyps are usually typical of chronic sinusitis. Osteitis is usually a long-term consequence.

2. **A.** Acute sinusitis in a patient undergoing bone marrow transplantation has direct effect on long-term prognosis. Hence clinicians often scan the patient before bone marrow transplantation and treat sinusitis as needed.

3. **C.** Frontal sinuses drain to the frontal recess; the maxillary sinus drains to the ostium and infundibulum and then to the middle meatus, posterior ethmoid, and sphenoid sinus via the sphenoethmoidal recess. The anterior ethmoids also drain to the middle meatus.

4. **A.** An air-fluid level is a finding indicative of an acute process. Mucosal thickening can occur in acute or chronic sinusitis. Osteitis, mucous retention cysts, and polyps occur in chronic sinusitis.

Comment

Imaging Findings

The imaging findings that imply acute sinusitis include new mucosal thickening, air-fluid levels (Figure S1-1), and air bubbles in sinus secretions (Figure S1-2) even in the absence of an air-fluid level. The misconception that mucosal edema/ thickening occurs only in chronic sinusitis is rampant, but this author, who underwent serial imaging of himself during the course of 14 days of antibiotics and intranasal steroid therapy, demonstrated that mucosal thickening appears and resolves over that period of time along with symptoms.

Sites of Obstruction

When reviewing cases of chronic and acute sinusitis, clinicians should note the potential obstructive sites that may be the underlying cause of the sinusitis. Radiologists should report on areas of mucosal thickening and narrowings of the maxillary sinus ostia, hiatus semilunaris, infundibulum, and middle meatus in cases of maxillary and ethmoid sinusitis. For frontal sinusitis, the frontal (ethmoidal) recess and middle meatus should be scrutinized. For posterior ethmoid and sphenoid sinusitis, the spheno-ethmoidal recess should be assessed for obstruction.

Pathogens

Viral and bacterial microorganisms are the usual culprits in an immunocompetent individual with acute sinusitis. Rhinoviruses, influenza virus, parainfluenza virus, and respiratory syncytial virus are the leading viral pathogens. *Streptococcus pneumoniae, Haemophilus influenzae, Moraxella catarrhalis, Streptococcus pyogenes,* and *Staphylococcus aureus* constitute the usual bacteria.

Reference

Wittkopf ML, Beddow PA, Russell PT, Duncavage JA, Becker SS. Revisiting the interpretation of positive sinus CT findings: a radiological and symptom-based review. *Otolaryngol Head Neck Surg.* 2009;140(3):306-311.

Cross-Reference

Neuroradiology: The Requisites, 3rd ed, 425.

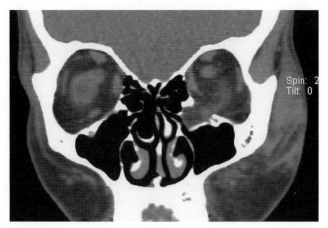

Figure 2-1

HISTORY: A young man complains of eye pain and has contusions after being punched in the left side of the face.

1. Which facial bone or bones appear to be fractured in Figure 2-1? (Choose all that apply.)
   A. Orbital floor
   B. Lamina papyracea
   C. Anterior maxillary spine
   D. Zygomatic arch

2. With regard to orbital fractures, which of the follow is *true?*
   A. The lamina papyracea is fractured more commonly than the orbital floor.
   B. The orbital floor is fractured more commonly than the orbital rim.
   C. The orbital roof is fractured more commonly than the lateral orbital wall.
   D. The orbital septum is fractured more commonly than the orbital spine.

3. What is the difference between a trap door deformity (single fracture swinging downward) and Bombay door deformity (two fracture fragments swinging downward) of the orbital floor?
   A. The number of fragments depressed
   B. The incidence of diplopia
   C. The coincidence of medial orbital wall fracture
   D. The age of the fracture

4. Which of the following is correlated with the degree of early and late enophthalmos?
   A. Orbital fracture volume
   B. Size of hematoma
   C. Concurrent hyperthyroidism
   D. Entrapment

See Supplemental Figures section for additional figures and legends for this case.

CASE 2

Facial Fracture

1. **A and B.** The orbital floor and its common wall with the medial orbit (the lamina papyracea) are fractured.

2. **B.** The orbital floor is fractured more commonly than the other walls. After fractures of the floor, the most common fractures are of the lamina papyracea, then the rim, and then the lateral orbital wall.

3. **A.** The incidence of diplopia is the same. There is no difference in the coincidence of medial orbital wall fracture or age of the fracture.

4. **A.** The orbital fracture volume and the degree of floor depression are well correlated with the presence of enophthalmos and/or hypoglobus.

Comment

Complications of Orbital Fractures

The long-term complications of orbital fracture include enophthalmos and diplopia. The former is more commonly associated with higher volume orbital fractures with greater displacement of orbital contents. Diplopia after repair of orbital fractures occurs at a higher frequency if the initial computed tomographic scan at the time of injury shows extraocular muscle enlargement. In this example, the orbital floor fragment rotates like a trap door (Figure S2-1).

Incidence of Facial Bone Fractures

In children, mandibular fractures outnumber orbital fractures, and motor vehicle accidents are the most common scenarios of injury. At all ages, nasal bone fractures predominate.

LeFort fractures include those that affect the maxilla (LeFort I), the orbital floor (LeFort II), and the lateral orbital walls (LeFort III). Fractures of the pterygoid plates consistently accompany these LeFort fractures.

Reference

Jin HR, Lee HS, Yeon JY, Suh MW. Residual diplopia after repair of pure orbital blowout fracture: the importance of extraocular muscle injury. *Am J Rhinol.* 2007;21(3):276-280. doi:10.2500/ajr.2007.21. 3024

Cross-Reference

Neuroradiology: The Requisites, 3rd ed, 188-189, 341-342.

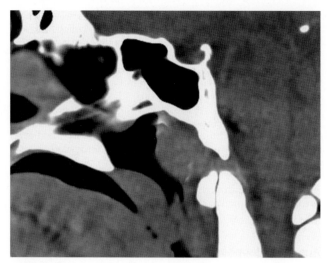

Figure 3-1

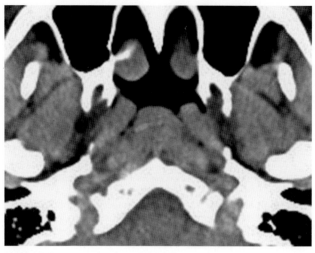

Figure 3-2

HISTORY: A 52-year-old woman presents with ear congestion.

1. Which of the following would be included in the differential diagnosis for the imaging findings presented? (Choose all that apply.)
   A. Lymphoid hyperplasia
   B. Lymphoma
   C. Tornwaldt cyst
   D. Juvenile nasopharyngeal angiofibroma (JNA)

2. What type of lymphoma has a predilection for the nasopharynx?
   A. Hodgkin lymphoma
   B. Burkitt lymphoma
   C. Undifferentiated carcinoma
   D. Non-Hodgkin lymphoma

3. What is the best imaging finding that suggests lymphoid hyperplasia rather than tumor?
   A. High signal on T2-weighted image
   B. Striated enhancement pattern
   C. Crenated nodularity
   D. Cyst formation

4. What is the most common cause of obstructive sleep apnea in children?
   A. Tonsillar enlargement
   B. Uvular hypertrophy
   C. Adenoidal hypertrophy
   D. Lingual thyroid glands

See Supplemental Figures section for additional figures and legends for this case.

CASE 3

Adenoidal Hypertrophy

1. **A and B.** Lymphoid hyperplasia and lymphoma may look alike, and both should be included in the differential diagnosis. Tornwaldt cysts are midline cysts of low density. Juvenile nasopharyngeal angiofibroma is more likely to occur in a teenaged boy and not in a 52-year-old woman.

2. **D.** The non-Hodgkin lymphoma has a predilection for the nasopharynx; it is usually a diffuse-type, large-cell cancer. Undifferentiated carcinoma is not a lymphoma.

3. **B.** High signal on T2-weighted image in lymphoid hyperplasia is uncommon, and so it would not help in determining lymphoid hyperplasia. The striated appearance suggests lymphoid hyperplasia.

4. **C.** Adenoidal hypertrophy can lead to cardiovascular complications, including pulmonary hypertension and right-sided heart failure. Although lingual thyroid glands can cause obstructive sleep apnea in children, it is a rare condition and not the most common cause.

Comment

Associations with Lymphoid Hyperplasia

Lymphoid hyperplasia (Figure S3-1 sagittal and Figure S3-2 axial) can affect the nasopharyngeal adenoidal tissue, the palatine tonsils, and the lingual tonsil tissue. It may be associated with lymph node enlargement as well. Most cases are reactive to adjacent inflammation, such as an upper respiratory or sinonasal tract infection; however, chronic illnesses such as human immunodeficiency virus (HIV) disease, collagen vascular diseases, and immunosuppressive conditions (such as that after organ transplantation) may also lead to such enlargements. Patients with atopic or seasonal allergies may have more lymphoid tissue present. Epstein-Barr virus (EBV) is the virus most closely associated with adenoidal hypertrophy, which is problematic because EBV also is associated with nasopharyngeal carcinoma. However, virtually all viruses can cause enlargement of the adenoidal pad in children and even in an adult whose adenoids had previously atrophied.

Effect of Lymphoid Hyperplasia

Adenoidal hypertrophy can lead to snoring, chronic mouth breathing, obstructive sleep apnea, and otitis media. Secondary right-sided heart failure and pulmonary hypertension may coexist.

Age and Nasopharyngeal Adenoidal Prominence

Adenoidal tissue enlarges in the first decade of life, but by the end of the second decade, it should regress. When tissue in the nasopharynx is enlarged in an adult, particularly if obstructing the eustachian tube, the clinician should consider the possibility of carcinoma and lymphoma. A linear striated enhancement pattern provides reassurance that the condition is simply adenoidal hypertrophy of a benign nature.

Reference

Rout MR, Mohanty D, Vijaylaxmi Y, Bobba K, Metta C. Adenoid hypertrophy in adults: a case series. *Indian J Otolaryngol Head Neck Surg.* 2013;65(3):269-274. doi:10.1007/s12070-012-0549-y

Cross-Reference

Neuroradiology: The Requisites, 3rd ed, 441-442.

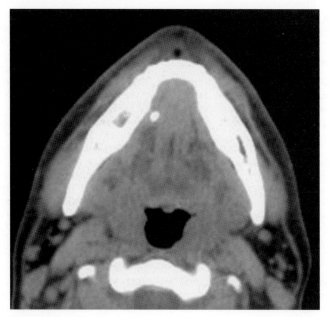

Figure 4-1

HISTORY: The patient is experiencing intermittent pain in the submandibular region while eating.

1. Which of the following would be included in the differential diagnosis for the imaging findings presented? (Choose all that apply.)
   A. Phlebolith
   B. Ectopic tooth
   C. Calculus
   D. Squamous cell carcinoma

2. What is the name of the main duct of the submandibular gland (SMG)?
   A. Stensen
   B. Rivinus
   C. Bartholin
   D. Wharton

3. Which of the following is *not* a rationale for why the SMG has more calculi than the parotid gland?
   A. Secretions of the SMG have a lower pH.
   B. Secretions of the SMG are more viscous.
   C. Secretions of the SMG drain in an uphill direction.
   D. The SMG has a wider duct.

4. Which of the following types of SMG stone is most common?
   A. Uric acid
   B. Calcium bicarbonate
   C. Calcium bisphosphonate
   D. Calcium oxalate

See Supplemental Figures section for additional figures and legends for this case.

CASE 4

Submandibular Gland Calculus

1. **C.** The phlebolith is not the right shape or consistency and an ectopic tooth would not be in this location. Squamous cell carcinoma does not manifest as a calcification. The calculus is located in the submandibular duct.

2. **D.** Wharton duct drains the SMG, whereas Stensen duct drains the parotid gland, and the ducts of Rivinus and Bartholin drain the sublingual glands.

3. **A.** The SMG secretes saliva that is more basic (higher pH) than secretions of the parotid gland, and therefore calcium oxalate or calcium phosphate stones are *more* likely to be created. The duct runs uphill, and the saliva is more viscous and therefore is more prone to stasis, which leads to stones.

4. **D.** Uric acid and calcium bicarbonate stones are rare, and calcium **bisphosphonate** stones are uncommon. Calcium oxalate stones are the second most common after **calcium phosphate.**

Comment

Imaging for Stones

Computed tomography (CT) is the most sensitive test for detection of salivary stones/calculi. Contrast enhancement is not necessary unless a coexistent abscess is suspected. Affected patients typically have pain on salivation and therefore when eating, particularly sour foods.

Higher Risk for Stones in the Submandibular Gland

Stones form four times as often in the SMG system as in the parotid gland; stones in the other salivary glands are not really represented to any degree. The reasons why the SMG has more stones have been elucidated above. The ductal orifice of the SMG is also somewhat tighter, which leads to stasis more commonly, and that duct is easily traumatized. Stones are most commonly calcium phosphate, and calcium hydroxyapatite/oxalate stones are second most common.

Site of Stones

Of all SMG stones, 85% are located in the Wharton duct (Figure S4-1), and 15% are in the gland parenchyma. The most common ductal site is in the proximal duct, close to the gland. Only 30% get stuck at the orifice in the anterior floor of the mouth. Usual sizes are less than 10 mm in diameter; those larger than 35 mm are considered "giant." All stones can lead to severe pain and disruption of the floor of the mouth in which the Wharton duct runs.

Systemic Diseases and Stones

Sjögren syndrome and sarcoidosis, as well as all forms of chronic sialadenitis, are associated with an increased rate of stone formation. A Küttner tumor is a pseudomass that simulates a neoplasm on palpation but is actually a complication of chronic sialadenitis with associated sclerosis, calcifications, and ductal dilatation.

Reference

Rai M, Burman R. Giant submandibular sialolith of remarkable size in the comma area of Wharton's duct: a case report. *J Oral Maxillofac Surg.* 2009;67(6):1329-1332. doi:10.1016/j.joms.2008.11.014

Cross-Reference

Neuroradiology: The Requisites, 3rd ed, 476-477, 478-479, 483-484.

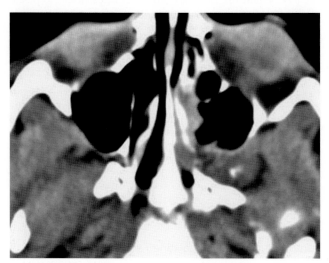

Figure 5-1

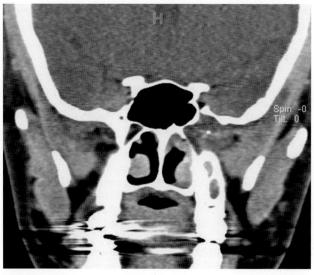

Figure 5-2

HISTORY: A 25-year-old woman has left-sided sinus pain.

1. Which of the following would be included in the differential diagnosis for the imaging findings presented? (Choose all that apply.)
   A. Schwannoma
   B. Meningioma
   C. Epidermoid
   D. Squamous cell carcinoma
   E. Chondrosarcoma

2. What is the cranial nerve intrinsic to the pterygopalatine fossa (PPF)?
   A. V_1
   B. V_2
   C. V_3
   D. VII

3. Which benign vascular tumor has a predilection for the PPF?
   A. Meningioma
   B. Hemangioma
   C. Juvenile nasopharyngeal angiofibroma
   D. Venous vascular malformation

4. For what malignancy is perineural spread most common?
   A. Squamous cell carcinoma
   B. Nasopharyngeal carcinoma
   C. Adenoid cystic carcinoma
   D. Melanoma

See Supplemental Figures section for additional figures and legends for this case.

CASE 5

Trigeminal Schwannoma

1. **A.** Meningioma would be unusual outside the central nervous system. Epidermoid would be cystic. Squamous cell carcinoma would have mucosal extension. Chondrosarcoma does not occur at this site. Schwannoma can occur in the PPF.

2. **B.** The second division (V$_2$) of the cranial nerve V (trigeminal nerve) is the maxillary nerve, and it is associated with the PPF (with a ganglion there). The mandibular nerve (V$_3$) is associated with foramen ovale, and the ophthalmic nerve (V$_1$) goes through the superior orbital fissure and branches into lacrimal, frontal, and nasociliary nerves.

3. **C.** Juvenile nasopharyngeal angiofibroma commonly infiltrates the PPF from its origin at the sphenopalatine foramen.

4. **C.** Squamous cell carcinoma and melanoma do not demonstrate perineural spread as commonly as adenoid cystic carcinoma, which has a 50% to 60% rate of perineural spread. Nasopharyngeal carcinoma grows here by direct spread, not perineural extension.

Comment

Anatomy of the Pterygopalatine Fossa

The main structures of the PPF are branches of the maxillary nerve, pterygopalatine ganglion, internal maxillary artery branches, and nerve of the pterygoid canal (Vidian nerve). It sits just behind the maxillary sinus but leads from the palate to the intracranial compartment. The Vidian nerve receives innervation from parts of the superficial petrosal branch of cranial nerve VII, and it receives parasympathetic innervation from the deep petrosal sympathetic plexus.

Exits from the Pterygopalatine Fossa

Exits from the pterygopalatine foramen include the greater and lesser palatine canals inferiorly, the Vidian canal and foramen rotundum posteriorly, the sphenopalatine foramen and palatovaginal canal medially, the inferior orbital fissure anterolaterally, and the pterygomaxillary fissure laterally. Spread to and from these regions by tumors that have a propensity for perineural spread (adenoid cystic carcinoma in particular) may fill the PPF. Skin lesions such as basal cell carcinoma or aggressive melanomas, mucosal squamous cell carcinomas of the pharynx and oral cavity, and nasopharyngeal carcinoma may also invade the PPF via the nerves.

Tumors of the Pterygopalatine Fossa

The most common primary tumors of the PPF are schwannomas (Figures S5-1 and S5-2). Juvenile nasopharyngeal angiofibromas frequently inhabit the same space. Secondary spread is usually either from perineural spread of tumors or directly from sinonasal, facial, or nasopharyngeal primary cancers.

Reference

Williams LS. Advanced concepts in the imaging of perineural spread of tumor to the trigeminal nerve. *Top Magn Reson Imaging.* 1999; 10(6):376-383. doi:10.1097/00002142-199912000-00004

Cross-Reference

Neuroradiology: The Requisites, 3rd ed, 357, 598.

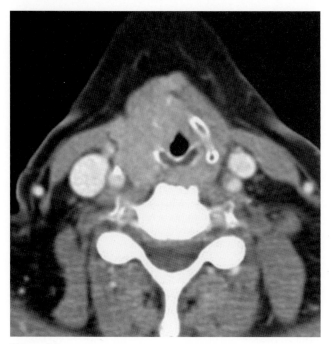

Figure 6-1

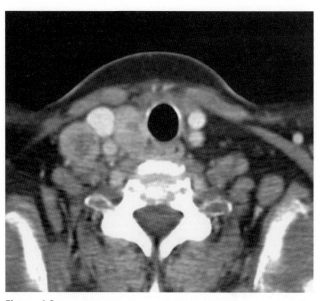

Figure 6-2

HISTORY: A middle-aged man presents with voice changes and a palpable neck mass.

1. Which of the following should be included in the differential diagnosis for the imaging findings presented? (Choose all that apply.)
   A. Laryngeal cancer
   B. Thyroid cancer
   C. Esophageal cancer
   D. Piriform sinus cancer

2. In how many cases does thyroid cancer erode the larynx?
   A. 1% to 5%
   B. 6% to 10%
   C. 11% to 15%
   D. >15%

3. In how many cases does thyroid cancer erode the trachea?
   A. 1% to 5%
   B. 6% to 10%
   C. 11% to 15%
   D. >15%

4. In how many cases does thyroid cancer erode the esophagus?
   A. 1% to 5%
   B. 6% to 10%
   C. 11% to 15%
   D. >15%

See Supplemental Figures section for additional figures and legends for this case.

CASE 6

Thyroid Cancer

1. **A, B, and D.** Thyroid cancer is invading the thyroid cartilage on the right and has right-sided nodal metastases. Laryngeal cancer and piriform sinus cancer can also be included in the differential diagnosis because they also may erode cartilage, but the site of esophageal cancer is too remote.

2. **B.** Thyroid cancer typically erodes the larynx in 6% to 10% of cases.

3. **B.** Thyroid cancer typically erodes the trachea in 6% to 10% of cases.

4. **A.** Thyroid cancer typically erodes the esophagus in 1% to 5% of cases. Esophageal erosion is less common than laryngotracheal invasion.

Comment

Invasion of Adjacent Structures by Thyroid Cancer

Laryngeal and tracheal invasion by thyroid cancer is uncommon because thyroid cancer is often detected while it is still indolent, often as an incidental finding. Imaging findings are most accurate for tracheal invasion when one identifies soft tissue in the cartilage (Figure S6-1), an intraluminal mass, and tumor encircling the trachea by 180 degrees or more. These findings, in combination, yield 100% sensitivity and 84% specificity. To detect esophageal invasion, the clinician should look for abnormal T2-weighted wall signal, enhancement in the esophageal wall, or circumferential involvement by greater than 180 degrees to suggest its invasion. The incidence of aerodigestive system invasion by thyroid cancer varies by the histologic subtype. Anaplastic carcinoma, although a very rare subtype, invades the airway in as many as 20% of cases, whereas the well-differentiated papillary and follicular cancers are much less likely to do so. Strap muscle involvement is the most common type of extrathyroidal spread, followed by involvement of the trachea, larynx, recurrent laryngeal nerve, and esophagus. These structures may be infiltrated by direct spread of the thyroid cancer or via metastatic lymph nodes (Figure S6-2), particularly those in a paratracheal location. When invasion occurs, hemoptysis, stridor, difficulty breathing as a result of aspiration of blood, and viscus perforation may lead to superimposed infection and other complications.

Neck Masses

Lymph nodes and thyroid nodules are the most common palpable abnormalities in the neck in adults, whereas reactive lymph nodes are the most common palpable neck abnormalities in children.

Reference

Honings J, Stephen AE, Marres HA, Gaissert HA. The management of thyroid carcinoma invading the larynx or trachea. *Laryngoscope.* 2010;120(4):682-689. doi:10.1002/lary.20800

Cross-Reference

Neuroradiology: The Requisites, 3rd ed, 508.

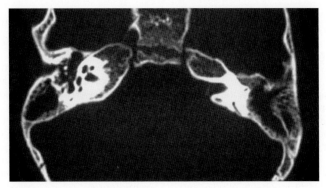

Figure 7-1

HISTORY: A young adult presents with fever, acute bilateral ear pain, and sensation of fullness in the ears in association with mild conductive hearing loss.

1. Which of the following should be included in the differential diagnosis for this case of temporal bone inflammatory disease? (Choose all that apply.)
   A. Otomastoiditis
   B. Isolated otitis media
   C. Coalescent mastoiditis
   D. Cholesteatoma

2. What is the importance of coalescence in mastoiditis?
   A. Destruction of the bony septa effectively creates osteomyelitis and intramastoid empyema.
   B. It can lead to an extramastoid collection and spread of infection.
   C. It necessitates more aggressive antibiotic therapy and, potentially, surgery.
   D. All of the above are important.

3. In an adult presenting with unexplained serous otitis media and or mastoid effusions, which of the following conditions must be primarily considered?
   A. Human immunodeficiency virus (HIV) infection
   B. Incompetent eustachian tube
   C. Cerebrospinal fluid (CSF) leak
   D. Nasopharyngeal carcinoma

4. Which of the following statements is *not* true?
   A. The Macewen triangle is the space between the posterior wall of the external acoustic meatus and the posterior zygomatic process.
   B. Griesinger's sign is erythema and edema over the mastoid process as a result of septic thrombosis of the mastoid emissary vein.
   C. A Bezold abscess is a complication of mastoiditis in which fluid collects just below the mastoid.
   D. Tuberculous mastoiditis is manifested by the classic triad of multiple tympanic membrane perforations, brightly erythematous bloody inflammatory tympanic membrane thickening, and facial paralysis.

See Supplemental Figures section for additional figures and legends for this case.

CASE 7

Otomastoiditis and Coalescent Mastoiditis

1. **A and C.** The image shows opacification of both mastoid antra with erosion of the septa of the mastoid air cells, which are consistent with coalescent mastoiditis and otomastoiditis. Otitis media is middle ear disease, and a cholesteatoma would not manifest acutely in this way, although it may erode bone.

2. **D.** If there is coalescence, the prognosis is worse and more aggressive treatment is required. It is analogous to osteomyelitis.

3. **D.** A nasopharyngeal carcinoma can obstruct the eustachian tube at the torus tubarius. A CSF leak is very rare.

4. **D.** Tuberculous inflammation is colorless or pale.

Comment

Importance of Diagnosing Coalescent Mastoiditis

Coalescent mastoiditis is rare as long as children and parents are compliant with administration of prescribed antibiotics. Once coalescence of otomastoiditis—depicted as loss of mastoid air cell septations (Figure S7-1)—occurs, the infection is much more serious and may necessitate surgery and/or intravenous antibiotics. A trial of myringotomy and drainage with parenteral antibiotics may be initiated; mastoidectomy is reserved for cases in which the response is inadequate.

Complications of Otomastoiditis

The propensity for developing subperiosteal or extramastoid (i.e., Bezold) abscesses or persistent infection is a known complication of coalescent mastoiditis. Intracranial spread of disease can lead to epidural abscesses, as well as venous sinus thrombosis. Although mastoid emissary veins may be involved initially (hence Griesinger's sign), the spread may lead to sigmoid or transverse sinus thrombosis.

Pathogens

Pathogens usually include *Streptococcus pneumoniae, Streptococcus pyogenes, Staphylococcus aureus,* and *Pseudomonas aeruginosa.*

Middle Ear/Mastoid Fluid Implications

In adults, the presence of otomastoiditis or noninflamed effusions should prompt the examination of the nasopharynx to confirm or rule out an obstructing lesion. Because nasopharyngeal carcinoma can be a disease of young adulthood, particularly in the Southeast Asian population, such examinations should be performed in all affected individuals past childhood.

Reference

Vazquez E, Castellote A, Piqueras J, Mauleon S, Creixell S, Pumarola F, et al. Imaging of complications of acute mastoiditis in children. *Radiographics.* 2003;23(2):359-372.

Cross-Reference

Neuroradiology: The Requisites, 3rd ed, 394.

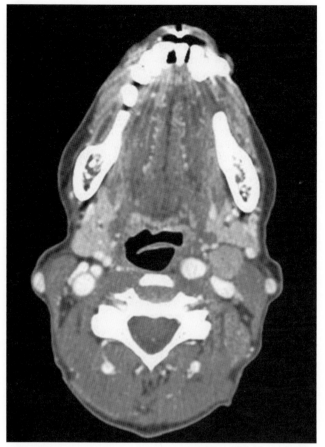

Figure 8-1

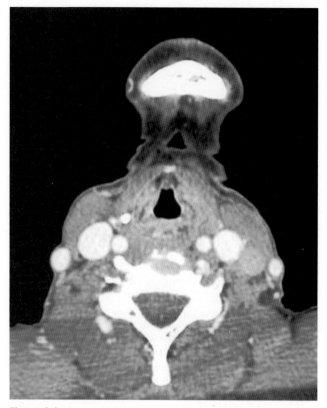

Figure 8-2

HISTORY: The patient presents with left-sided neck mass and has a history of head and neck cancer.

1. Which of the following should be included in the differential diagnosis? (Choose all that apply.)
   A. Recurrent cancer
   B. Benign adenopathy
   C. Schwannoma
   D. Meningioma

2. What size criterion would provide a 90% assurance that the node is nonneoplastic, according to the landmark Radiology Diagnostic Oncology Group (RDOG) study?
   A. 15 mm
   B. 12 mm
   C. 10 mm
   D. 8 mm
   E. None of the above

3. What is the expected accuracy of fine-needle aspiration (FNA) for metastatic lymph nodes?
   A. 0% to 20%
   B. 21% to 40%
   C. 41% to 60%
   D. 61% to 80%
   E. >80%

4. Which is *not* a possible source of an enhancing node?
   A. Thyroid cancer
   B. Castleman disease
   C. Kimura disease
   D. Lymphoma
   E. None of the above

See Supplemental Figures section for additional figures and legends for this case.

CASE 8

Lymph Node in Setting of Prior History of Cancer

1. **A.** Given the size of the nodes in the presence of obvious radiation changes, recurrent or residual cancer has to be the top diagnosis.

2. **E.** To achieve 90% negative predictive value, the criterion for size should be 5 mm.

3. **E.** FNA generally has 80% to 85% accuracy in evaluation of lymph nodes.

4. **E.** All four of the diagnoses listed are possible, so E (none of the above) is correct. Of the four diagnoses provided, lymphoma is the least likely to produce highly enhancing lymph nodes.

Comment

Radiology Diagnostic Oncology Group Landmark Study

The RDOG study revealed that with the 10-mm cutoff, computed tomography (CT) was only 39% specific and 88% sensitive for detecting disease, and magnetic resonance imaging (MRI) did not perform much better (48% and 81%, respectively). The RDOG study demonstrated that a 5-mm cutoff was needed to achieve a 90% rate of correctly predicting a negative node, but that left a false-positive rate of 56%. For the evaluation of nodes, most clinicians favor CT (Figures S8-1 and S8-2) over MRI because the presence of necrosis and extracapsular spread is more evident with CT.

Nodal Evaluation: Positron Emission Tomography versus Fine-Needle Aspiration

FNA has been supplanted by positron emission tomography (PET) for evaluation of nodes after treatment. However, during the initial period immediately after radiation therapy, radiation changes can cause false-positive results; therefore, PET should be performed after a 3-month delay. PET is highly accurate. PET may also help detect a primary tumor when a metastatic node is present and no mucosal lesion is evident.

Thyroid Cancer Adenopathy

Thyroid carcinoma is the most mystical as far as nodal disease. A patient can have cystic, calcified, avidly enhancing, retropharyngeal, necrotic, solid, and colloid-containing lymph nodes from thyroid cancer. The size criteria described previously apply only to squamous cell carcinoma. Thus nodes in the presence of thyroid cancer should be described fully even if smaller than 10 mm in diameter. The average size of thyroid cancer metastatic nodes in the central portion of the neck (level VI) is about 3 to 4 mm.

Reference

Curtin HD, Ishwaran H, Mancuso AA, Dalley RW, Caudry DJ, McNeil BJ. Comparison of CT and MR imaging in staging of neck metastases. *Radiology.* 1998;207(1):123-130.

Cross-Reference

Neuroradiology: The Requisites, 3rd ed, 439-440, 444, 447, 470-471, 471-472, 472.

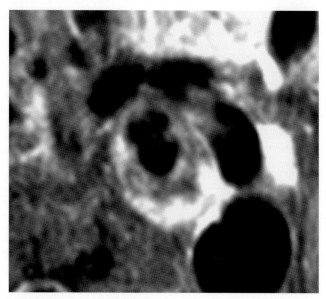

Figure 9-1

HISTORY: An elderly man has a carotid bruit and a history of a transient ischemic attack.

1. Which of the following should be included in the differential diagnosis for the imaging findings presented? (Choose all that apply.)
   A. Carotid atherosclerotic plaque
   B. Carotid dissection
   C. Carotid pseudoaneurysm
   D. Carotid occlusion

2. Which of the following is most thrombogenic?
   A. Intimal calcification
   B. Exposed lipid core
   C. Exposed muscularis
   D. Carotid wall vasa vasorum

3. Which of these percentages of stenosis is an indication for carotid endarterectomy according to the North American Symptomatic Carotid Endarterectomy Trial (NASCET) criteria?
   A. 25%
   B. 50%
   C. 75%
   D. 100%

4. Which of the following is *not* a risk factor for stroke?
   A. Thin ruptured fibrous cap
   B. Intraplaque hemorrhage
   C. Carotid stenosis of more than 70%
   D. Calcified plaque

See Supplemental Figures section for additional figures and legends for this case.

CASE 9

Carotid Atherosclerotic Plaque

1. **A.** This is an atherosclerotic plaque. There is no flap (dissection), outpouching (aneurysm), or luminal clot (occlusion).

2. **B.** The lipid core of an atherosclerotic plaque is highly thrombogenic. Therefore, thinning or rupture of the fibrous cap, which causes exposure of the lipid core, is a high-risk event.

3. **C.** Most clinicians prefer medical treatment for 50% to 70% stenosis, but for more than 70% stenosis, carotid endarterectomy is the preferred treatment option. The role of stents has not been adequately determined.

4. **D.** The presence of hemorrhage in the plaque, the ruptured fibrous cap of the plaque, and the high degree of stenosis are the factors that increase the risk of stroke, not the presence of calcification.

Comment

North American Symptomatic Carotid Endarterectomy Trial

The NASCET criterion of more than 70% stenosis as an indication for carotid endarterectomy surgery to prevent subsequent stroke has been used for decades. NASCET showed a significant benefit of endarterectomy in patients with 70% to 99% symptomatic stenosis; the medically treated group had a 2-year risk for ipsilateral stroke of 26%, whereas in patients treated with carotid endarterectomy, the risk was only 9%. Although some clinicians believe that, in men, 60% stenosis is important and a surgical indication, most still base the decision of surgery on a 70% value. However, using only stenosis as an indication is increasingly considered a simplistic approach to managing carotid plaque.

Plaque Composition

Wasserman and colleagues showed the value of contrast-enhanced magnetic resonance imaging (MRI) of plaques. When the circulating cells are exposed to lipid core, particularly necrotic cores, thrombi often develop. What overlies the lipid core is the fibrous cap, which enhances on MRI (Figure S9-1). Therefore, thinning or rupture of the fibrous cap increases the risk for thrombi and subsequent stroke. Also, intraplaque hemorrhage is a risk factor for subsequent stroke and leads to increased volumes of the wall and the lipid-rich necrotic core. Another risk factor, seemingly independent of stenosis, is adventitial enhancement circumferentially of more than 50%.

Ultrasonography and Plaque

On ultrasonography, intima-media thicknesses of the internal carotid artery and common carotid artery and carotid plaque volumes have been shown to be helpful in predicting the risk of subsequent stroke.

References

Etesami M, Hoi Y, Steinman DA, Gujar SK, Nidecker AE, Astor BC, et al. Comparison of carotid plaque ulcer detection using contrast-enhanced and time-of-flight MRA techniques. *AJNR Am J Neuroradiol.* 2013;34(1):177-184. Epub 2012 May 24. doi:10.3174/ajnr. A3132

Wasserman BA, Wityk RJ, Trout HH III, Virmani R. Low-grade carotid stenosis: looking beyond the lumen with MRI. *Stroke.* 2005;36(11):2504-2513.

Cross-Reference

Neuroradiology: The Requisites, 3rd ed, 105-107.

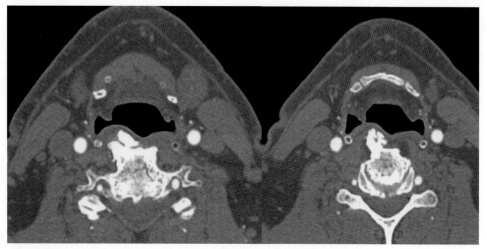

Figure 10-1

HISTORY: An elderly woman experiences pain when swallowing, but endoscopy reveals no abnormality.

1. Which of the following should be included in the differential diagnosis? (Choose all that apply.)
   A. Diffuse idiopathic skeletal hyperostosis (DISH)
   B. Osteophyte
   C. Osteoma
   D. Submucosal osteosarcoma

2. Which is a criterion for DISH?
   A. Flowing calcifications and ossifications along the anterolateral aspect of at least two contiguous vertebral bodies
   B. Decrease in disk height in the involved areas with excessive disk disease
   C. Sacroiliac erosions and sclerosis
   D. Flowing calcifications and ossifications along the anterolateral aspect of at least four contiguous vertebral bodies

3. Osteophytic compression of the submucosa of the aerodigestive system most commonly results in what complaint?
   A. Obstructive sleep apnea
   B. Stridor
   C. Reflux
   D. Dysphagia

4. Aspiration with dysphagia is associated with an anterior osteophyte of what size?
   A. 0 to 4 mm
   B. 5 to 8 mm
   C. 9 to 12 mm
   D. No specific size

See Supplemental Figures section for additional figures and legends for this case.

CASE 10

Osteophyte Compressing Pharynx

1. **A and B.** DISH requires flowing osteophytes across four vertebral body levels. On this axial image, it is not possible to assess extent.

2. **D.** Flowing calcifications and ossifications along the antero-lateral aspect of at least four contiguous vertebral bodies, without significant decrease in disk and absence of sacro-iliac erosions and sclerosis, are suggestive of DISH.

3. **D.** Most osteophytes are asymptomatic, but if a patient does have a symptom, it is dysphagia.

4. **C.** The larger the osteophyte, the higher is the risk for dysphagia and aspiration. They are usually larger than 1 cm when symptomatic.

Comment

Osteophytes and Dysphagia

Anterior osteophytes from the cervical spine (Figure S10-1) are very common. They occur in 20% of patients older than 70. However, they account only rarely for patients' complaint of dysphagia. Osteophytes account for symptoms in only 1% to 3% of patients with dysphagia. Patients with DISH may have the highest risk. However, older patients with concurrent disease and osteophytes larger than 10 mm are at higher risk for aspiration in association with DISH or degenerative osteophytosis.

DISH Criteria

Donald Resnick's criteria for DISH are listed as follows:
- The presence of flowing calcification and ossification along the anterolateral aspect of at least four contiguous vertebral bodies with or without associated localized pointed excrescences at the intervening vertebral body-intervertebral disc junctions
- The presence of relative preservation of intervertebral disk height in the involved vertebral segment and the absence of extensive radiographic changes of "degenerative" disk disease, including vacuum phenomena and marginal sclerosis of vertebral bodies
- The absence of apophyseal joint bony ankylosis and sacroiliac joint erosion, sclerosis, or intra-articular osseous fusion

Treatment

When dysphagia, aspiration, or obstructive sleep apnea is attributed to osteophytes, surgical removal may be useful. The success rate is higher than 80%, but there are antecedent risks of vocal cord paralysis, bleeding, infection, and vascular injury. Nonetheless, it is not difficult surgery.

Reference

Fuerderer S, Eysel-Gosepath K, Schröder U, Delank KS, Eysel P. Retro-pharyngeal obstruction in association with osteophytes of the cervical spine. *J Bone Joint Surg Br.* 2004;86(6):837-840.

Cross-Reference

Neuroradiology: The Requisites, 3rd ed, 531-533.

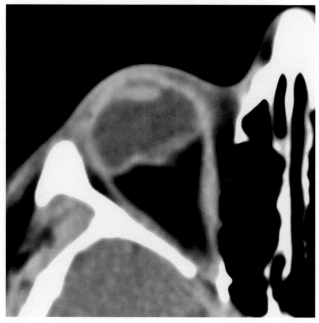

Figure 11-1

HISTORY: The patient presents with orbital trauma and monocular blindness, and the ophthalmologist cannot see beyond the anterior chamber.

1. Which of the following should be included in the differential diagnosis? (Choose all that apply.)
   A. Anterior chamber rupture
   B. Anterior hyphema
   C. Vitreous rupture
   D. Ocular hypotony

2. Which part of the globe ruptures most commonly?
   A. The vitreous
   B. The posterior chamber
   C. The anterior chamber
   D. The choroid

3. What is the normal intraocular pressure, and what defines ocular hypotony?
   A. Normal pressure is between 10 and 20 mm Hg, and ocular hypotony is pressure less than 5 mm Hg.
   B. Normal pressure is between 20 and 30 mm Hg, and ocular hypotony is pressure less than 10 mm Hg.
   C. Normal pressure is between 5 and 10 mm Hg, and ocular hypotony is pressure less than 2 mm Hg.
   D. Normal pressure is between 100 and 120 mm Hg, and ocular hypotony is pressure less than 50 mm Hg.

4. What is wrong with the patient's lens?
   A. Traumatic cataract and dislocation
   B. Traumatic cataract
   C. Lens dislocation
   D. Nothing (it is normal)

See Supplemental Figures section for additional figures and legends for this case.

CASE 11

Globe Rupture

1. **A, B, C, and D.** The patient exhibits increased density in the anterior chamber (anterior hyphema) with a shallow anterior chamber (anterior chamber rupture) and a flattened vitreous (rupture and ocular hypotony).

2. **C.** The anterior chamber ruptures most commonly because it is the first defense against trauma, being most superficial.

3. **A.** Normal ocular pressure is between 10 and 20 mm Hg, and in ocular hypotony, pressure is less than 5 mm Hg. This can lead to the flattened appearance of the vitreous when it ruptures.

4. **A.** The lens has abnormal density (cataract) and is slightly medial to its normal location (dislocation). Acute traumatic cataracts are less dense than the normal lens.

Comment

Ocular Trauma

Ocular trauma (Figure S11-1) is usually directed more to the anterior structures than to the vitreous, retina, and choroid, which are the structures that radiologists tend to focus on. Blood in the anterior chamber of the eye is called an *anterior hyphema*. This blood usually prevents the ophthalmologist from getting a good look behind it to check for choroidal or retinal detachments or even blood in the vitreous. The anterior chamber can also be ruptured: in fact, it is ruptured more commonly than the vitreous (both of which are present here). An open wound to the globe is accompanied by a high rate of endophthalmitis, which can lead to phthisis bulbi at its end stage. Therefore, treatment of open globes is aggressive, with antibiotics, cleansing, and shielding.

Traumatic Cataract

In the acute setting, injury to the lens may lead it to imbibe water, lose its normal high proteinaceous intrinsic architecture, or both. Therefore, its density may decrease when disruption occurs *(traumatic cataract)*. Whereas senescent cataracts may be more dense than normal lenses, traumatic cataracts are less dense. In many cases, the suspensory ligaments of the lens may also be disrupted (as in this case), and the lens seems malpositioned. This condition, *lens dislocation* or *subluxation,* is caused by injury to the region of the ciliary body and these ligamentous fixation points.

Ocular Hypotony

Ocular hypotony, in which intraocular pressure falls below 5 mm Hg, may result from (1) decreased production of aqueous humor, (2) leakage from trauma, (3) iridocyclitis, (4) tractional ciliary body detachment, (5) retinal detachments, (6) ciliary body infections that impair aqueous humor production, (7) ocular surgery, or (8) overtreatment of glaucoma (trabeculectomy).

Reference

Kubal WS. Imaging of orbital trauma. *Radiographics.* 2008;28: 1729-1739. doi:10.1148/rg.286085523

Cross-Reference

Neuroradiology: The Requisites, 3rd ed, 326.

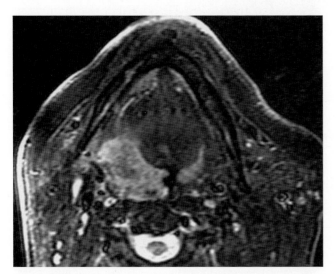

Figure 12-1

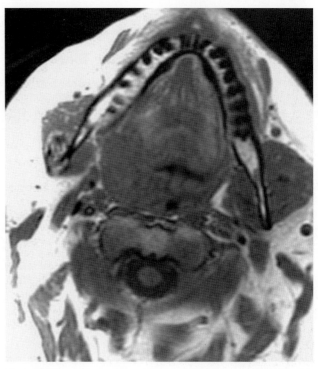

Figure 12-2

HISTORY: An elderly man with a 25-pack/year smoking history has lost 20 pounds of weight in 6 months.

1. Which of the following should be included in the differential diagnosis? (Choose all that apply.)
   A. Squamous cell carcinoma of the floor of mouth
   B. Oral cavity cancer
   C. Retromolar trigone cancer
   D. Squamous cell carcinoma of the tonsil

2. Which is the most common direction of spread of tonsil cancer?
   A. Across the midline to the contralateral tonsil
   B. Across the midline via the posterior pharyngeal wall
   C. Across the midline via the buccal space
   D. Across the midline via the base of the tongue

3. What is the most common risk factor for tonsil squamous cell carcinoma in a 35-year-old?
   A. Smoking cigarettes
   B. Smoking marijuana
   C. Chewing tobacco
   D. Oral sex

4. Why is the prognosis for tonsil cancer worse than the prognosis for floor-of-mouth cancer?
   A. Higher rate of coincidental presence of a second primary cancer
   B. Higher rate of human papillomavirus (HPV) cancers
   C. Higher rate of mandibular involvement
   D. Increased rate of nodal spread

See Supplemental Figures section for additional figures and legends for this case.

CASE 12

Squamous Cell Carcinoma of the Tonsil

1. **D.** The location of the lesion is in the tonsil, which is a part of the oropharynx.

2. **D.** When tonsillar cancer crosses the midline, it usually does so via the tongue base rather than via the contralateral tonsil, posterior pharynx, or buccal space (Figures S12-1 and S12-2).

3. **D.** HPV exposure increases with the number of sexual partners with whom a person has oral sex. This is a risk factor for oropharyngeal carcinoma.

4. **D.** The high incidence of nodal spread by oropharyngeal cancer dramatically affects the prognosis because nodal disease decreases the rate of 5-year survival by 50%. HPV-positive cancers have a better prognosis than do HPV-negative ones.

Comment

HPV-Positive Oropharyngeal Cancer

The incidence of tonsil cancer has risen dramatically in a younger age group that is not smoking or drinking excessively. This is thought to be due to HPV-positive squamous cell carcinomas of the oropharynx predominantly affecting the tongue base and tonsil. While oral cavity and laryngeal cancers have been declining with the lower incidence of smoking, these cancers have been rising in prevalence. The increase has been attributed to increased oral sex engaged in at younger ages and with multiple partners. The spread of HPV may be abated with the vaccination against HPV in teenage males and females.

HPV Types

There are different HPV types that have high and low risks:
- High-risk HPV types: 16, 18, 31, 33, 35, 52, 58, 59, 68, 73, 82
- Low-risk HPV types: 6, 11, 40, 42, 43, 44, 54, 61, 70, 72, 81

HPV 16 is the most prevalent and, unfortunately, the most virulent type observed with oropharyngeal cancer. More men than women are affected. The disease spreads more readily to nodes, which are more commonly cystic. HPV type 16 tumors are, however, more responsive to all therapeutic maneuvers than are other types.

Risk Factors for HPV-Positive Cancers

The risk factors include higher numbers of sex partners for vaginal intercourse (>26) and for oral sex (>6) and intercourse with a sexual partner known to have a history of HPV-associated cancer. These factors increase the risk for subsequent HPV-positive cancer. Anal-oral sex, sexual intercourse with a partner with an abnormal finding on Papanicolaou smear, and HPV type 16 oral infection are also risk factors.

References

Corey AS, Hudgins PA. Radiographic imaging of human papillomavirus related carcinomas of the oropharynx. *Head Neck Pathol.* 2012;6(Suppl 1):S25-S40.

D'Souza G, Kreimer AR, Viscidi R, Pawlita M, Fakhry C, Koch WM, et al. Case-control study of human papillomavirus and oropharyngeal cancer. *N Engl J Med.* 2007;356(19):1944-1956.

Cross-Reference

Neuroradiology: The Requisites, 3rd ed, 388-389, 435-436, 457-471, 486, 492, 494.

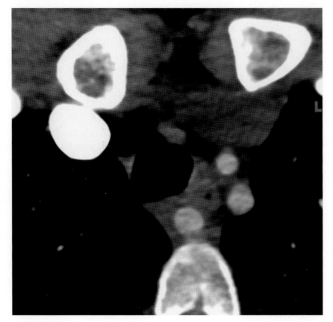

Figure 13-1

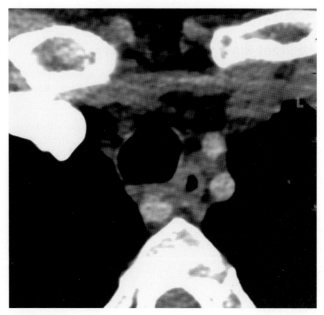

Figure 13-2

HISTORY: The patient is being evaluated for a palpable left thyroid nodule.

1. Which of the following should be included in the differential diagnosis? (Choose all that apply.)
   A. Aneurysm of the aorta
   B. Aberrant right subclavian artery
   C. Right-sided aortic arch
   D. Aberrant left subclavian artery

2. From which embryologic vascular arch does the normal right proximal subclavian artery derive?
   A. Arch number 1
   B. Arch number 2
   C. Arch number 3
   D. Arch number 4

3. What is the most common anomaly of the aortic arch vessels?
   A. Bifid aorta
   B. Aberrant right subclavian artery
   C. Right-sided aortic arch
   D. Aberrant left subclavian artery

4. What is the most common symptom with this anomaly?
   A. Nothing
   B. Vocal cord paralysis
   C. Zenker diverticulum
   D. Reflux esophagitis

See Supplemental Figures section for additional figures and legends for this case.

CASE 13

Aberrant Right Subclavian Artery (Arteria Lusoria)

1. **B.** The figure shows a vessel coursing behind the esophagus. This is an aberrant right subclavian artery.

2. **D.** Arch 4 is the origin of the aberrant right subclavian artery. Arch 1 is associated with the maxillary artery, arch 2 with the stapedial artery, and arch 3 with the carotid artery.

3. **B.** The aberrant right subclavian artery is the most common anomaly of the primitive arch.

4. **A.** In most cases, this anomaly is asymptomatic. When patients do complain, the symptoms are of difficulty swallowing (dysphagia lusoria).

Comment

Congenital Vascular Anomalies

Coarctation of the aorta, tetralogy of Fallot, and interrupted aortic arches may coexist with an aberrant right subclavian artery. These more dangerous cardiac disorders and their impact on cardiopulmonary function obviously overshadow any complaints caused by the impression of the aberrant subclavian artery on the esophagus. When an aberrant subclavian artery coexists with a coarctation of the aorta, the aberrant artery may arise proximal or distal to the coarctation. Aberrant right subclavian artery is a vascular lesion that used to be diagnosed on barium swallow studies; now it is more commonly an incidental finding on a cross-sectional imaging study performed for other reasons (Figures S13-1, S13-2, and S13-3). A prevalence rate of 0.5% to 2% has been reported.

Treatment of Aberrant Subclavian Artery

Treatment of aberrant subclavian artery (if required) usually consists of transposition of the vessel to the right common carotid artery; a cervical approach is favored over a median sternotomy. Aneurysms of the aberrant subclavian artery may occur and can be difficult to diagnose because of their unusual location. Rupture of such an aneurysm into the esophagus can be catastrophic. The right recurrent laryngeal nerve is often absent because the laryngeal nerve descends directly from the vagus nerve without looping under the right subclavian artery. At surgery for correction of the aberrant subclavian artery, the surgeon must identify and protect the vagus and recurrent laryngeal nerves.

Reference

Atay Y, Engin C, Posacioglu H, Ozyurek R, Ozcan C, Yagdi T, et al. Surgical approaches to the aberrant right subclavian artery. *Tex Heart Inst J.* 2006;33(4):477-481.

Cross-Reference

Neuroradiology: The Requisites, 3rd ed, 110.

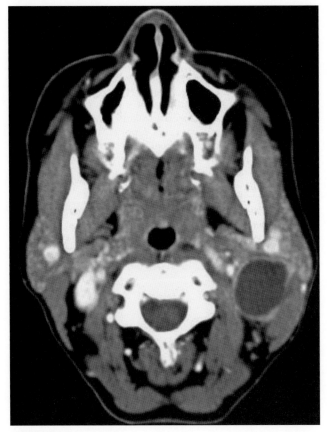

Figure 14-1

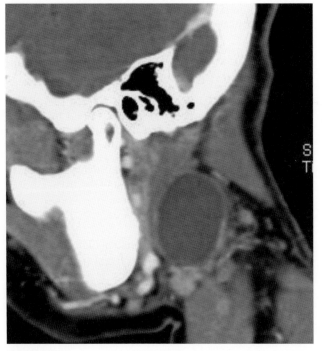

Figure 14-2

HISTORY: A young patient has a long history of left-sided neck swelling.

1. Which of the following should be included in the differential diagnosis? (Choose all that apply.)
    A. Branchial cleft cyst (BCC)
    B. Cystic nodal mass
    C. Jugular lymphatic sac
    D. Tornwaldt cyst

2. Which primary tumor is most commonly associated with a cystic lymph node?
    A. Papillary carcinoma of the thyroid
    B. Lymphoma
    C. Human papillomavirus (HPV)–negative squamous cell carcinoma of the larynx
    D. Melanoma

3. Where is a Bailey type 3 second BCC?
    A. Deep to the sternocleidomastoid muscle
    B. Superficial to the sternocleidomastoid muscle (SCM)
    C. Deep to the carotid sheath
    D. Insinuating in the carotid bifurcation, like a carotid body tumor

4. Which neck cyst has a strong predilection for the left side of the neck?
    A. Thyroglossal duct cyst
    B. Second BCC
    C. Jugular lymphatic sac
    D. Zenker diverticulum

See Supplemental Figures section for additional figures and legends for this case.

CASE 14

Second Branchial Cleft Cysts

1. **A and B.** This cystic mass may be a BCC or a cystic nodal mass. Tornwaldt cysts occur in the nasopharynx, and jugular lymphatic sacs occur in the lower neck.

2. **A.** Thyroid cancer and tonsil cancers, particularly ones that are HPV-positive, have a strong association with cystic nodes.

3. **D.** Bailey type 1 second BCCs are superficial to the SCM, type 2 are between the SCM and the carotid bifurcation, type 3 insinuate between the carotid arteries, and type 4 are deep to the carotid bifurcation.

4. **C.** Jugular lymphatic sacs and thymopharyngeal cysts have a predilection for the lower left side of the neck.

Comment

Bailey Classification of Second Branchial Cleft Cysts

Bailey classified second BCCs in 1929. He defined them as follows:

Type I: along the anterior surface of the SCM, deep to the platysma muscle

Type II: along the anterior margin of the SCM, deep to it, and posterior to the submandibular gland

Type III: invaginating into the carotid bifurcation

Type IV: deep to the carotid bifurcation along the lateral pharyngeal wall or parapharyngeal space

Appearance of Second BCCs

Second BCCs usually develop in the second and third decade of life with an enlarging neck mass (Figures S14-1 and S14-2). The mass may be traumatized or infected, which may lead to a less-than-pure cystic anechoic ultrasound appearance. In fact, in more than half the cases reported by Ahuja and colleagues (2000), there was internal debris, a complex heterogeneous echo pattern, or a uniformly homogeneous pseudosolid appearance. Thick walls were present in 12% of cases.

Differential Diagnosis

The differential diagnosis includes cystic nodal disease, which also is uncommonly anechoic. Lymphatic low flow malformations and cystic hygromas may simulate second BCCs when they are lower in location in the neck. Lymphatic malformations tend to appear in the posterior triangle and axilla and manifest earlier in life.

Reference

Ahuja AT, King AD, Metreweli C. Second branchial cleft cysts: variability of sonographic appearances in adult cases. *AJNR Am J Neuroradiol.* 2000;21(2):315-319.

Cross-Reference

Neuroradiology: The Requisites, 3rd ed, 445, 479t, 487, 495, 496f

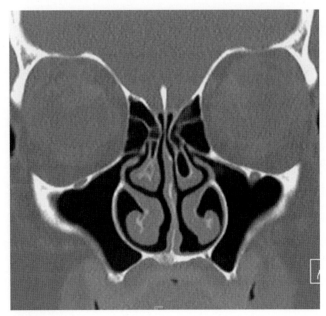

Figure 15-1

HISTORY: The patient has a long history of sinus congestion.

1. Which of the following normal variants are seen in the left sinonasal cavity? (Choose all that apply.)
   A. Paradoxical turbinate
   B. Haller cell
   C. Sinus lateralis
   D. Concha bullosa

2. What are the two main attachments of the middle turbinate?
   A. Middle meatus and hiatus semilunaris
   B. Cribriform plate and nasal septum
   C. Cribriform plate and lamina papyracea
   D. Ethmoid bulla and lamina papyracea

3. What is the incidence of a concha bullosa?
   A. 0% to 20%
   B. 21% to 40%
   C. 41% to 60%
   D. >60%

4. What other sinonasal variant is most closely correlated with a concha bullosa?
   A. Haller cell
   B. Uncinate bullosa
   C. Maxillary sinus hypoplasia
   D. Septal deviation

See Supplemental Figures section for additional figures and legends for this case.

CASE 15

Concha Bullosa

1. **D.** A concha bullosa represents aeration of the middle turbinate. When the vertical segment is aerated, it may be called a *lamellar cell.*

2. **C.** The attachments of the middle turbinate are the cribriform plate and lamina papyracea. This puts the orbit and intracranial contents at risk when the turbinate is removed at endoscopy.

3. **C.** After septal deviation, the concha bullosa is the most common normal variant in the sinonasal cavity.

4. **D.** Concha bullosa and septal deviation often coexist.

Comment

Middle Turbinate Anatomy

When the vertical cribriform plate attachment of the middle turbinate (the vertical lamella) is aerated, it is sometimes called a *lamellar cell.* When that vertical aeration extends to the inferior bulbous portion of the middle turbinate, it is more formally called a *concha bullosa* (Figure S15-1). The lateral attachment to the lamina papyracea is sometimes called the *ground,* or *basal, lamella.* The incidence of cerebrospinal fluid leakage and orbital hematoma associated with functional endoscopic sinus surgery may have been high initially because of overvigorous removal of the middle turbinate, which led to "trauma" at the vertical and ground lamella.

Concha Bullosa

Conchae bullosa are very common. The incidence has been reported as 44% for at least one concha bullosa; 23% of the general population have a unilateral concha, and 21% have bilateral conchae bullosa. Nasal septal deviation has a close association with concha bullosa. However, sinusitis occurs equally among people with or without a concha bullosa. The larger the concha, the greater is the likelihood of obstruction of the osteomeatal unit and the greater is the likelihood of nasal septal deviation. Nasal septal deviation occurs in about 25% of the population.

Sinonasal Normal Variants

A *Haller cell* is an infraorbital maxilloethmoidal cell. When large, it may obstruct the maxillary sinus ostium. Such cells are reported in about one third of all patients. Onodi cells—ethmoidal air cells that lie posterior and sometimes superior to the sphenoidal sinus—are present in 25% of patients. Agger nasi cells—anterior ethmoidal air cells that lie anterior lateral and inferior to the frontoethmoidal recess and anterior and above the attachment of the middle turbinate—are present in nearly 90% of patients presenting for sinus CTs.

Reference

Stallman JS, Lobo JN, Som PM. The incidence of concha bullosa and its relationship to nasal septal deviation and paranasal sinus disease. *AJNR Am J Neuroradiol.* 2004;25(9):1613-1618.

Cross-Reference

Neuroradiology: The Requisites, 3rd ed, 420.

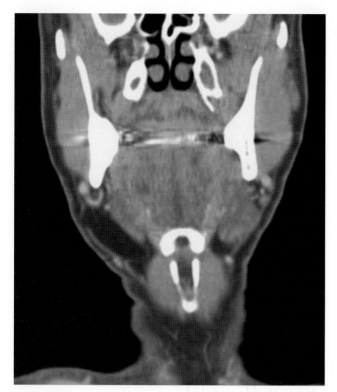

Figure 16-1

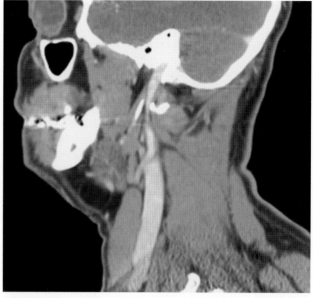

Figure 16-2

HISTORY: A patient presents with a right-sided fluctuant neck mass.

1. Which of the following would be included in the differential diagnosis for the imaging findings presented? (Choose all that apply.)
   A. Hibernoma
   B. Dermoid
   C. Epidermoid
   D. Lipoma
   E. None of the above

2. In what depth of the neck do lipomas occur most commonly?
   A. Skin
   B. Subcutaneous tissue
   C. Muscle
   D. Bone
   E. Mucosa

3. Which statement is *true* of hibernomas?
   A. Hibernomas are tumors of immature brown fat.
   B. Hibernomas have a higher rate of conversion to liposarcomas than do lipomas.
   C. Hibernomas enlarge in the wintertime rather than in the summertime.
   D. Hibernomas do not take up tracer on fluorodeoxyglucose positron emission tomography (PET).

4. Which is *not* true of lipomas?
   A. They can look just like liposarcomas.
   B. They may grow or regress with overall body habitus.
   C. They have a predilection for the posterior aspect of the neck.
   D. They are associated with Maffucci syndrome.
   E. None of the above.

See Supplemental Figures section for additional figures and legends for this case.

CASE 16

Lipoma

1. **A, B, and D.** All these lesions contain fat and may simulate lipomas. Epidermoid is usually more cystic.

2. **B.** Lipomas can occur in all sites specified, but they occur most often in subcutaneous tissue.

3. **A.** Hibernomas are tumors of immature brown fat. They may be a source of confusion on PET because they take up fluorodeoxyglucose. They do not have potential for malignancy.

4. **D.** Maffucci syndrome is the association of multiple enchondromas with multiple hemangiomas and occasional lymphangiomas, not lipomas.

Comment

Locations

Lipomas are the most common benign mesenchymal tumors of the head and neck. Of all lipomas, 13% occur in the head and neck (Figures S16-1 and S16-2), and of all mesenchymal benign masses, 43% are lipomas. They are usually found in the subcutaneous tissue. In 5% of cases, multiple lipomas are found. The differential diagnosis may include Madelung disease (benign symmetric lipomatosis) and liposarcoma. The ratio of benign lipomas to liposarcomas is greater than 100:1, but these malignancies are rare in the head and neck, occurring more commonly in the extremities and retroperitoneum.

Imaging Findings

Lipomas may occur as part of a familial lipomatosis syndrome and are also more common in patients with Gardner syndrome.

Lipomas demonstrate typical fat density and intensity on computed tomography and magnetic resonance imaging (MRI). Fat-suppression techniques eliminate confusion with epidermoids or cysts. Enhancement should raise suspicion of liposarcoma. Additional tissue of nonfatty origin might suggest dermoid or teratoma.

Symptoms of Hibernomas

Hibernomas are uncommon, benign, slow-growing soft-tissue tumors consisting of brown fat similar to that in hibernating animals. These tumors usually arise from areas in which vestiges of brown fetal fat persist beyond fetal life, such as the neck, axilla, back, and mediastinum. Hibernomas usually develop between the ages of 20 and 40 and are slightly more common in women. They grow slowly and usually manifest with painless enlargement. Symptoms related to the compression of adjacent structures rarely develop.

Hibernomas are typically fatty, hypervascular lesions that are grossly similar to lipomas. They are well-defined, encapsulated, and mobile masses. On imaging, hibernomas are usually depicted as heterogeneous masses with marked contrast enhancement. The computed tomographic and MRI examinations show a well-demarcated mass with signal intensity intermediate between those of subcutaneous fat and muscle, and it enhances after injection of contrast material. The treatment of hibernomas consists of complete surgical resection, and local recurrence does not develop. There are no reports of metastases or malignant transformation.

Reference

Ahuja AT, King AD, Kew J, King W, Metreweli C. Head and neck lipomas: sonographic appearance. *AJNR Am J Neuroradiol.* 1998; 19(3):505-508.

Cross-Reference

Neuroradiology: The Requisites, 3rd ed, 288, 293, 317-318, 373, 484, 494, 564-565

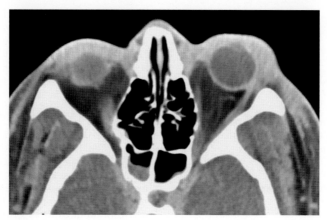

Figure 17-1

HISTORY: A young patient presents with a 1-week history of left eye swelling after an insect bite.

1. Which of the following would be included in the differential diagnosis for the imaging findings presented? (Choose all that apply.)
   A. Periorbital cellulitis
   B. Orbital cellulitis
   C. Periorbital abscess
   D. Periosteal abscess

2. What is the structure that distinguishes periorbital cellulitis from orbital cellulitis?
   A. The globe
   B. The periosteum
   C. The sclera
   D. The septum

3. Which of the following is more common in periorbital cellulitis than in orbital cellulitis?
   A. Ophthalmoplegia
   B. Eyelid swelling
   C. Loss of vision
   D. Pain on eye movement

4. Why is distinguishing periorbital from orbital cellulitis important?
   A. Periorbital cellulitis increases the risk for optic neuritis.
   B. Orbital cellulitis may lead to periorbital cellulitis.
   C. Orbital cellulitis is a disease that must be treated surgically with incision and drainage, whereas periorbital cellulitis is not treated surgically.
   D. Orbital cellulitis must be treated with intravenous antibiotics, whereas periorbital cellulitis is treated with oral antibiotics.

See Supplemental Figures section for additional figures and legends for this case.

CASE 17

Periorbital Cellulitis

1. **A.** The inflammation is limited to the superficial tissues around the left eye.

2. **D.** The orbital septum is the structure that is violated when a periorbital cellulitis spreads to become an orbital cellulitis. Once the orbital septum has been violated, the infection is much more dangerous.

3. **B.** Ophthalmoplegia, visual loss, pain on eye movement, and ischemic optic neuropathy may complicate orbital cellulitis.

4. **D.** The treatment of orbital cellulitis requires intravenous antibiotics.

Comment

Symptoms of Periorbital Cellulitis

Periorbital cellulitis is best termed *preseptal cellulitis* to indicate that the infection remains anterior to the orbital septum (Figure S17-1). Orbital cellulitis, or *postseptal cellulitis,* is a more dangerous infection that can infiltrate the intraconal structures, including the optic nerve and sheath, and can lead to vascular complications as well. Visual loss, ophthalmoplegia, pain on eye movement, and proptosis may be clinical indications of orbital cellulitis, whereas periorbital cellulitis may manifest with eyelid swelling, superficial pain, and erythema.

Causes of Periorbital Cellulitis

The orbital septum is usually a fairly good barrier to the spread of infection. It is a membranous septum of fibrous tissue that is continuous with the periosteum in both a transverse direction and a craniocaudal direction. Periorbital cellulitis is usually caused by superficial pathogens such as puncture wounds, insect bites, dog bites, trauma, dermatitis, acne, or conjunctivitis, whereas the most common cause of orbital cellulitis is sinusitis. Sinusitis also occasionally causes periorbital cellulitis.

Treatment of Periorbital Cellulitis

Periorbital cellulitis is nearly 10 times more common than orbital cellulitis and is a milder infection, usually treated with oral antibiotics. The antibiotics prescribed cover the most common pathogens, usually *Staphylococcus aureus* (including methicillin-resistant *S. aureus* [MRSA]), *Streptococcus pneumoniae,* other streptococci, and anaerobes. If the patient does not respond in 24 to 48 hours after administration of antibiotics, imaging may be necessary to confirm or rule out spread from a preseptal location.

Complications of Sinusitis

This is the Chandler classification of orbital infections (derived from complications of sinusitis):
Group I: preseptal cellulitis
Group II: orbital cellulitis
Group III: subperiosteal abscess
Group IV: orbital abscess
Group V: cavernous sinus thrombosis

Reference

Botting AM, McIntosh D, Mahadevan M. Paediatric pre- and post-septal peri-orbital infections are different diseases. A retrospective review of 262 cases. *Int J Pediatr Otorhinolaryngol.* 2008;72:377.

Cross-Reference

Neuroradiology: The Requisites, 3rd ed, 324, 339.

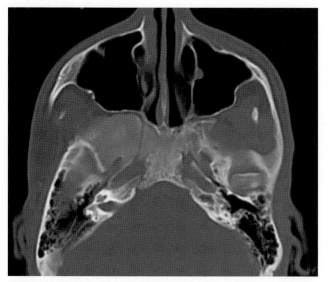

Figure 18-1

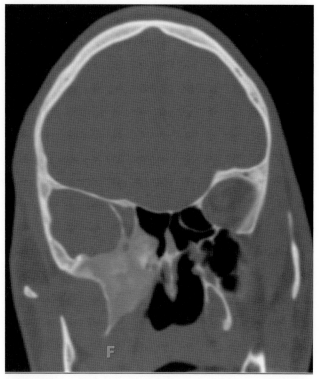

Figure 18-2

HISTORY: This 24-year-old patient has headaches in the right midface.

1. Which of the following would be included in the differential diagnosis for the imaging findings presented? (Choose all that apply.)
   A. Metastasis
   B. Paget disease
   C. Camurati-Engelmann disease
   D. Caffey disease
   E. Fibrous dysplasia

2. What head and neck bone is most commonly affected by Paget disease?
   A. Maxilla
   B. Mandible
   C. Calvaria
   D. Sphenoid bone
   E. Temporal bone

3. What head and neck bone is most commonly affected by fibrous dysplasia?
   A. Maxilla
   B. Mandible
   C. Calvaria
   D. Sphenoid bone
   E. Temporal bone

4. What are the incidences of malignant change in Paget disease and in fibrous dysplasia?
   A. Paget disease: 5%; fibrous dysplasia: 1%
   B. Paget disease: 1%; fibrous dysplasia: 5%
   C. Paget disease: 5%; fibrous dysplasia: 5%
   D. Paget disease: 1%; fibrous dysplasia: 1%
   E. Both: <1%

See Supplemental Figures section for additional figures and legends for this case.

CASE 18

Fibrous Dysplasia

1. **E.** Paget disease can be considered from the standpoint of the imaging findings, but not in a 24-year-old patient. Camurati-Engelmann disease affects long bones, and Caffey disease occurs in infancy, although both can have sclerotic appearances.

2. **C.** The skull is most commonly affected by Paget disease.

3. **A.** The maxilla, followed by the mandible, are the bones most commonly affected by fibrous dysplasia. The other bones mentioned are far less common to be affected.

4. **E.** Malignant change is uncommon in both fibrous dysplasia and Paget disease, especially in the craniofacial region.

Comment
Points of Differentiation

The differentiation of fibrous dysplasia from other bone conditions that cause hyperostosis may be problematic. Many of the conditions affect the mandible as a flat bone in particular, and affected patients may include infants (Caffey disease), young adults (Camurati-Engelmann disease and fibrous dysplasia), and older adults (Paget disease and metastases). On imaging, fibrous dysplasia may be recognized by the ground-glass appearance of the bone, as opposed to the homogeneous appearance in the lytic form or even the sclerotic form of Paget disease.

Symptoms

When these diseases affect the skull base, headache or facial pain is usually associated, particularly if the neural foramina are affected with narrowings. In the latter case, narrowing of the Vidian canal (Figure S18-1) and of the foramen rotundum (Figure S18-2) on the right side is apparent on imaging, which accounts for the patient's facial pain. The Vidian nerve is involved in the sinonasal secretions and symptoms of vasomotor neuritis. Sectioning of the Vidian nerve causes anesthesia in the nasal mucosa.

Types

Fibrous dysplasia may be monostotic (affecting only one bone) or polyostotic (affecting more than one bone). The incidence of malignant bone tumors in the polyostotic form of fibrous dysplasia is estimated at 1%, which is less than that with the monostotic form. The polyostotic variety is less common except in such syndromes as McCune-Albright syndrome, in which it may be associated in female patients with café au lait spots, usually on the back, and precocious puberty. McCune-Albright syndrome is caused by mutations in the *GNAS1* gene. Hyperthyroidism and acromegaly may also manifest in McCune-Albright syndrome.

Reference

Cheng J, Wang Y, Yu H, Wang D, Ye J, Jiang H, et al. An epidemiological and clinical analysis of craniomaxillofacial fibrous dysplasia in a Chinese population. *Orphanet J Rare Dis.* 2012;7:80.

Cross-Reference

Neuroradiology: The Requisites, 3rd ed, 343, 411, 434, 435f, 487-488.

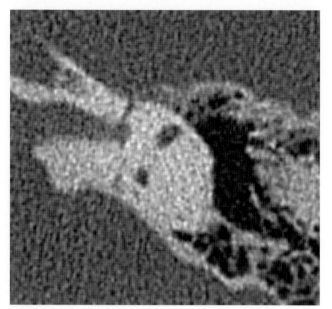

Figure 19-1

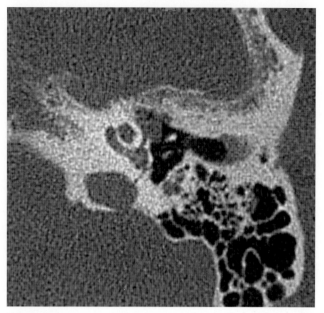

Figure 19-2

HISTORY: A patient presents with head trauma and hearing loss.

1. Which of the following would be included in the differential diagnosis for the imaging findings presented? (Choose all that apply.)
   A. Vertical fracture of the temporal bone
   B. Horizontal fracture of the temporal bone
   C. Oblique fracture of the temporal bone
   D. Longitudinal fracture of the temporal bone

2. What is the most common complication of this type of fracture?
   A. Hearing loss
   B. Facial nerve dysfunction
   C. Otorrhea
   D. Perilymphatic fistula

3. What is the most common cause of temporal bone fractures?
   A. Falls
   B. Penetrating trauma
   C. Motor vehicle collisions
   D. Assaults

4. Which are the four main parts of the temporal bone?
   A. Sphenoid, squamosal, tympanic, and petrous
   B. Sphenoid, mastoid, squamosal, and petrous
   C. Styloid, sphenoid, squamosal, and petrous
   D. Tympanic, mastoid, squamosal, and petrous

See Supplemental Figures section for additional figures and legends for this case.

CASE 19

Vertical Temporal Bone Fracture

1. **A.** This fracture extends across the inner ear structures in a vertical direction. Previously this was termed a *transverse fracture,* and the current description includes *otic capsule–violating* or *otic capsule–sparing.*

2. **A.** Because this fracture crosses the otic capsule (i.e., the cochlea), the risk is for hearing loss.

3. **C.** Blunt trauma from motor vehicle collisions is the most common cause of temporal bone fractures. Falls are the second most common cause. Penetrating trauma is a relatively rare cause of temporal bone fractures, and assaults are also uncommon causes.

4. **D.** Tympanic, mastoid, squamosal, and petrous are the four main parts of the temporal bone. Some authorities also include the styloid process as the fifth part.

Comment

Classifications of Temporal Bone Fractures

Most temporal bone fractures are more oriented in the longitudinal/horizontal direction, along the long axis of the temporal bone, than in the vertical/transverse direction, along the short axis. Because the fractures are not truly across the bone, most authorities refer to temporal bone fractures as being oblique or characterize the fracture according to the main axis of the fracture. Other classifications describe the fractures as otic capsule–violating (involving the inner ear components—the cochlea (Figures S19-1 and S19-2), vestibule, and semicircular canals) or as otic capsule–sparing. The fractures that do not involve the inner ear components usually course lateral and anterior to those structures. The facial nerve is involved in 50% of the vertical fractures and 20% of the horizontal fractures. Sensorineural hearing loss is more common in vertical fractures, otic capsule–violating fractures.

Complications

Both otorrhea and rhinorrhea can occur after temporal bone fracture as cerebrospinal fluid (CSF) leaks into the middle ear from disruption of the common walls with the intracranial contents. CSF can leak into the nasal cavity to cause rhinorrhea via the eustachian tube or out the external auditory canal through a violated tympanic membrane.

Surgical Emergencies

Two surgical emergencies may occur with temporal bone fractures: (1) brain herniation through a fracture site, which can lead to seizures, encephalitis, and meningitis (particularly with an open wound), and (2) laceration of the carotid artery, which can lead to severe hemorrhage. Early intervention to repair facial nerves that have been lacerated or show progressive dysfunction is also suggested. Children with temporal bone fractures have a much lower rate of facial nerve injury than do adults with these fractures, but affected children have a higher rate of transient hearing loss.

Reference

Patel A, Groppo E. Management of temporal bone trauma. *Craniomaxillofac Trauma Reconstr.* 2010;3(2):105-113.

Cross-Reference

Neuroradiology: The Requisites, 3rd ed, 414-416, 415f, 415t, 416f.

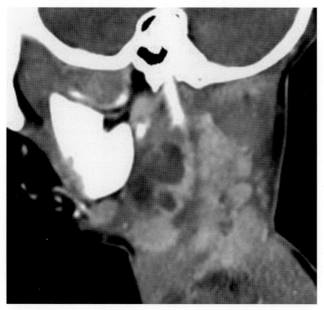

Figure 20-1

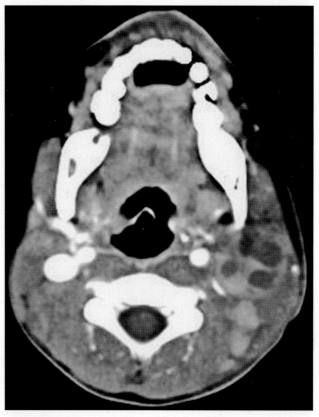

Figure 20-2

HISTORY: A child presents with neck swelling and tenderness and with fever.

1. Which of the following would be included in the differential diagnosis for the imaging findings presented? (Choose all that apply.)
   A. Necrotizing adenitis
   B. Infected lymphatic malformation
   C. Abscess
   D. Rhabdomyosarcoma

2. What percentage of lymphatic malformations manifest before age 3?
   A. <25%
   B. 26% to 50%
   C. 51% to 75%
   D. >75%

3. In children, for which space in the neck do lymphatic malformations have a predilection?
   A. Submandibular space
   B. Visceral space
   C. Posterior triangle
   D. Masticator space

4. In which infections do lymph nodes commonly become necrotic?
   A. Epstein-Barr virus (EBV)
   B. Cat scratch disease
   C. Toxoplasmosis
   D. Tuberculosis

See Supplemental Figures section for additional figures and legends for this case.

CASE 20

Necrotizing Adenitis

1. **A, B, and C.** All of these lesions could cause an inflamed multiloculated "mass" in a child. In an adult, the differential diagnosis would probably not include a lymphatic malformation.

2. **D.** The classical teaching is that 90% of lymphatic malformations manifest before the age of 2. Some are being diagnosed nowadays through fetal magnetic resonance imaging (MRI).

3. **C.** Lymphatic malformations tend to develop in the posterior triangle and the axilla. They also develop in the orbits.

4. **D.** Tuberculosis is the infection that classically causes necrotic infectious adenopathy. However, any of the mycobacterial infections can also do so. Because staphylococcal and streptococcal infections are more common than TB in America, they are also common sources of necrotizing adenitis.

Comment

Types of Necrotic Masses

In a child with a necrotic mass in the soft tissues of the neck that is unassociated with the mucosa or the Waldeyer ring and that appears to be inflammatory, the clinician should consider several entities. The most common lesion is necrotizing adenitis. Children have a propensity for necrotic adenopathy, which is often seen with pharyngitis and classically may be located in the retropharyngeal space. Staphylococcal and streptococcal infections, by virtue of being so common, are the pathogens most commonly associated with necrotic adenopathy. Nonetheless, the clinician should also assess for mycobacterial and fungal infections, which cause a high rate of lymph node necrosis.

Differential Diagnosis

In this case, the debate was whether this infection had an underlying lesion because of the multiloculated nature of the process. The clinician should consider underlying lymphatic malformation, although most such malformations are located in the posterior triangle of the neck or extend to the axilla (Figures S20-1 and S20-2). Another alternative would be an infected second branchial cleft cyst (BCC), but necrotic adenopathy usually has more solid tissue associated with it than classic Bailey's type 2 BCC. To call this an abscess with associated lymphadenopathy is not wrong, but it does not clarify the source. Most pediatric abscesses are associated with pharyngitis, tonsillitis, dental lesions, or puncture wounds; otherwise, there is no reason for an infection to develop de novo in the soft tissues of the neck. The clinician should therefore investigate the possibility of an underlying lesion unless there is a puncture wound, a fistula, a dermal appendage infection, and so forth. That is why most of these infections are thought to represent necrotizing adenitis.

Lymphatic Malformations

Of all lymphatic malformations, 90% manifest before the age of 3. Microcytic and macrocytic (spaces > 2 cm large) varieties exist. Treatment of the macrocytic varieties may include sclerotherapy with bleomycin, alcohol (which can be painful), doxycycline, or OK-432. Laser therapy and radiofrequency ablation may also be an option. In some cases, surgery is the best option and is curative. Radiofrequency ablation has also been tried for the microcytic varieties.

Reference

Perkins JA, Manning SC, Tempero RM, Cunningham MJ, Edmonds JL Jr, Hoffer FA, et al. Lymphatic malformations: current cellular and clinical investigations. *Otolaryngol Head Neck Surg.* 2010;142(6): 789-794.

Cross-Reference

Neuroradiology: The Requisites, 3rd ed, 444.

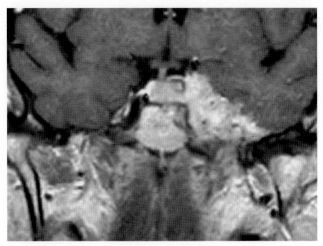

Figure 21-1

HISTORY: A 42-year-old woman has had headaches for 2 years with deep left-sided discomfort.

1. Which of the following would be included in the differential diagnosis for the imaging findings presented? (Choose all that apply.)
   A. Meningioma
   B. Sarcoidosis
   C. Lymphoma
   D. Plasmacytoma

2. What is *not* included in the differential diagnosis of a calcified mass at the skull base?
   A. Meningioma
   B. Chordoma
   C. Chondrosarcoma
   D. Plasmacytoma

3. With what entity is there an increase in the frequency of meningiomas?
   A. Neurofibromatosis type 1
   B. Neurofibromatosis type 2
   C. Sturge Weber syndrome
   D. Tuberous sclerosis

4. What is the most common radiation-induced neoplasm of the central nervous system?
   A. Meningioma
   B. Glioblastoma multiforme
   C. Sarcomas
   D. None of the above

See Supplemental Figures section for additional figures and legends for this case.

CASE 21

Skull Base Meningioma

1. **A, B, C, and D.** All of these lesions may affect the skull base and manifest with a dural mass.

2. **D.** Plasmacytomas are usually lytic and do not manifest with a calcified or chondroid lesion.

3. **B.** Meningiomas are one of the components of MISME (multiple inherited schwannomas, meningiomas, and ependymomas), which is the other name for neurofibromatosis type 2.

4. **A.** Radiation-induced meningiomas are more aggressive, recur more frequently, grow faster, undergo malignant degeneration more commonly, and have more mitoses and a higher metabolic rate than de novo meningiomas. Sarcomas are most common in patients with retinoblastomas.

Comment

Imaging Findings

Meningiomas exist in many different varieties, including—in order of increasing aggressiveness—the fibroblastic, transitional, syncytial, angioblastic, and malignant anaplastic types. Atypical meningiomas (7.2%) and malignant meningiomas (2.4%) are encountered fairly commonly in a busy practice. The apparent diffusion coefficient (ADC) values of these more ominous meningiomas are typically lower than those of benign meningiomas. On T2-weighted scans, the syncytial and angioimmunoblastic types often appear brighter than the fibroblastic and transitional types. Meningiomas are the most common type of nonglial brain tumor and are usually well managed surgically. They have dural tails on enhanced scans that are characteristic (Figure S21-1). Recurrent or primary meningiomas at the skull base for which conventional surgical therapy has failed may be treated successfully with radiation therapy with or without brachytherapy with interstitial iodine-125 seeds.

Types of Scans

The skull base is one of the locations where scanning lesions with both computed tomography (CT) and magnetic resonance imaging (MRI) is justified. The soft tissue resolution of MRI (Figure S21-1) enables surgeons to see the relationship between lesions and the cranial nerves, the brain, and the nearby vascular structures. CT is most useful for viewing bony landmarks and anatomic variants that guide or hinder surgery. In addition, angiography with embolization or interventional management of the arterial and venous structures may be necessary. Magnetic resonance angiography and computed tomographic arteriography enable diagnostic imaging of the relationship between masses and the vascular structures. Three-dimensional imaging may even guide surgery with intraoperative localization. Relationships may be more easily displayed with three-dimensional data sets.

Reference

Filippi CG, Edgar MA, Uluğ AM, Prowda JC, Heier LA, Zimmerman RD. Appearance of meningiomas on diffusion weighted images: correlating diffusion constants with histopathologic findings. *AJNR Am J Neuroradiol.* 2001;22(1):65-72.

Cross-Reference

Neuroradiology: The Requisites, 3rd ed, 59-62.

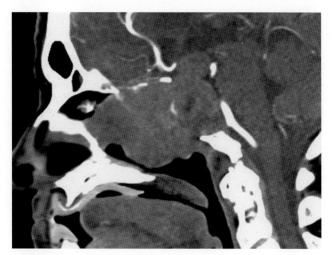

Figure 22-1

HISTORY: An adult presents with persistent headache and nasal congestion and does not have sinusitis.

1. Which of the following would be included in the differential diagnosis for the imaging findings presented? (Choose all that apply.)
   A. Metastasis
   B. Nasopharyngeal carcinoma
   C. Carcinoid tumor
   D. Pituitary adenoma

2. Of all benign skull base masses, which is the most common?
   A. Meningioma
   B. Pituitary adenoma
   C. Nasopharyngeal carcinoma
   D. Schwannoma

3. What is a normal prolactin level?
   A. <25 ng/mL
   B. 26 to 50 ng/mL
   C. 51 to 100 ng/mL
   D. >100 ng/mL

4. What size distinguishes microadenomas from macroadenomas?
   A. 10 mm
   B. 10 mL
   C. Prolactin level of >25 ng/mL
   D. 12 mm

See Supplemental Figures section for additional figures and legends for this case.

CASE 22

Pituitary Adenoma

1. **A, B, and D.** These are lesions that affect the skull base. When carcinoid tumor affects the skull base, it usually appears on imaging as a blastic bone lesion.

2. **B.** Meningiomas are the most common intracranial masses, but pituitary adenomas are the most common skull base lesions. Meningiomas occur all over the dural surfaces of the brain, not just the skull base.

3. **A.** Pituitary macroadenomas have prolactin levels in the hundreds to thousands. Lesions that compress the pituitary or stalk may mildly elevate prolactin.

4. **A.** The threshold between microadenomas and macroadenomas is 10 mm.

Comment

Differential Diagnosis

This case of a pituitary adenoma (Figure S22-1) is a reminder that such lesions can have many different appearances. Whenever a sphenoethmoidal mass, a nasopharyngeal mass, a sellar mass, a clival mass, a suprasellar mass, an orbital mass, a condylar mass, or an anterior cranial fossa floor mass is considered, one should check for the normal pituitary gland. If it is not visible, one must strongly suspect that the lesion may be a pituitary adenoma. It is the most common central skull base tumor, and it can grow in a variety of different ways and mimic many other tumors. Another skull base lesion that can infiltrate widely is nasopharyngeal carcinoma. This lesion can erode bone and grow widely in many directions. The tumor staging of nasopharyngeal carcinoma provides guidance for the various modes of spread:

- **T1:** Tumor is confined to the nasopharynx or extends to the oropharynx and/or nasal cavity but not to the parapharyngeal space.
- **T2:** Tumor extends to the parapharyngeal space.
- **T3:** Tumor involves sphenoid bone bony structures and/or the paranasal sinuses.
- **T4:** Tumor extends intracranially and/or involves cranial nerves, the infratemporal fossa, the hypopharynx, the orbit, or the masticator space.

Prolactin Levels

The level of prolactin indicates that the lesion does not secrete prolactin (<25 ng/mL), that the lesion is merely compressing the gland or not actively secreting prolactin (25 to 100 ng/mL), that the lesion is a prolactinoma (hundreds of nanograms per milliliter) or that the lesion is a prolactinoma that has invaded the cavernous sinus (possibly thousands of nanograms per milliliter).

Management

After surgery and hormonal treatment for aggressive pituitary adenomas, temozolomide and radiation therapy may be employed. Carcinomatous change is decidedly uncommon. Metastases usually are the proof that a pituitary mass is a carcinoma.

Reference

Buchfelder M. Management of aggressive pituitary adenomas: current treatment strategies. *Pituitary*. 2009;12(3):256-260.

Cross-Reference

Neuroradiology: The Requisites, 3rd ed, 364-366.

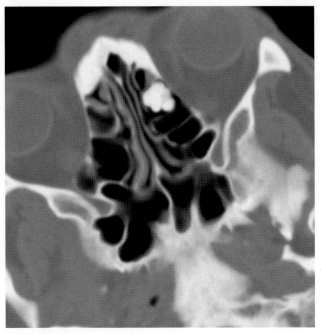

Figure 23-1

HISTORY: A patient with chronic sinusitis has pain in the left frontal region.

1. Which of the following would be included in the differential diagnosis for the imaging findings presented? (Choose all that apply.)
   A. Enchondroma
   B. Sinus osteoma
   C. Ossifying fibroma
   D. Fibrous dysplasia
   E. None of the above

2. Which syndrome is associated with sinus osteomas?
   A. Gardner syndrome
   B. Paget disease
   C. Gorlin syndrome
   D. Peutz-Jeghers syndrome
   E. All of the above

3. What is the classic history in frontal sinus osteomas?
   A. No history, they are most commonly found incidentally
   B. Headache pain
   C. Facial asymmetry
   D. Leontiasis ossea
   E. All of the above

4. Which sinus has the highest rate of osteoma?
   A. Maxillary
   B. Sphenoid
   C. Ethmoid
   D. Sinus of Morgagni
   E. None of the above

See Supplemental Figures section for additional figures and legends for this case.

CASE 23

Sinus Osteoma

1. **B.** Sinus osteoma is the most common tumor and the diagnosis. Enchondromas, fibrous dysplasia, and ossifying fibromas are possible but much less likely and usually have density other than bone.

2. **A.** The association is with Gardner syndrome (familial colonic polyps). Thyroid cancer, epidermoid cysts, fibromas, and sebaceous cysts may also occur in Gardner syndrome.

3. **A.** Most frontal sinus osteomas are found incidentally as part of a work up for sinusitis or facial trauma. If they cause symptoms, it is usually headache pain, which classically is exacerbated by flying and relieved by aspirin.

4. **E.** The frontal sinus is most commonly affected.

Comment

Incidence of Sinus Osteoma

Osteomas of the nose and paranasal sinuses are the most common benign tumors of these regions, occurring in as many of 3% of patients who undergo evaluation by computed tomography for symptomatic sinusitis. The frontal sinus is the most common site for osteomas, followed by the ethmoid sinus (Figure S23-1). Complications of sinus osteomas include postobstructive sinusitis, mucocele formation, orbital invasion, intracranial spread, pneumocephalus, and meningeal irritation. Osteomas manifest in the second to fifth decades of life, and male patients outnumber female patients by 2:1. The preponderance in male patients may be attributable to the possibility that osteomas may be precipitated by trauma.

Treatment of Sinus Osteoma

Indications for surgery include the following:
- Rapid enlargement
- Extension beyond the sinus into the orbit or intracranial space
- Involvement of 50% of the volume of the sinus
- Recurrent sinusitis/headache
- Meningitis
- Cosmesis
- Sphenoid sinus osteomas because of the risk to optic nerves

Gardner Syndrome

Gardner syndrome is a rare, inherited autosomal dominant disorder characterized by multiple colonic polyps; supernumerary teeth; osteomas of the sinuses and skull; and fatty/epithelial cysts or fibrous tumors, or both, in the skin. Desmoid tumors, dental abnormalities, carcinoma of the ampulla of Vater, and thyroid carcinoma have also been reported. Linkage to marker C11p11 on chromosome 5q22, which is part of the adenomatosis polyposis coli (APC) tumor suppressor gene, has been demonstrated. The APC protein affects cell division, cellular attachment, and cell migration. In the Wnt signaling pathway, the APC protein helps control β-catenin, which suppresses genes that stimulate cell division.

Reference

Eller R, Sillers M. Common fibro-osseous lesions of the paranasal sinuses. *Otolaryngol Clin North Am.* 2006;39(3):585-600.

Cross-Reference

Neuroradiology: The Requisites, 3rd ed, 433-434.

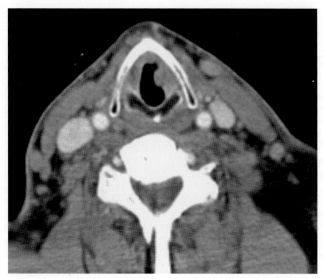

Figure 24-1

HISTORY: The patient presents with a change in voice after a smoking history of 40 pack years.

1. Which of the following would be included in the differential diagnosis for the imaging findings presented? (Choose all that apply.)
   A. Chondrosarcoma of the cricoid cartilage
   B. Rhabdomyosarcoma
   C. Squamous cell carcinoma
   D. Vocal cord polyp

2. Of what part of the head and neck is the retromolar trigone?
   A. Supraglottic larynx
   B. Oral cavity
   C. Oropharynx
   D. Glottic larynx
   E. None of the above

3. Which is the significance of the anterior commissure involvement by this mass?
   A. It means the tumor is transglottic.
   B. It means the patient's options are limited to a total laryngectomy.
   C. It means the staging is T3B.
   D. It means the surgery required may be an extended vertical hemilaryngectomy.
   E. None of the above.

4. What structure must be tumor free if a supracricoid laryngectomy is to be performed?
   A. The vocal cords
   B. The thyroid cartilage
   C. The epiglottis
   D. The false vocal cord
   E. Interarytenoid area

See Supplemental Figures section for additional figures and legends for this case.

CASE 24

True Vocal Cord Squamous Cell Carcinoma

1. **C and D.** Both of these cause a soft tissue mass that affects the true vocal cord. There is no chondroid matrix or involvement of the cricoid cartilage. Rhabdomyosarcomas occur in children and not in older patients.

2. **B.** The oral cavity includes the lips, oral tongue, floor of mouth, alveolar ridges, and retromolar trigone.

3. **D.** The extended vertical hemilaryngectomy allows removal of one third of the contralateral vocal cord but preserves voice.

4. **E.** The arytenoids must be mobile for the larynx to function. If the arytenoids are immobilized by tumor, a total laryngectomy is the only surgical option.

Comment

Management

This is a glottic cancer which has spread from the left true vocal cord to the anterior commissure (Figure S24-1). Once the anterior commissure has become involved, possible spread may occur anteriorly through the soft tissues to the strap muscles, to the top of the thyroid cartilage, and to the Delphian node anterior to the larynx/trachea. It also means that the surgeon cannot perform a *simple* vertical hemilaryngectomy, which is one of the preferred procedures for bulky cancers of the true vocal cord that are not amenable to primary laser or cordectomy surgery or to radiation therapy. However, the *extended* vertical hemilaryngectomy, in which a sizable portion of the contralateral vocal cord is resected, would still be an option for this patient. If the arytenoids are mobile, and if the cricoid cartilage, the base of the tongue, and the hyoid bone are free of tumor, another surgical option is the supracricoid laryngectomy with cricohyoidopexy. Because of the valvelike effect of the epiglottis, it would be preferable for the epiglottis to be incorporated into the reconstruction, in a cricohyoidoepiglottopexy, but this is not essential.

Tumor Staging of Glottis Cancer

Glottis cancer is staged as follows:
- **T1:** Tumor is limited to one or both vocal cords (may involve anterior or posterior commissure) with normal mobility.
- **T1a:** Tumor is limited to one vocal cord.
- **T1b:** Tumor involves both vocal cords.
- **T2:** Tumor extends to supraglottis and/or subglottis, with or without impaired vocal cord mobility.
- **T3:** Tumor is limited to the larynx with vocal cord fixation and/or invades paraglottic space, with or without minor erosion of the thyroid cartilage (e.g., inner cortex).
- **T4a:** Tumor invades through the thyroid cartilage and/or invades tissue beyond the larynx (e.g., trachea; soft tissues of the neck, including the deep extrinsic muscle of the tongue, strap muscles, thyroid, or esophagus).
- **T4b:** Tumor invades prevertebral space, encases carotid artery, or invades mediastinal structures.

Reference

Tufano RP. Organ preservation surgery for laryngeal cancer. *Otolaryngol Clin North Am.* 2002;35(5):1067-1080.

Cross-Reference

Neuroradiology: The Requisites, 3rd ed, 465-467.

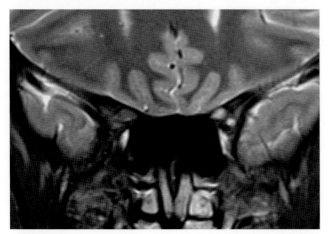

Figure 25-1

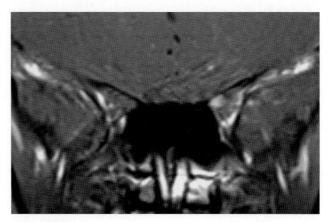

Figure 25-2

HISTORY: A young woman has blurred vision with some color discrepancy.

1. Which are possible causes of optic neuritis? (Choose all that apply.)
   A. Multiple sclerosis
   B. Herpesvirus infection
   C. Sarcoidosis
   D. Devic syndrome

2. In how many cases do intracranial demyelinating plaques occur concomitantly with optic neuritis?
   A. 0% to 20%
   B. 21% to 40%
   C. 41% to 60%
   D. 61% to 80%
   E. >80%

3. In what percentage of cases is optic neuritis centered in the intracranial prechiasm or chiasm region of the optic nerve (as opposed to the orbital portion)?
   A. 0% to 10%
   B. 11% to 30%
   C. 31% to 50%
   D. 51% to 70%
   E. >70%

4. What percentage of patients presenting with optic neuritis develop multiple sclerosis?
   A. 0% to 20%
   B. 21% to 40%
   C. 41% to 60%
   D. 61% to 80%
   E. >80%

See Supplemental Figures section for additional figures and legends for this case.

CASE 25

Optic Neuritis

1. **A, B, C, and D.** Optic neuritis has numerous causes, including vascular (ischemic optic neuropathy), inflammatory, infectious, demyelinating, metabolic, nutritional, and iatrogenic (e.g., radiation damage) entities.

2. **C.** Because multiple sclerosis is a common cause of optic neuritis in young adults, the clinician must always look for characteristic demyelinating plaques in the brain of such a patient.

3. **A.** Most cases of optic neuritis are in the orbit, not outside the orbit. The optic canal is frequently involved.

4. **C.** Eighty percent of patients with multiple sclerosis have an episode of optic neuritis in their lifetime. Of patients presenting with optic neuritis, 50% eventually receive the diagnosis of multiple sclerosis after 10 years.

Comment

Differential Diagnosis

The most common cause of optic neuropathy is ischemic. Atherosclerosis with or without diabetes in elderly patients leads to transient or permanent visual loss. The worst cases involve retinal artery occlusion and severe visual field cut. The differential diagnosis for optic neuropathy is vast and includes infectious causes—most commonly viral, such as herpes simplex virus, human immunodeficiency virus (HIV), and measles, but also bacterial tuberculosis, syphilis, and toxoplasmosis)—and noninfectious inflammatory conditions such as sarcoidosis, radiation neuritis, collagen vascular diseases, and iatrogenic conditions that result from retrobulbar injections.

Incidence of Optic Neuritis

In 20% to 35% of patients with optic neuritis, the condition recurs, again at a higher rate among patients who also have multiple sclerosis. With demyelinating optic neuritis, vision is recovered slowly, over the course of weeks to months, but may be close to complete. Of patients with multiple sclerosis, 80% have an episode of optic neuritis at some point in their lives, and 50% to 60% of patients with optic neuritis carry a diagnosis of multiple sclerosis by 10 years. The figures show the characteristic high signal in the optic nerve (Figure S25-1) and enhancement of the "plaque" (Figure S25-2). However, one finding can exist without the other.

Optic Neuritis Associations

Devic syndrome, also known as *neuromyelitis optica* (NMO), has been associated with a specific serum autoantibody marker, NMO–immunoglobulin G, that targets the water channel protein aquaporin 4. The syndrome is associated with a monophasic relatively fulminant case of optic neuritis and transverse myelitis. The titer of aquaporin 4 antibody is correlated with the length of spinal cord lesions and the relapse rate of transverse myelitis.

Reference

Smith MM, Strottmann JM. Imaging of the optic nerve and visual pathways. *Semin Ultrasound CT MR.* 2001;22(6):473-487.

Cross-Reference

Neuroradiology: The Requisites, 3rd ed, 233, 234f, 332b, 345-347, 346f.

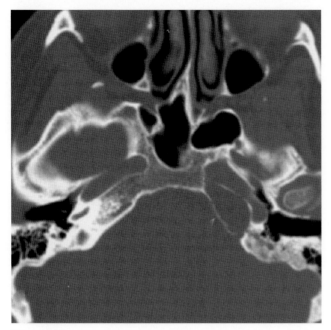

Figure 26-1

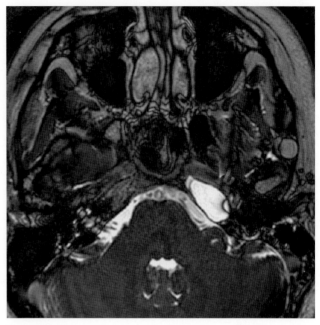

Figure 26-2

HISTORY: A patient presents with ear and facial pain and with left abducens palsy. CN IV

1. Which of the following would be included in the differential diagnosis for the imaging findings presented? (Choose all that apply.)
   A. Cholesterol granuloma
   B. Epidermoid
   C. Petrous apex mucocele
   D. Petrous apicitis

2. In what percentage of cases is the petrous apex aerated?
   A. 0% to 20%
   B. 21% to 40%
   C. 41% to 60%
   D. >60%

3. Which of these conditions would *not* show high signal on fast spin echo T2- and T1-weighted images?
   A. Petrous apex fat
   B. Cholesterol granuloma
   C. Petrous apex mucocele
   D. Petrous apicitis

4. Which is *not* a component of Gradenigo syndrome?
   A. Fifth nerve palsy
   B. Fifth nerve pain
   C. Sixth nerve palsy
   D. Otitis media with otorrhea

See Supplemental Figures section for additional figures and legends for this case.

CASE 26

Petrous Apicitis

1. **C and D.** Cholesterol granulomas are expansile lesions that show blood products, most often with bright signal on T1-weighted images. Epidermoids usually appear bright on diffusion-weighted imaging. High signal on T2-weighted imaging is invariable in the choices provided.

2. **B.** The petrous apex is aerated in 33% of cases. Only in these cases are both petrous apicitis and cholesterol granuloma present.

3. **D.** Fast spin echo T2-weighted images may be bright because of fat, inflammation, and, often, blood. But petrous apicitis usually does not appear bright on T1-weighted images.

4. **A.** Gradenigo syndrome includes facial pain, sixth nerve palsy, and otorrhea.

Comment

Characteristics of Petrous Apicitis

Fewer than half of the patients described in Giuseppe Gradenigo's original publication on petrous apicitis had all components of the triad named after him. In petrous apicitis, the area most commonly affected is the ophthalmic division of the trigeminal nerve. Since the advent of modern antibiotics, fewer patients have been affected by the full syndrome, and most cases do not necessitate the definitive therapy of mastoidectomy needed previously to eradicate the infection. Nowadays patients with petrous apicitis are admitted for intravenous antibiotic therapy. The most common pathogens are, in order of frequency, *Staphylococcus aureus, Pseudomonas aeruginosa, Streptococcus pneumoniae,* other streptococcal species, and *Mycobacterium tuberculosis.*

Imaging Findings

Imaging of petrous apex inflammation (Figures S26-1, S26-2, S26-3, and S26-4) should include fat-suppressed sequences because, per the question above, normal petrous apex fat can simulate mucoceles and cholesterol granulomas and epidermoids. Diffusion-weighted imaging sequences are useful for the latter, but cholesterol granulomas, by virtue of blood products, can obscure the findings. Expansion of the air cells is indicative of mucoceles and cholesterol granulomas. Enhancement helps define abscesses and the walls of mucoceles. Petrous carotid aneurysms, depending on whether they are thrombosed completely or partially, exhibit flow-related artifact or normal-flow signal voids that may simulate many lesions of the petrous apex. Petrous apicitis usually develops after an episode of otitis media. Complications may also include petrosal sinus thrombosis.

Reference

Connor SE, Leung R, Natas S. Imaging of the petrous apex: a pictorial review. *Br J Radiol.* 2008;81(965):427-435.

Cross-Reference

Neuroradiology: The Requisites, 3rd ed, 411-412.

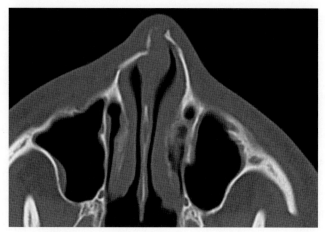

Figure 27-1

HISTORY: A patient presents to the emergency department with facial trauma after an altercation.

1. What bone or bones are fractured in Figure 27-1?
   A. Ethmoid bone
   B. Maxillary spine
   C. Orbital floor
   D. Frontal bone
   E. Nasal bone

2. What percentage of facial bone fractures affect the nasal bones?
   A. 0% to 30%
   B. 31% to 60%
   C. 61% to 90%
   D. >90%
   E. The nasal bone is not considered a facial bone.

3. Complications of nasal bone fractures include all except which of the following? (Choose all that apply.)
   A. Epistaxis
   B. Airway compromise
   C. Internal carotid artery (ICA) pseudoaneurysm
   D. Rhinorrhea

4. Indications for surgical correction include all except which of the following? (Choose all that apply.)
   A. Septal hematoma
   B. Cosmesis
   C. Incomplete fractures
   E. Airway compromise

See Supplemental Figures section for additional figures and legends for this case.

CASE 27

Nasal Bone Fracture

1. **E.** The nasal bone is the only bone shown to be fractured here. This is a common posttraumatic finding.

2. **B.** The nasal bones represent about 40% of facial fractures. The mandible and orbit are also commonly fractured.

3. **C.** Epistaxis, airway compromise, and rhinorrhea may complicate nasal bone fractures. The nose is relatively far from the carotid arteries.

4. **C.** Incomplete fractures usually do not necessitate surgical management and may heal without cosmetic deformity.

Comment

Computed Tomographic Scans of Nasal Bone Fractures

Nasal bone fractures are common findings in patients with facial trauma because of the protruding nature of the nose. Unfortunately, the face has sutures that can simulate fractures; thus evaluation with plain radiographs of the face and selective nasal bone films may be difficult. Computed tomography may seem like overkill, but important concurrent findings warrant this type of detailed study:

- Concurrent fractures of the orbits and nasoethmoidal struts
- Nasal septum hematoma, which can lead to ischemia of the cartilage and to autonecrosis and collapse of the nasal architecture
- Cerebrospinal fluid leakage at the anterior skull base from the cribriform plate
- Fracture dislocations (Figure S27-1)
- Involvement of the frontal recess and/or the nasolacrimal duct

Because of the capacious vascular plexus in the nasal region, nasal bone fractures can cause significant blood loss. In rare cases, the anterior ethmoidal artery may be traumatized, which may even necessitate embolization to arrest bleeding.

Repairing Nasal Bone Fractures

Reduction of the nasal bone fractures may be closed or open. Open reduction is done in fewer than 5% of cases. Unilateral minimally displaced fractures may be approached with a closed manipulation while the patient is under sedation or local anesthesia. Open reduction of comminuted fractures is difficult for the distal fractures, but it may be required when the bridge of the nose is traumatized and for fracture dislocations, open fractures, and marked nasal septal deviation. It is important to address the septal hematoma because it can lead to ischemic necrosis of the nasal cartilage and saddle nose deformity. In most cases, nasal bone fractures are addressed after acute swelling has subsided, 5 to 10 days after injury. Septorhinoplasty, performed by otorhinolaryngologists or plastic surgeons, may be deferred for weeks to months to provide the best reconstructive cosmetic result. Open wounds and cases with concurrent foreign matter in the wound are other situations in which careful treatment with debridement and irrigation may be required.

Reference

Hwang K, You SH, Kim SG, Lee SI. Analysis of nasal bone fractures; a six-year study of 503 patients. *J Craniofac Surg.* 2006;17(2): 261-264.

Cross-Reference

Neuroradiology: The Requisites, 3rd ed, 187, 189, 414-416.

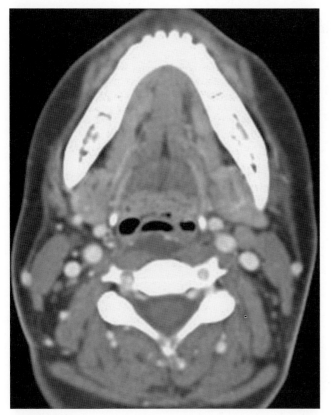

Figure 28-1

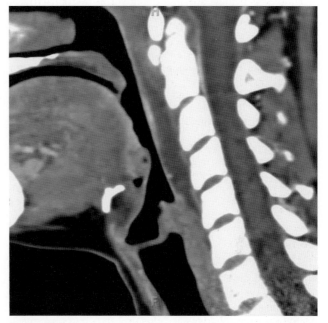

Figure 28-2

HISTORY: A young adult presented with a 24-hour history of neck pain and stiffness.

1. Which of the following would be included in the differential diagnosis for the imaging findings presented? (Choose all that apply.)
   A. Normal
   B. Phlegmon
   C. Edema
   D. Abscess

2. Which of the following is most likely to cross the midline?
   A. Retropharyngeal course of carotid arteries
   B. Necrotizing retropharyngeal adenitis
   C. Tonsil cancer
   D. Retropharyngeal abscess

3. How is a retropharyngeal abscess distinguished from phlegmon or edema?
   A. Degree/character of enhancement
   B. Density of collection
   C. Crossing of the midline
   D. Necrotizing adenitis

4. What is not a cause of retropharyngeal edema?
   A. Lymphoma
   B. Calcific longus tendonitis
   C. Radiation therapy
   D. Pharyngitis

See Supplemental Figures section for additional figures and legends for this case.

CASE 28

Retropharyngeal Edema

1. **C and B.** In the absence of peripheral enhancement, the choices generally are phlegmon versus retropharyngeal edema, although the former may show faint enhancement.

2. **D.** Nodes and vessels very rarely cross the midline. The abscess may cross the midline if it represents coalescent adenitis, or it may develop de novo.

3. **A.** Edema, phlegmon, and abscesses may cross the midline and have low density, but abscesses typically exhibit peripheral well-defined enhancement.

4. **A.** Lymphoma does not present as low density edema (but the other entities might). It appears as a solid mass that may occur in the retropharyngeal space either as a primary tumor or as a metastasis from the aerodigestive system lymphoid tissue.

Comment

Distinction Between Retropharyngeal Edema and Other Lesions

The distinction among the four entities of retropharyngeal edema (Figures S28-1 and S28-2), retropharyngeal phlegmon, necrotizing retropharyngeal adenitis, and retropharyngeal abscess is a difficult one that many head and neck radiologists ponder. Although this may be a personal approach, two lesions can be ruled out for the following reasons:

1. A patient with unilateral abnormalities that are in the expected location of the medial or lateral retropharyngeal lymph nodes without extension across the midline probably has necrotizing adenitis. They should have an intact nodal capsule. Whether those necrotic, purulent nodes need to be drained depends on early response to therapy and surgical philosophy.

2. A patient with a ring-enhancing collection that crosses the midline and shows mass effect has a retropharyngeal abscess. This probably necessitates percutaneous or surgical drainage, although for small abscesses in older patients, antibiotics may be tried for 24 to 48 hours.

The following two entities are more difficult to determine:

3. An amorphous collection without enhanced, well-defined borders is phlegmon, with adjacent edema and inflammatory changes in the nearby tissues.

4. Retropharyngeal edema usually has no inflammatory component evident, crosses the midline, and is not drainable. It is usually symmetric and fills the space.

Gray Zones

Unfortunately there *are* abscesses that do not enhance in a rim manner. If a large collection has distinct borders without enhancement, it is probably a purulent drainable collection (i.e., abscess). Some phlegmons are as drainable as abscesses and may show faint rim enhancement. Sometimes necrotizing adenitis coalesces and, in fact, may be the cause of the abscess. Pharyngitis and longus tendinitis, both inflammatory conditions, may cause retropharyngeal edema.

Reference

Hoang JK, Branstetter BF 4th, Eastwood JD, Glastonbury CM. Multiplanar CT and MRI of collections in the retropharyngeal space: is it an abscess? *AJR Am J Roentgenol.* 2011;196(4):W426-W432.

Cross-Reference

Neuroradiology: The Requisites, 3rd ed, 499-500.

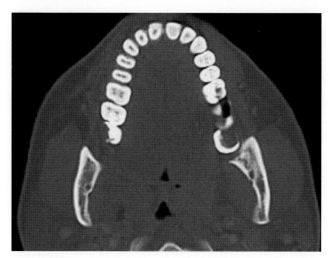

Figure 29-1

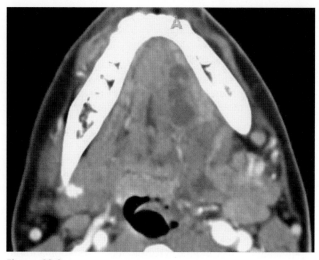

Figure 29-2

HISTORY: The patient is a 29-year-old woman complaining of "bad teeth," seen in the emergency department.

1. Which of the following would be included in the differential diagnosis for the imaging findings presented? (Choose all that apply.)
   A. Odontogenic abscess
   B. Sublingual space abscess
   C. Ludwig angina
   D. Bartholin duct cyst

2. What is the most likely source of infection in the floor of the mouth?
   A. Dental infection
   B. Sialolithiasis
   C. Folliculitis
   D. Mucocele

3. How does abscess spread from the submandibular space to the sublingual space?
   A. Through the congenital defects between the muscle fibers of the mylohyoid muscle
   B. By stripping the mylohyoid muscle from its attachment site along the inner surface of mandible
   C. Through the natural opening along the posterior margin of the mylohyoid muscle
   D. Separately from the submandibular abscess

4. What are the anatomic boundaries of the sublingual space?
   A. Mylohyoid muscle medially, mandible laterally
   B. Mylohyoid muscle laterally, hyoglossus muscle medially
   C. Hyoglossus muscle laterally, genioglossus muscle medially
   D. Submandibular gland inferiorly, parotid gland superiorly

See Supplemental Figures section for additional figures and legends for this case.

CASE 29

Sublingual Abscess

1. **A, B, and C.** This was an abscess that arose from an odontogenic origin and spread to the sublingual space in the floor of the mouth, which is characteristic of Ludwig angina.

2. **A.** The condition originated from an infected tooth.

3. **C.** The same mylohyoid muscle opening that may allow a ranula to plunge inferiorly into the submandibular space may be a conduit for spread of infection.

4. **B.** The sublingual space is a part of the floor of the mouth under the tongue. It is bounded by mylohyoid muscle laterally and hyoglossus muscle medially and contains the sublingual gland and the Wharton duct of the submandibular gland.

Comment

Diagnosis

This patient has a sublingual space abscess, seen as the low-density collection between the mylohyoid muscle and the hyoglossus muscle with peripheral enhancement (Figures S29-1 and S29-2). It originated from the carious teeth in the mandible on the left side in the region of the second molar (Figure S29-3). This route of spread—from tooth to submandibular space to sublingual space—is not uncommon; it is known as *Ludwig's angina* when it leads to a cellulitis of the space, and it may compromise the airway. In the era of modern antibiotics, it is a rare disease, and early recognition is the key to prevent the historically high rates of mortality.

Sublingual Abscess Symptoms

Once in the sublingual space, infection creates mass effect on the tongue with posterior displacement of the tongue base and oropharyngeal airway compromise. Cellulitis can further dissect along the facial planes into the parapharyngeal and retropharyngeal spaces and into the mediastinum. About 25% of cases are observed in the pediatric population.

Imaging Findings

Computed tomography may show a low-density collection, as in this sublingual abscess, or it may show more typical features of cellulitis and fasciitis.

Reference

Yonetsu K, Izumi M, Nakamura T. Deep facial infections of odontogenic origin: CT assessment of pathways of space involvement. *AJNR Am J Neuroradiol.* 1998;19(1):123-128.

Cross-Reference

Neuroradiology: The Requisites, 3rd ed, 477.

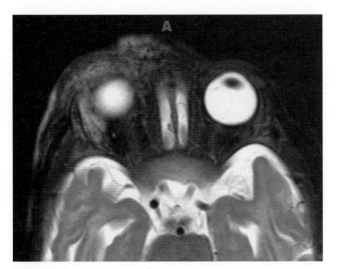

Figure 30-1

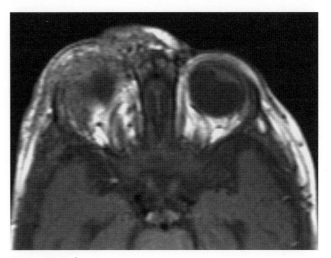

Figure 30-2

HISTORY: An infant presents with purplish swelling of the orbital eyelid.

1. Which of the following would be included in the differential diagnosis for the imaging findings presented? (Choose all that apply.)
   A. Infantile hemangioma
   B. Rhabdomyosarcoma
   C. Giant cell tumor
   D. Blue rubber bleb syndrome

2. Which of the following is the best description of PHACE?
   A. **P**olymicrogyria, **H**emangioma, **A**rterial lesions (blood vessel abnormalities in the head or neck), **C**ardiac (heart) abnormalities/aortic coarctation, and **E**ye abnormalities
   B. **P**osterior fossa brain malformations, **H**emangioma, **A**genesis of the corpus callosum, **C**ardiac (heart) abnormalities/aortic coarctation, and **E**ye abnormalities
   C. **P**osterior fossa brain malformations, **H**emangioma, **A**rterial lesions (blood vessel abnormalities in the head or neck), **C**loacal extrophy, and **E**ye abnormalities
   D. **P**osterior fossa brain malformations, **H**emangioma, **A**rterial lesions (blood vessel abnormalities in the head or neck), **C**ardiac (heart) abnormalities/aortic coarctation, and **E**ye abnormalities

3. What is the natural history of infantile hemangiomas?
   A. They slowly enlarge with age.
   B. They slowly decrease in size after birth.
   C. They remain stable over time.
   D. They enlarge and then involute.

4. What is the vascular malformation of blue rubber bleb nevus syndrome?
   A. Arteriovenous malformations
   B. Venous vascular malformations
   C. Lymphatic malformations
   D. Hemangiomas

See Supplemental Figures section for additional figures and legends for this case.

Infantile Hemangioma of the Orbit

1. **A.** Infantile hemangiomas are the vascular neoplasms of infancy that grow and regress and would be "purplish."

2. **D.** PHACE stands for Posterior fossa brain malformations, Hemangioma, Arterial lesions (blood vessel abnormalities in the head or neck), Cardiac (heart) abnormalities/aortic coarctation, and Eye abnormalities.

3. **D.** Infantile hemangiomas have a growth phase and then a regression (involution) phase. The involution phase may be rapid.

4. **B.** Blue rubber bleb nevus syndrome is characterized by numerous venous malformations of the skin and gastrointestinal viscera.

Comment
Associations with Hemangiomas

Infantile hemangiomas are tumors that have a growth-proliferative phase and an involutional regression phase. Venous vascular malformations, in comparison, enlarge slowly over time. Infantile hemangiomas are the most common childhood tumors of the orbits. They most often affect girls and premature infants and manifest at a mean age just less than 1 year old. They may appear in the skin, the subcutaneous tissues, and elsewhere in the face and neck (Figures S30-1, S30-2, and S30-3). They involute between the ages of 2 and 8; during involution, they may undergo fibrofatty change.

Imaging Findings

The scans often show an artery feeding this lesion, and the lesion is opacified in the arterial phase of a dynamic magnetic resonance–enhanced scan. Venous malformations, by contrast, become visible in the later venous phase. Congenital hemangiomas are visible at birth, whereas infantile hemangiomas appear after a few weeks of life. The former may take the form of a rapidly involuting congenital hemangioma (RICH) or a noninvoluting congenital hemangioma (NICH).

PHACE

PHACE syndrome refers to posterior fossa brain malformations, such as Dandy-Walker syndrome; hemangioma; arterial lesions (blood vessel abnormalities in the head or neck, such as cerebral aneurysms, stenosis, and anomalous primitive connections); cardiac anomalies, such as ventricular septal defects, patent ductus arteriosus, and aortic coarctation; and eye abnormalities, such as retinal vascularity, bilateral retinal hyperemia, and Horner syndrome. In addition, sternal clefting is often present (and thus the eponym is *PHACES*). Hemangiomas associated with PHACE often affect the face in the distribution of cranial nerve branch V_1.

Reference

Kavanagh EC, Heran MK, Peleg A, Rootman J. Imaging of the natural history of an orbital capillary hemangioma. *Orbit*. 2006;25(1): 69-72.

Cross-Reference

Neuroradiology: The Requisites, 3rd ed, 491-492.

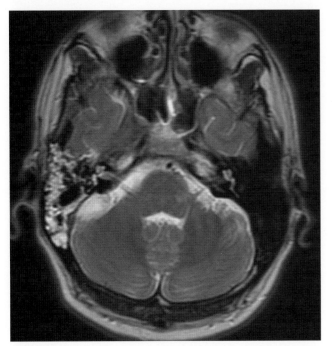

Figure 31-1

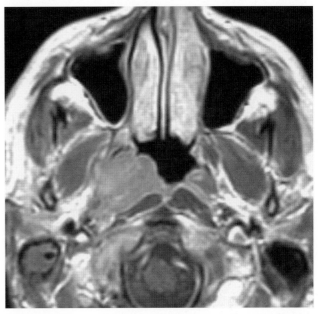

Figure 31-2

HISTORY: The patient presents with right-sided hearing loss and a sensation of fullness in the right ear.

1. Which of the following should be included in the differential diagnosis? (Choose all that apply.)
   A. Nasopharyngeal carcinoma
   B. Malignant otitis externa
   C. Calcific tendinitis of the longus colli musculature
   D. Otomastoiditis

2. Which of the following is most likely to occur?
   A. A mucosal lesion of the nasopharynx growing into the skull base
   B. A skull base tumor growing into the nasopharynx
   C. A sinonasal tumor growing into the nasopharynx
   D. A temporal bone lesion growing into the nasopharynx

3. Through which orifice might this lesion spread into the cavernous sinus?
   A. Through the foramen rotundum (via the second division of the fifth cranial nerve)
   B. Via the sinus of Morgagni
   C. Via the torus tubarius
   D. All of the above

4. Which of the following is *not* a World Health Organization (WHO) 2005 histologic subtype of nasopharyngeal carcinoma?
   A. Keratinizing squamous cell carcinoma
   B. Nonkeratinizing carcinomas
   C. Basaloid squamous cell carcinoma
   D. Lymphoepithelioma

See Supplemental Figures section for additional figures and legends for this case.

CASE 31

Nasopharyngeal Carcinoma

1. **A.** There is a mass in the posterolateral right nasopharynx.

2. **A.** A mucosal lesion of the nasopharynx grows into the skull base.

3. **A.** Nasopharyngeal carcinoma may spread directly with contiguous tumor growth or along the nerves. The route to the cavernous sinus may be through the foramen rotundum.

4. **D.** The WHO recognizes keratinizing squamous cell carcinoma, nonkeratinizing carcinoma (differentiated and undifferentiated type), and basaloid squamous cell carcinoma. The term *lymphoepithelioma* is no longer used.

Comment

Incidence of Nasopharyngeal Carcinoma

The incidence of nasopharyngeal carcinoma in the native or immigrant Asian population is about 20 times greater than in the white U.S. population. Polymerase chain reaction with the Epstein-Barr virus is positive in the nonkeratinizing carcinoma and undifferentiated carcinomas but not in the keratinizing squamous cell tumors and adenocarcinomas. Smoking and alcohol use do not appear to be significant risk factors. Nasopharyngeal carcinoma is not treated surgically; a cure relies on radiation therapy and/or chemotherapy. Once disease has spread intracranially or outside the nasopharynx, the prognosis is poor, mainly because of the higher incidence of hematogenous metastases and poor local control rates.

Imaging Findings After Treatment

After radiotherapy (and chemotherapy), fibrotic changes that resemble persistent tumor often occur. The presence of a defined mass and enhancing focal tissue, rather than mucosal asymmetry, suggests persistent or recurrent disease. Lobulation is an ominous sign; smoothness is benign. Magnetic resonance imaging (MRI) is superior to computed tomography for both the initial and the follow-up evaluations of nasopharyngeal carcinoma (Figures S31-1 and S31-2). Because nasopharyngeal tumors often burrow submucosally, imaging and nasopharyngoscopy play complementary roles in evaluation. For diagnosing spread to the lymph nodes (retropharyngeal lymph nodes in 50% of cases), imaging is superior to clinical evaluation. The mechanism of spread through the skull base may be through the fascial planes and bone or via perineural extension.

The Sinus of Morgagni

The sinus of Morgagni lies between the superior pharyngeal constrictor muscle and the skull base. It is a defect in the pharyngobasilar fascia through which the eustachian tube and levator veli palatini muscle gain access to the nasopharynx. It is a route for the spread of carcinoma from the nasopharynx to the skull base, especially via the mandibular nerve. Trotter syndrome or sinus of Morgagni syndrome consists of a clinical triad of unilateral deafness, trigeminal neuralgia, and soft palate dysmotility.

Reference

Hyare H, Wisco JJ, Alusi G, Cohen M, Nabili V, Abemayor E, et al. The anatomy of nasopharyngeal carcinoma spread through the pharyngobasilar fascia to the trigeminal mandibular nerve on 1.5 T MRI. *Surg Radiol Anat.* 2010;32(10):937-944.

Cross-Reference

Neuroradiology: The Requisites, 3rd ed, 439, 458-459.

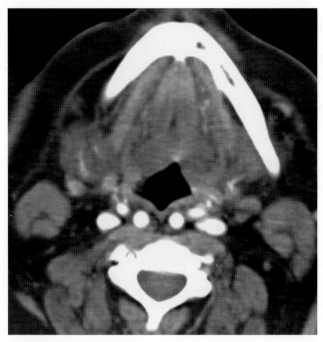

Figure 32-1

HISTORY: A patient presents with neck pain and fever.

1. Which of the following should be included in the differential diagnosis? (Choose all that apply.)
   A. Carotid dissection
   B. Carotid aneurysm
   C. Normal variation of retropharyngeal internal carotid artery
   D. Abscess
   E. Retropharyngeal lymphadenopathy

2. What are the symptoms of a retropharyngeal course of carotid arteries?
   A. Dysphagia
   B. Tinnitus
   C. Stroke
   D. No symptoms
   E. A, B, and C

3. What part of the cervical fascia is incompetent in the presence of a retropharyngeal carotid artery?
   A. Alar fascia
   B. Superficial layer of deep cervical fascia
   C. Platysma
   D. Retropharyngeal fat
   E. None of the above

4. What are "kissing carotid arteries"?
   A. Carotid arteries that extend to the sublabial region
   B. Carotid arteries that are superficial and can be visualized in the neck as pulsatile masses
   C. Bilateral retropharyngeal carotid arteries that appose each other
   D. Carotid arteries that meet in the submandibular triangle
   E. None of the above

See Supplemental Figures section for additional figures and legends for this case.

CASE 32

Retropharyngeal Carotid Artery

1. **C.** This is a normal variant.

2. **D.** Affected patients have no symptoms. However, on endoscopy, a submucosal mass may appear. Usually it appears pulsatile.

3. **A.** The retropharyngeal space is enclosed in deep cervical fascia, but the alar fascia's common wall with the carotid space may be incompetent and allow the carotid artery to migrate in.

4. **C.** "Kissing carotid arteries" are ones in the retropharyngeal space that appose each other.

Comment

Imaging Findings

Common carotid arteries and internal carotid arteries occasionally migrate into the retropharyngeal space as a result of incompetence of the alar fascia (Figure S32-1). Although this is an asymptomatic finding, it may be associated with tortuosity of the carotid arteries that results from hypertension and other atherosclerotic risk factors. Serial scanning has demonstrated that the retropharyngeal course may be a transient phenomenon that can change within hours to days. On magnetic resonance imaging (MRI), serial scans obtained hours apart may show that the carotid arteries may move in and out of this retropharyngeal location.

Implications of Findings

What are the implications for this asymptomatic finding? Identifying the presence of this normal variant would be critical in the following situations:

- To prevent unnecessary biopsy, because of the suggestion of a pulsatile mass in the pharynx
- In cases in which an anterior approach for cervical fusion is contemplated
- In cases of traumatic intubation
- With anterior approaches to pin correction of odontoid fractures
- When anesthesia of skull base foramina is contemplated
- For anterior chordoma surgery
- As a potential surgical risk in adenoidectomy, tonsillectomy, velopharyngeoplasty, and drainage of peritonsillar and retropharyngeal abscesses

Reference

Cohen SR, Briant TD. Anomalous course of the internal carotid artery—a warning. *J Otolaryngol.* 1981;10(4):283-286.

Cross-Reference

Neuroradiology: The Requisites, 3rd ed, 499.

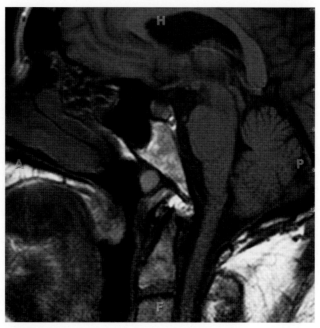

Figure 33-1

HISTORY: The patient has a long-standing history of low-grade headaches.

1. Which of the following should be included in the differential diagnosis? (Choose all that apply.)
   A. Mucous retention cyst
   B. Dermoid cyst
   C. Tornwaldt cyst
   D. Adenoid cystic carcinoma

2. What is the treatment of the lesion shown in Figure 33-1?
   A. Benign neglect
   B. Antibiotics
   C. Marsupialization
   D. Aspiration

3. What is the incidence of hyperintensity of these lesions on T1-weighted imaging?
   A. <25%
   B. 26% to 50%
   C. 51% to 75%
   D. >76%

4. What anatomic structure is associated with the development of the Tornwaldt cyst?
   A. The craniopharyngeal duct
   B. The primitive stomodeum
   C. The Rathke pouch
   D. The thyroglossal duct
   E. None of the above

See Supplemental Figures section for additional figures and legends for this case.

CASE 33

Tornwaldt Cyst

1. **A and C.** Tornwaldt cysts are classically bright on T1-weighted images; mucous retention cysts with high protein content could appear the same but are usually off midline.

2. **A.** Tornwaldt cysts are incidental lesions (unrelated to this patient's headaches) and do not need to be treated. In rare cases, they cause halitosis.

3. **B.** As stated previously, they may appear bright on T1-weighted images. On T2-weighted images, however, they are nearly always bright.

4. **E.** Tornwaldt cysts are associated with the ascension of notochord tissue, where the mucosal retraction encysts.

Comment

Incidence and Implications of Tornwaldt Cysts

The Tornwaldt cyst develops because of a persistent attachment of the notochord to the pharyngeal endoderm as it passes through the skull base. If invagination of the pharyngeal mucosa occurs, a bursa may be formed that can become obstructed with retained hyperproteinaceous secretions (Figure S33-1). In a large series, Tornwaldt cysts were observed in 0.06% of magnetic resonance imaging and computed tomographic studies; according to reports of autopsy studies, however, the incidence is between 2% and 4%, which implies that it is the most common of the congenital lesions of the head and neck.

Symptoms of Tornwaldt Cysts

Tornwaldt **disease** is the uncommon condition in which the cyst becomes infected and may obstruct the eustachian tube, cause halitosis, emit its secretions, and cause pharyngitis with concomitant throat pain. The possibility of a nasopharyngeal craniopharyngioma is explained by remnants of the obliterated craniopharyngeal duct arising along the migration of the Rathke pouch in the vomer, nasopharynx, clivus, basisphenoid, and sella turcica. In contrast to Tornwaldt cysts, which are left alone, nasopharyngeal craniopharyngiomas should be removed in their entirety.

Reference

Miyahara H, Matsunaga T. Tornwaldt's disease. *Acta Otolaryngol Suppl.* 1994;517:36-39.

Cross-Reference

Neuroradiology: The Requisites, 3rd ed, 446, 449.

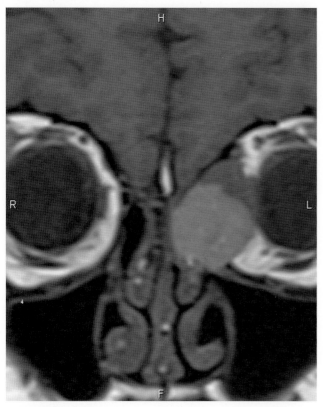

Figure 34-1

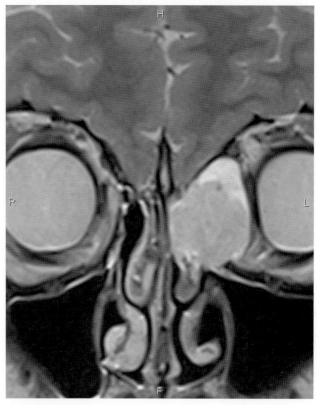

Figure 34-2

HISTORY: A 30-year-old patient presents with headache in the frontal region.

1. Which of the following should be included in the differential diagnosis? (Choose all that apply.)
   A. Melanoma
   B. Mucocele
   C. Aspergilloma
   D. Inverted papilloma

2. Which is not a cause of hyperintensity on a T1-weighted image?
   A. Hemorrhage
   B. Hyperproteinaceous secretions
   C. Melanin
   D. Cholesterol granuloma
   E. None of the above

3. What is the most common site for sinonasal melanoma?
   A. Nasal cavity
   B. Maxillary sinus
   C. Ethmoid sinus
   D. Frontal sinus
   E. Sphenoid sinus

4. What is the least common site for a mucocele?
   A. Maxillary sinus
   B. Ethmoid sinus
   C. Frontal sinus
   D. Sphenoid sinus

See Supplemental Figures section for additional figures and legends for this case.

CASE 34

Mucocele

1. **A, B, and C.** These entities may appear bright on a T1-weighted image without contrast medium. Inverted papilloma may be associated with calcifications but does not usually appear bright on T1-weighted images.

2. **E.** Hemorrhage, hyperproteinaceous secretions, melanin, and cholesterol granuloma could appear bright on a T1-weighted image.

3. **A.** Melanomas are often detected as pigmented lesions on the turbinates. The nasal cavity accounts for 70% of melanomas and the sinuses for 30%.

4. **D.** Frontoethmoidal areas are the most common sites for mucoceles. The sphenoid sinus is the least.

Comment

Imaging Findings

Imaging reveals an expansile lesion in the anterior ethmoid air cell (Figures S34-1 and S34-2). The signal intensity characteristics—bright appearance on the T1-weighted image and darkish appearance on the T2-weighted image—suggest that the most likely diagnosis is a mucocele. In the periphery, there are secretions that have low intensity on T1-weighted image and high intensity on T2-weighted image. These combinations of intensities indicate low protein in the periphery and high protein centrally. At the extremes of high protein, there may be concretions in which the signal intensity on both T1-weighted image and T2-weighted image is low.

Sinonasal Melanoma

The differential diagnosis includes melanoma, which can also appear bright on T1-weighted images and may appear dark on T2-weighted images; however, melanoma is usually even more invasive, with bone destruction. Melanoma is more commonly found in the nasal cavity or along the nasal septum and is characterized clinically by a pigmented lesion that is visible endoscopically. When a black eschar is seen, the differential diagnosis includes fungal sinusitis.

Cholesterol Granuloma

Cholesterol granulomas are much more common in the petrous apex than in the ethmoid air cells. In fact, they are uncommon in the paranasal sinuses. Expansion of the air cells is also characteristic of a cholesterol granuloma in the petrous apex.

Reference

Yousem DM, Li C, Montone KT, Montgomery L, Loevner LA, Rao V, et al. Primary malignant melanoma of the sinonasal cavity: MR imaging evaluation. *Radiographics*. 1996;16:1101-1110.

Cross-Reference

Neuroradiology: The Requisites, 3rd ed, 339, 431.

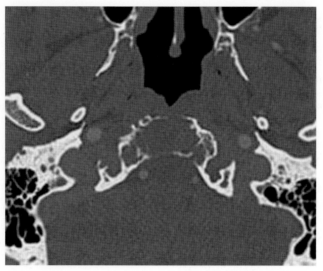

Figure 35-1

HISTORY: The patient is experiencing headaches with esotropia of the left globe.

1. Which of the following should be included in the differential diagnosis? (Choose all that apply.)
   A. Metastasis
   B. Myeloma
   C. Chordoma
   D. Osteoblastoma

2. Which of the following is correct in regard to diffusion-weighted imaging of skull base lesions?
   A. Chondrosarcoma has a higher mean apparent diffusion coefficient (ADC) than does chordoma.
   B. Chordoma has a higher mean ADC than does chondrosarcoma.
   C. Chordomas and chondrosarcomas cannot be distinguished on imaging.
   D. Chondrosarcoma and chordomas have higher ADCs than do arachnoid cysts.

3. Which is characterized by the lowest survival rate?
   A. Chordoma
   B. Chondrosarcoma
   C. Chondroma
   D. Arachnoid cyst

4. What is the typical range of ages of patients with poorly differentiated chordomas?
   A. 0 to 15 years
   B. 16 to 30 years
   C. 31 to 45 years
   D. >45 years

See Supplemental Figures section for additional figures and legends for this case.

CASE 35

Chordoma

1. **A, B, and C.** Whereas these three lesions commonly appear in the clivus, the location is decidedly uncommon for osteoblastoma (even though it may be a lytic lesion).

2. **A.** Chondrosarcoma has a higher mean ADC than does chordoma; this may help distinguish between the two, inasmuch as they otherwise may look very similar.

3. **A.** Chordomas have the worst prognosis. Chondrosarcomas in this location are very low grade, and affected patients do well over time.

4. **A.** Poorly differentiated chordomas typically occur in patients aged 2 to 10 years. Most chordomas affect people aged 40 to 60. Only 5% of chordomas occur in people younger than 20; childhood chordomas, which are usually poorly differentiated, are very rare.

Comment

Imaging Findings

To distinguish chordomas from chondrosarcomas, radiologists rely on the midline location in the clivus for chordomas and the off-midline petrooccipital fissure origin of chondrosarcomas. Unfortunately, the lesions in the different locations very often overlap, or the tumor is so big at presentation that it is not possible to suggest one diagnosis over the other on the basis of location. Moreover, both can appear very bright on T2-weighted images, both can show moderate contrast enhancement, and both can contain matrix protein (Figure S35-1). The median age at diagnosis for both is the late 30s. Less common, poorly differentiated chordomas may occur in the first decade of life and may not appear bright on T2-weighted images. For that reason, ADC values from the diffusion-weighted imaging scans are used to distinguish the two. Chondrosarcomas have higher mean ADC values (approximately 2000 mm^2/second) than do classic chordomas (1474 mm^2/second) and poorly differentiated chordomas (875 mm^2/second), but the latter two cannot be distinguished from each other. The higher ADC of chondrosarcomas may result from the cartilaginous stroma that has more free water available and increases diffusivity.

Reference

Yeom KW, Lober RM, Mobley BC, Harsh G, Vogel H, Allagio R, et al. Diffusion-weighted MRI: distinction of skull base chordoma from chondrosarcoma. *AJNR Am J Neuroradiol.* 2013;34(5):1056-1061.

Cross-Reference

Neuroradiology: The Requisites, 3rd ed, 383, 502, 567

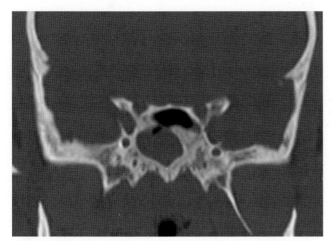

Figure 36-1

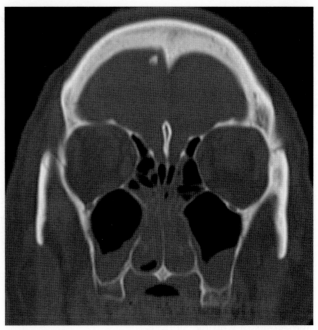

Figure 36-2

HISTORY: The patient complains of having had congestion and nasal stuffiness for years.

1. Which of the following should be included in the differential diagnosis? (Choose all that apply.)
   A. Chronic sinusitis mucosal thickening
   B. Chronic osteitis
   C. Polyps
   D. Mucocele

2. What sinonasal neoplasm is associated with intracranial cysts?
   A. Sinonasal undifferentiated carcinoma
   B. Adenocarcinoma
   C. Inverted papilloma
   D. Olfactory neuroblastoma

3. How many patients with sinusitis experience intracranial complications?
   A. 1% to 5%
   B. 6% to 10%
   C. 11% to 15%
   D. 16% to 20%

4. In how many patients with chronic sinusitis is chronic bony thickening seen on computed tomography (CT)?
   A. 0% to 25%
   B. 26% to 50%
   C. 51% to 75%
   D. >75%

See Supplemental Figures section for additional figures and legends for this case.

CASE 36

Chronic Sinusitis

1. **A and B.** The presence of bony thickening in the walls of the sphenoid sinus and of mucosal thickening without air-fluid levels or air bubbles implies chronic sinusitis and osteitis.

2. **D.** Olfactory neuroblastoma, also known as *esthesioneuroblastoma,* may be accompanied by intracranial cysts.

3. **A.** Among all the patients who show chronic sinusitis on imaging, intracranial complications are incredibly rare.

4. **B.** In chronic sinusitis, the bone is usually not considered infected. This condition is not analogous to osteomyelitis. The bone does show reactive hyperostosis that may be asymptomatic.

Comment

Symptoms of Chronic Sinusitis

The most commonly reported symptoms of chronic sinusitis are nasal obstruction, nasal congestion, discharge, fatigue, headache, sensation of facial pressure, and dysosmia. There are various methods to grade the degree of sinusitis.

LUND-MACKAY SCORING SYSTEM: In the Lund-Mackay scoring system, the opacification of the sinus system and the osteomeatal complex is rated on a scale of 0 to 2. This scoring system yields a maximum score of 12 per side:

LUND-MACKAY SCORING SYSTEM

Sinus System	Score* Left	Score* Right
Maxillary	0-2	0-2
Anterior ethmoid	0-2	0-2
Posterior ethmoid	0-2	0-2
Sphenoid	0-2	0-2
Frontal	0-2	0-2
Osteomeatal complex	0-2	0-2
Total	0-12	0-12

*0 = absence of opacification, 1 = partial opacification, 2 = complete opacification.

ZINREICH MODIFICATION* OF LUND-MACKAY SCORING SYSTEM

Score	Opacification of Affected Sinus
0	0%
1	25%
2	26%-50%
3	51%-75%
4	76%-99%
5	100%

*The involvement of the osteomeatal complex is scored 0 for absence of opacification, 1 for partial opacification, and 2 for complete opacification.

Imaging Findings

In up to 40% of affected individuals without symptoms (depending on the season and where they live), changes compatible with acute or chronic sinusitis are evident on CT (Figures S36-1 and S36-2) or magnetic resonance imaging (MRI). Moreover, in approximately 15% to 20% of patients with sinus symptoms, imaging studies yield negative findings. In approximately 10% of patients determined to be "totally normal" by imaging studies, however, endoscopy reveals significant sinus mucosal findings. Most cases of sinusitis do not necessitate imaging of any kind except through the endoscope. Imaging is used predominantly to guide surgery or to assess for intraorbital or intracranial extension of the infection. Intraorbital infection is probably evaluated equally well with either CT or MRI, but certainly MRI is the "gold standard" for evaluating intracranial and optic nerve abnormalities related to sinusitis.

Neurologic Complications Associated with Sinusitis

Besides meningitis and abscess formation (periosteal, epidural, or subdural empyemas), venous and dural sinus thrombosis and thrombophlebitis are possible causes of neurologic complications of sinusitis. Arteritis and mycotic aneurysm formation are not commonly observed except in cases of the most virulent fungal infection.

Reference

Lee JT, Kennedy DW, Palmer JN, Feldman M, Chiu AG. The incidence of concurrent osteitis in patients with chronic rhinosinusitis: a clinicopathological study. *Am J Rhinol.* 2006;20(3):278-282.

Cross-Reference

Neuroradiology: The Requisites, 3rd ed, 417-440.

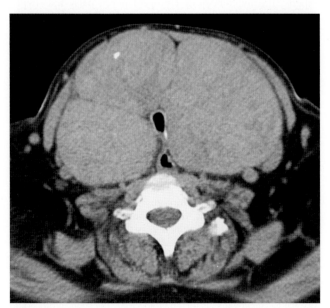

Figure 37-1

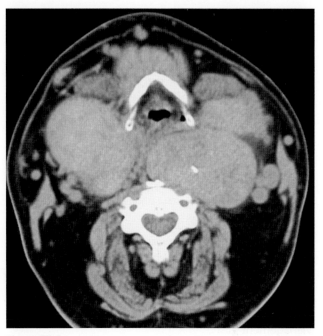

Figure 37-2

HISTORY: A 50-year-old woman presents with a palpable neck mass and inspiratory stridor.

1. Which of the following should be included in the differential diagnosis of the mass shown in Figures 37-1 and 37-2? (Choose all that apply.)
   A. Massive lymphadenopathy
   B. Metastasis
   C. Thyroid goiter
   D. Thyroid cancer

2. What is the greatest risk to the trachea with long-standing goiter?
   A. Acute compression
   B. Invasion
   C. Tracheomalacia
   D. Recurrent laryngeal nerve palsy

3. In specimens of total thyroidectomy performed for multinodular goiter, what is the approximate incidence of thyroid cancer?
   A. 1% to 15%
   B. 16% to 30%
   C. 31% to 45%
   D. >45%

4. What is the surgical treatment of choice for multinodular goiter?
   A. Partial thyroidectomy
   B. Subtotal thyroidectomy
   C. Total thyroidectomy
   D. Lumpectomy
   E. None of the above

See Supplemental Figures section for additional figures and legends for this case.

CASE 37

Goiter

1. **C.** A lesion that crosses the midline and encircles the airway is almost always a goiter, although an occult cancer cannot be totally ruled out.

2. **C.** The chronic compression of the walls of the trachea by the thyroid goiter can lead to pressure erosion of the cartilage and to tracheomalacia.

3. **A.** Multiple studies have shown the incidence to be between 3% and 15%. However, these findings may be small cancers that are incidental.

4. **C.** A goiter, when symptomatic, is treated by removal of the entire thyroid gland. Substitution hormone therapy helps prevent recurrence.

Comment

Management

Total thyroidectomy is the procedure of choice for benign multinodular goiter, partly because of the low rate of recurrence and also because the rate of incidental thyroid cancers is relatively high. Patients with thyroid cancer who have undergone incomplete thyroidectomies then require total thyroidectomies in follow-up. When surgery is performed by experts, the incidences of laryngeal nerve palsy and hypoparathyroidism are less than 2%, which is considered an acceptable rate of complications.

Symptoms of Thyroid Goiters

Airway compromise may occur with thyroid goiters (Figures S37-1 and S37-2), but **substernal** thyroid goiters account for most cases of compressed airway, perhaps because of the tighter confines of the upper chest. Esophageal compromise occurs at a rate of 33% that of tracheal compromise, but the two may coexist. Although otorhinolaryngologic surgeons should be notified when the tracheal diameter is narrowed to less than 1 cm, the chronic nature of goitrous narrowing may not necessitate emergency therapy. A nodule that acutely bleeds or a cyst that acutely grows in a goiter, however, may cause more precipitous symptoms. Clinical evaluation in that case is very important. In the long term, patients are at risk for tracheomalacia, which may lead to collapse of the trachea even after surgical management/removal of the thyroid gland.

Reference

Agarwal G, Aggarwal V. Is total thyroidectomy the surgical procedure of choice for benign multinodular goiter? An evidence-based review. *World J Surg.* 2008;32(7):1313-1324.

Cross-Reference

Neuroradiology: The Requisites, 3rd ed, 506-507.

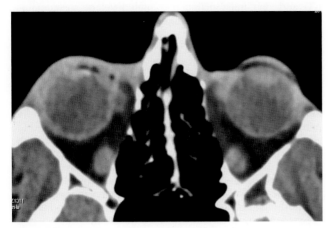

Figure 38-1

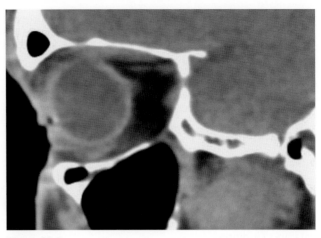

Figure 38-2

HISTORY: A patient sustained a penetrating injury to the globe while drilling in the workshop.

1. Which of the following should be included in the differential diagnosis? (Choose all that apply.)
   A. Phthisis bulbi
   B. Sudden pupillary dilation and fixation
   C. Retinal detachment
   D. Presence of foreign body

2. What does a balsa wood foreign body look like on computed tomography (CT)?
   A. Air
   B. Blood
   C. Calcification
   D. Metal

3. What does a leaded glass foreign body look like on CT?
   A. Air
   B. Blood
   C. Calcification
   D. Metal

4. What does a pencil point foreign body look like on CT?
   A. Air
   B. Blood
   C. Calcification
   D. Metal

See Supplemental Figures section for additional figures and legends for this case.

CASE 38

Orbital Foreign Body

1. **D.** A tiny radiopaque foreign body present. The patient also appears to have rupture of the anterior chamber of the globe. It is very shallow.

2. **A.** Light wood looks like air and can be easily overlooked.

3. **C.** Leaded glass is very dense.

4. **C.** Lead from a pencil is very dense as well.

Comment

Imaging Findings

This patient shows evidence of anterior hyphema with anterior chamber rupture. A laceration leading to the globe is an open wound; hence the term *open globe*. The patient had a wood foreign body, identified at surgery, that accounted for the small radiodensity indicated by the arrows (Figures S38-1, S38-2, S38-3, and S38-4). Light-weight woods (as opposed to pencils with lead in them) may have density similar to air on CT, and one must maintain a high level of suspicion for unusual-appearing orbital emphysema.

Treatment of Open Globes

Treatment of an open globe requires topical antibiotics, intravitreal antibiotics, and operative exploration. Usually intravitreal antibiotics are given as part of the preoperative treatment, especially in cases of posttraumatic endophthalmitis. If not treated immediately, open globes often lead to endophthalmitis. The end stage of this infection is phthisis bulbi, and the acute infection is often quite painful. *Bacillus cereus* is the most common pathogen implicated in posttraumatic endophthalmitis, but staphylococcal infection after cataract surgery is the most common cause of endophthalmitis. Risk factors for the development of endophthalmitis after trauma include metal foreign bodies, retained intraocular foreign bodies, disrupted lens, and delay in operative treatment.

Reference

Durand ML. Endophthalmitis. *Clin Microbiol Infect.* 2013;19(3):227-234.

Cross-Reference

Neuroradiology: The Requisites, 3rd ed, 341-342.

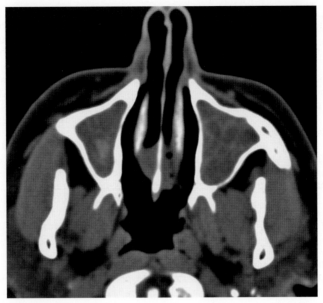

Figure 39-1

HISTORY: A 32-year-old patient presents with long-standing sinus congestion and mucoid discharge.

1. Which of the following should be included in the differential diagnosis? (Choose all that apply.)
   A. Inspissated secretions
   B. Polyps
   C. Squamous cell carcinoma
   D. Fungus

2. What signal intensity of secretions represents the highest level of protein?
   A. Bright on T1- and T2-weighted images
   B. Dark on T1-weighted images, bright on T2-weighted images
   C. Bright on T1-weighted images, dark on T2-weighted images
   D. Dark on T1- and T2-weighted images

3. What sinonasal tumor characteristically has high signal intensity on T1-weighted images?
   A. Squamous cell carcinoma
   B. Melanoma
   C. Chondroma
   D. Sinonasal undifferentiated carcinoma

4. On computed tomography (CT), how are inspissated secretions differentiated from inflammatory polyps?
   A. Polyps fill the sinus.
   B. Polyps are more dense.
   C. Polyps show mass effect.
   D. Polyps enhance solidly.

See Supplemental Figures section for additional figures and legends for this case.

CASE 39

Inspissated Secretions

1. **A, B, and D.** All of these conditions can cause hyperdensity in the sinus. All may be bilateral. Squamous cell carcinoma is not hyperdense. It has the density of muscle.

2. **D.** As the protein concentration increases, the signal intensity changes from dark on T1-weighted images and bright on T2-weighted images to bright on T1- and T2-weighted images, to bright on T1-weighted images and dark on T2-weighted images, and to dark on T1- and T2-weighted images.

3. **B.** The melanin in melanoma causes the bright signal on T1-weighted images.

4. **C.** Whereas dense secretions and polyps may appear bright on CT, polyps are distinguished by the presence of mass effect. Polyps are often present on the turbinates as well as in the sinuses, widening passageways.

Comment

Differential Diagnosis of the Dense Sinus

When density is increased in a paranasal sinus on CT, the differential diagnosis is narrow. In a nonexpanded sinus, the most likely diagnosis is inspissated secretions, which may not fill the sinus and are fairly common with chronic sinusitis (Figure S39-1). If the sinus is completely opacified and hyperdense, the differential diagnosis may include a mucocele, polyps, or fungal sinusitis (usually allergic fungal sinusitis with eosinophilic mucin). Mucoceles may expand a sinus and thin its walls, but they usually do not have the same level of lobulation and contour observed with polyps or fungi. With mucoceles, the density is usually more homogeneous across the filled sinus air cell. With polyps, more than one sinus is often affected (although antrochoanal polyps may be the exception), and the nasal cavity is also usually involved (not typical of mucoceles or inspissated secretions). On contrast-enhanced imaging, inspissated secretions and mucoceles have thin peripheral enhancement, whereas polyps and allergic fungal sinusitis produce a more rippled effect and a crenated appearance. Tumors enhance in a solid manner. The definitive diagnosis of allergic fungal rhinosinusitis can be made only with histologic examination that demonstrates fungal hyphae in the allergic eosinophil-containing mucin (which corresponds to hyperattenuating or hypointense material on T2-weighted images) and lack of mucosal invasion.

Sinus Volume

Inspissated secretions alone do not change the volume of the paranasal sinus. Once a sinus is expanded, clinicians should consider mucoceles, polyps, or, in rare cases, neoplasms. Decreased volume of the affected sinus may be a result of hypoplasia (with or without opacification) or silent sinus syndrome (sinus atelectasis).

Reference

Fatterpekar GM, Delman BN, Som PM. Imaging the paranasal sinuses: where we are and where we are going. *Anat Rec (Hoboken).* 2008;291(11):1564-1572.

Cross-Reference

Neuroradiology: The Requisites, 3rd ed, 386, 477.

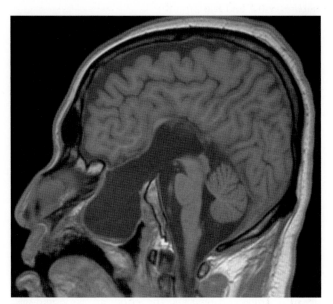

Figure 40-1

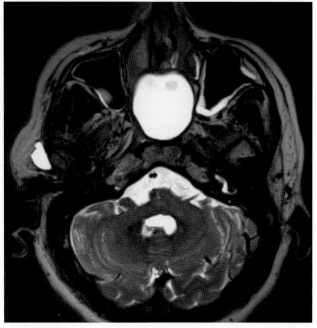

Figure 40-2

HISTORY: The patient is a young child with developmental delay and blindness.

1. Which of the following should be included in the differential diagnosis? (Choose all that apply.)
   A. Arachnoid cyst
   B. Epidermoid
   C. Cephalocele
   D. Arnold-Chiari malformation
   E. Meningoencephalocele

2. What is the most common site for cephaloceles in white people in the United States?
   A. Frontonasal
   B. Sphenobasal
   C. Parietal
   D. Temporal
   E. Occipital

3. Which congenital lesion is unique to the Arnold-Chiari type III malformation, as opposed to other Chiari malformations?
   A. Nasal glioma
   B. Schizencephaly
   C. Heterotopia
   D. Occipital cephalocele
   E. None of the above

4. What is the difference between a sincipital cephalocele and a basal cephalocele?
   A. Size
   B. Association with Dandy-Walker syndrome
   C. Presence of a stalk
   D. External appearance
   E. None of the above

See Supplemental Figures section for additional figures and legends for this case.

CASE 40

Transsphenoidal Cephalocele

1. **C and E.** *Cephalocele* is a generic term. *Meningoencephalocele* implies that meninges and brain are herniating through the skull defect. Sometimes *meningocystocele* is used to imply a cerebrospinal fluid (CSF) cyst herniation. This lesion shows communication of the CSF intensity lesion with the intracranial compartment. An epidermoid would not have this feature and the hindbrain is normal, eliminating Arnold-Chiari malformation. The location through the skull base is unlikely for an arachnoid cyst.

2. **E.** People of Southeast Asian descent tend to develop frontonasal, ethmoidal, and basal encephaloceles, but in white Americans, occipital encephaloceles are more common, as are atretic parietal cephaloceles. The cephaloceles in Africans are more commonly anterior ones.

3. **D.** Occipital (or high cervical) cephaloceles are characteristic of Arnold-Chiari type III malformations.

4. **D.** Sincipital cephaloceles project outwardly and produce cosmetic deformity externally. Basal ones may be invisible and/or cause internal bony structural abnormalities far below the skin surface.

Comment

Characteristics of Cephaloceles

Cephaloceles may contain only CSF and meninges (meningoceles), brain matter (encephaloceles), or both (meningoencephaloceles). They may be visible to the clinicians by virtue of protruding from the skull or face (sincipital), or they may be unapparent (basal). They may occur in nearly every location in the skull and have a predilection for the midline (Figures S40-1 and S40-2).

Incidence of Cephaloceles

The incidence is reported as 1 per 4000 live births. The basal and frontoethmoidal cephaloceles are most prevalent in people of Southeast Asian descent, whereas the North American population has a preponderance of occipital cephaloceles, which accompany Arnold-Chiari III malformation and other neural tube defects. Of the frontoethmoidal cephaloceles, the frontonasal type is twice as common as the nasoethmoidal type; the nasoorbital type is a distant third. Of the basal cephaloceles, the classification includes transsphenoidal, sphenoethmoidal, sphenoorbital, and transethmoidal. Transsphenoidal cephaloceles are also called *sphenopharyngeal cephaloceles,* in part because of a presumed association with the craniopharyngeal canal, which leads from the intracranial space to the pharynx via the sphenoid bone. Transsphenoidal cephaloceles like the one shown are strongly associated with pituitary and hypothalamic hormonal deficiencies (57%) as well as visual disturbances (60%), including optic nerve hypoplasia. Herniation of these tissues through the skull base defect may accompany the anterior cerebral arteries and render reconstruction dangerous. The lesions are associated with callosal dysgenesis in 60% to 80% of cases. Cleft lip, cleft palate, and hypertelorism may occur as well. Of all affected patients, 67% have some facial anomaly.

Reference

Koral K, Geffner ME, Curran JG. Transsphenoidal and sphenoethmoidal encephalocele: report of two cases and review of the literature. *Australas Radiol.* 2000;44(2):220-224.

Cross-Reference

Neuroradiology: The Requisites, 3rd ed, 380, 445.

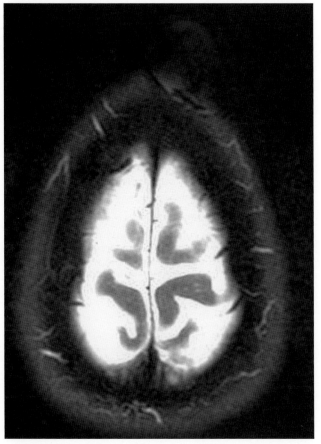

Figure 41-1

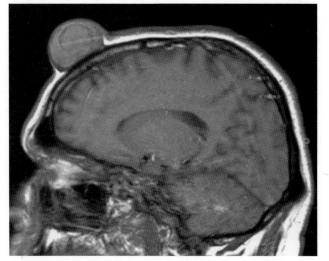

Figure 41-2

HISTORY: A patient presents with a soft tissue mass protruding from the left frontal aspect of the scalp.

1. Which of the following should be included in the differential diagnosis? (Choose all that apply.)
   A. Lipoma
   B. Neurofibroma
   C. Sebaceous cyst
   D. Chloroma
   E. None of the above

2. What is the most common subcutaneous mass of the scalp?
   A. Lipoma
   B. Neurofibroma
   C. Sebaceous cyst
   D. Chloroma
   E. None of the above

3. What accounts for the low signal intensity on the T2-weighted image in this case?
   A. Hemorrhage
   B. Keratin debris
   C. Fat
   D. Melanin
   E. Cholesterol

4. How do ruptured sebaceous cysts differ from unruptured cysts?
   A. Their borders are less distinct, and they have more septations.
   B. They have fewer septations and appear brighter on T2-weighted images.
   C. They appear bright on T1-weighted images, whereas unruptured ones do not.
   D. They are identical.

See Supplemental Figures section for additional figures and legends for this case.

CASE 41

Sebaceous Cyst

1. **C.** The signal on the T2-weighted image would not be dark for any of the other entities except a lipoma, and the sagittal T1-weighted image excludes the diagnosis of a lipoma.

2. **C.** Sebaceous cysts are more common than lipomas. Infected hair follicles and skin lesions are also very common.

3. **B.** The dark signal on T2-weighted image, sometimes so dark that the lesion is barely visible, is a feature of sebaceous cysts because of their keratin content.

4. **A.** The ruptured cysts are indistinct and more commonly septated. They may lead to local inflammation.

Comment

Terminology

The terminology for epidermal/subcutaneous cysts is imprecise. *Epidermal inclusion cyst* is a term that usually implies that the lesion results from arrests of epidermal elements in the subcutaneous tissue (Figure S41-1), either occurring on a congenital basis or acquired from trauma. In this way, they are like classic epidermoids in the extra-axial space of the brain. Some authorities consider sebaceous cysts a form of epidermal inclusion cysts. In this text, however, the term *sebaceous cyst* is used for the entity caused by occlusion of the pilosebaceous unit. The signal intensity of sebaceous cysts has a more varied appearance than that of epidermoids, and sebaceous cysts do not appear bright on diffusion-weighted imaging in the way many epidermoids do. It would be distinctly unusual for an epidermoid to be as dark as this lesion on T2-weighted images (Figure S41-2).

Characteristics of Sebaceous Cysts

Sebaceous cysts are benign, slow growing, and noninvasive. They do not enhance on imaging and do not erode the bone. They are common in the head and neck. The differential diagnosis also includes cutaneous neoplasms, and the lack of enhancement helps in that way, especially to exclude skin malignancies and neurofibromas. The rate of malignant degeneration of sebaceous cysts to squamous cell carcinomas is less than 1%.

Complications of Sebaceous Cysts

When sebaceous cysts rupture, they may demonstrate irregular margins, septations, and inflammatory-like enhancement. Fluid-fluid levels are occasionally visible within a sebaceous cyst, another finding that is different from the appearance of classic epidermoids.

Reference

Hong SH, Chung HW, Choi JY, Koh YH, Choi JA, Kang HS. MRI findings of subcutaneous epidermal cysts: emphasis on the presence of rupture. *AJR Am J Roentgenol.* 2006;186(4):961-966.

Cross-Reference

Neuroradiology: The Requisites, 3rd ed, 69-71, 280-282, 352, 371-373, 391-392, 445, 552

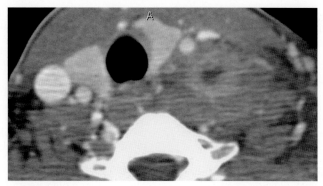

Figure 42-1

HISTORY: A patient who abuses intravenous drugs complains of neck pain and swelling and of fever.

1. Possible sources of this abscess include which of the following? (Check all that apply.)
   A. Infected lymph node
   B. Direct puncture abscess from attempt at venous access
   C. Infected branchial cleft cyst
   D. Fistula from piriform sinus

2. Which of these is the muscle immediately behind the lesion?
   A. Levator scapulae
   B. Sternocleidomastoid
   C. Anterior scalene
   D. Posterior scalene
   E. None of the above

3. Which lymph node chain(s) are between the hyoid bone and the cricoid cartilage (Choose the best answer.)?
   A. II
   B. III
   C. IV
   D. V
   E. III and V

4. What structure is at risk from an abscess in this location?
   A. The recurrent laryngeal nerve
   B. The jugular vein
   C. The aberrant subclavian artery
   D. The brachial plexus

See Supplemental Figures section for additional figures and legends for this case.

CASE 42

Neck Abscess

1. **A, B, C, and D.** All of these lesions may become a necrotic mass in the neck. The presence of edema in the nearby fat could be from inflammation or extracapsular spread from a necrotic metastatic lymph node. Sometimes the presence of a primary tumor in the same scan is the most useful feature.

2. **C.** The anterior scalene muscle is behind this lesion. This muscle borders the brachial plexus, which passes behind it.

3. **E.** Both the midjugular chain (chain III) and the upper posterior triangle (chain Va) chain of nodes are between the hyoid bone and cricoid cartilage.

4. **D.** Behind the anterior scalene muscle is the brachial plexus. Infected lymph nodes may cause a brachial plexitis. This is more common with tuberculous adenitis.

Comment

Differential Diagnosis

An abscess in this location is usually a result of necrotizing adenitis and occurs more commonly in children than in adults. The primary infectious process may emanate from pharyngitis, otitis media, mastoiditis, or a tooth infection. In adults, the differential diagnosis should include a necrotic node from squamous cell carcinoma, and a search for a primary tumor is initiated if the patient lacks the typical symptoms of pain, swelling and erythema. In this location, the lesion abuts the anterior scalene muscle (Figure S42-1). In fact, the patient had a brachial plexopathy.

Implications of Brachial Plexus Involvement

Involvement of the anterior scalene muscle leads to inflammation of the trunks of the brachial plexus and results in arm and hand discomfort, paresthesias, and motor weakness. Surgery on a lesion in this location is risky because of its proximity to the brachial plexus; hence percutaneous sampling and/or drainage may be necessary.

Imaging Findings

This location would be unusually low for a second branchial cleft cyst, the most common type. Its borders are thick and shaggy, and it does not have cystic components. For this to be related to the branchial cleft system, clinicians must consider the possibility of a third or fourth fistula, which could connect to the piriform sinus and result in an infection. Even in that case, this lesion seems lower than expected. In an inpatient population, the most common primary (nonnodal) origin of a lesion like this would be an infection acquired through an attempt at venous access, whereby the jugular vein or subclavian vein would be missed. Alternatively, a drug addict attempting jugular access may present with this type of lesion.

Reference

Krautsevich L, Khorow O. Clinical aspects, diagnosis and treatment of the phlegmons of maxillofacial area and deep neck infections. *Otolaryngol Pol.* 2008;62(5):545-548.

Cross-Reference

Neuroradiology: The Requisites, 3rd ed, 192, 197-201, 447, 543-546.

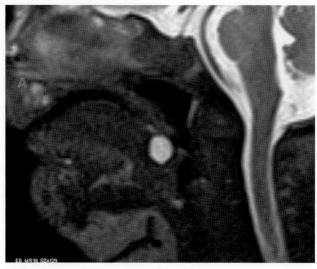

Figure 43-1

HISTORY: A child has a clinical history of "failure to thrive and developmental delay."

1. Which of the following should be included in the differential diagnosis? (Choose all that apply.)
   A. Ranula
   B. Branchial cleft cyst
   C. Epidermoid
   D. Thyroglossal duct cyst (TGDC)

2. What technique might be helpful in distinguishing an epidermoid cyst from a TGDC?
   A. Diffusion-weighted magnetic resonance imaging
   B. Iodine-131 nuclear medicine scans
   C. Ultrasonography
   D. Computed tomographic angiography combined with perfusion study

3. What location virtually confirms that a lesion is a TGDC?
   A. In the midline infrahyoid level
   B. In the midline in the tongue
   C. Off midline, abutting the thyroid gland
   D. In the strap muscle

4. What percentage of TGDCs are infrahyoid?
   A. 0% to 25%
   B. 26% to 50%
   C. 51% to 75%
   D. >75%

See Supplemental Figures section for additional figures and legends for this case.

CASE 43

Thyroglossal Duct Cyst

1. **C and D.** A lesion within the base of the tongue should be considered a TGDC or a dermoid/epidermoid cyst. This location is too high in the tongue for a ranula, which usually occurs in the floor of the mouth below the tongue.

2. **A.** Epidermoids usually appear bright on diffusion-weighted imaging (DWI). Abscesses, but not TGDCs, also appear bright on DWI.

3. **D.** TGDCs may be embedded in the strap muscles anterior to the hyoid bone, thyroid gland, or cricoid cartilage. Extremely few lesions are located there.

4. **C.** The majority of TGDCs are infrahyoid; 75% are in the midline.

Comment
Differential Diagnosis

When a child has a tongue lesion, one should consider a few characteristics: Is it cystic or solid? In a child, a solid lesion may be a hemangioma or a venous vascular malformation if it is reddish or purple; a teratoma if it is mixed in appearance; or a rhabdomyosarcoma if it is aggressive. A lingual thyroid gland has density and intensity characteristics of thyroid tissue and therefore appears bright on computed tomography without contrast and accumulates iodine-123, iodine-131, and technetium pertechnetate. If the lesion is cystic, as in this case, one should consider the epidermoid-dermoid line. These two embryologic rests can be distinguished by the presence of fat, calcification, hair, or other "dermal appendages" in the latter. Epidermoids, as with intracranial lesions, appear bright on DWI scanning by virtue of their high protein content, but dermoids could also be bright on DWI. Other cystic lesions in the tongue include mucous retention cysts and abscesses. Ranulas are in the floor of the mouth and are not really considered tongue cysts.

Locations of Thyroglossal Duct Cysts

TGDCs can occur anywhere along the path of the tract from the foramen cecum to the thyroid bed (Figure S43-1). The foramen cecum is at the upper surface of the tongue at the junction of the oral tongue (anterior two thirds) and the posterior base of the tongue (posterior third). This lesion is located close to the foramen cecum. Nonetheless, approximately 66% of TGDCs are infrahyoid, and 25% are off midline. If a lesion is embedded in strap muscles, TGDC should be the first diagnosis considered, with the caveat that this finding is specific but not sensitive for TGDCs. TGDCs only rarely contain thyroid tissue; therefore, they are not usually visible on nuclear medicine studies. Also for this reason, the occurrence of cancer in TGDCs is extremely rare.

Reference

Foley DS, Fallat ME. Thyroglossal duct and other congenital midline cervical anomalies. *Semin Pediatr Surg*. 2006;15(2):70-75.

Cross-Reference

Neuroradiology: The Requisites, 3rd ed, 446, 505, 512.

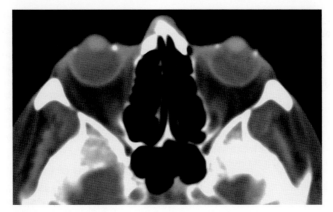

Figure 44-1

HISTORY: This patient presents with ocular pain.

1. Which of the following should be included in the differential diagnosis for these calcified lesions? (Choose all that apply.)
   A. Bilateral retinoblastoma
   B. Drusen
   C. *Toxocara* infection
   D. Senescent calcifications
   E. Human immunodeficiency virus (HIV) infection

2. Where are these ocular calcifications?
   A. In the choroid
   B. In the sclera
   C. In the retina
   D. In the muscle tendon
   E. In the uveal tract

3. Tumors associated with ocular calcification include which of the following? (Choose all that apply.)
   A. Retinoblastoma
   B. Hemangioblastoma
   C. Melanoma
   D. Cytomegalovirus-related retinitis
   E. Drusen

4. What diseases are associated with ocular calcifications?
   A. *Toxocara* infection
   B. Hyperparathyroidism
   C. Drusen
   D. Trauma and phthisis bulbi
   E. All of the above

See Supplemental Figures section for additional figures and legends for this case.

CASE 44

Senescent Calcifications of the Globe

1. **D.** In this location, the only diagnosis to suggest is senescent ocular calcifications. The other lesions may calcify, but not along the periphery of the globe in this way.

2. **B.** These ocular calcifications are located in the sclera. If they are in the choroid, one should consider osteoma. If they are in the retina, one should consider retinoblastoma.

3. **A.** Of the choices listed, retinoblastoma is the only calcified tumor. Cytomegalovirus-related retinitis and drusen are not tumors.

4. **E.** All of the lesions listed may be associated with calcifications for various reasons.

Comment

Incidence

This case is an example of senescent benign ocular calcification of the tendinous insertions of the sclera of the globe (Figure S44-1). The muscles involved are usually the medial and lateral recti (medial more common than lateral, and left more commonly than right), and this finding has no clinical significance. Bilateral involvement is present in more than 60% of affected patients. These calcifications occur frequently in older adults and, along with drusen, are the most common benign calcifications of the globe. The term *senile scleral plaque* has been used to describe the lesion. The median age at diagnosis is 84, and they are rare before the seventh decade of life. Their size varies between patients and in a single patient. Senescent calcifications of the globe occur more frequently in patients with primary and secondary hyperparathyroidism, hypervitaminosis D, chronic renal failure, and pseudohyperparathyroidism, which suggests that an influence of calcium-phosphorous dysmetabolism may increase the incidence.

Complications of Calcifications

Drusen are accumulations of proteinaceous debris usually seen at the insertion of the optic nerve head. They are a source of pseudopapilledema but appear white on ophthalmoscopy. Tumors that calcify in the globe include retinoblastomas (in infants, the rate of calcification is 90%), choroidal osteomas, and retinal hamartomas (an entity associated with tuberous sclerosis). Medulloepitheliomas of the uveal tract may also calcify. The lens, when traumatized or with severe cataract formation, may also calcify. Phthisis bulbi is usually associated with a small, shrunken, nonfunctional globe.

Reference

Alorainy I. Senile scleral plaques. *Neuroradiology.* 2000;42:145-148.

Cross-Reference

Neuroradiology: The Requisites, 3rd ed, 322f, 327.

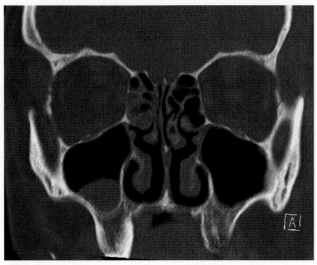

Figure 45-1

HISTORY: A young adult complains of sinus congestion.

1. Which of the following should be included in the differential diagnosis? (Choose all that apply.)
   A. Mucous retention cyst (MRC)
   B. Polyp
   C. Mucocele
   D. Antrochoanal polyp

2. What is the cause of an MRC?
   A. Degeneration of a polyp
   B. Obstruction of seromucinous glands
   C. Obstruction of osteomeatal unit
   D. Trauma

3. In which sinus are MRCs most prevalent?
   A. Frontal
   B. Ethmoid
   C. Maxillary
   D. Sphenoid

4. What feature on magnetic resonance imaging distinguishes an MRC from a polyp?
   A. Polyps enhance solidly; MRCs, peripherally.
   B. MRCs enhance solidly; polyps, peripherally.
   C. Polyps enhance in a crenated manner; MRCs, peripherally if at all.
   D. MRCs enhance in a crenated manner; polyps, peripherally if at all.

See Supplemental Figures section for additional figures and legends for this case.

CASE 45

Mucous Retention Cyst

1. **A and B.** When such a rounded excrescence is present in the maxillary antrum, it should be considered an MRC or a polyp.

2. **B.** There are multiple small minor salivary glands throughout the sinonasal cavity that account for the MRCs.

3. **C.** MRCs are most common in the maxillary sinus. They are hard to define in the ethmoid sinuses because of the small space.

4. **C.** Both polyps and MRCs appear dark on T1-weighted images and bright on T2-weighted images. However, with contrast, it would be very unusual for a polyp not to enhance, as opposed to MRCs. A curvilinear enhancement is typical of polyps.

Comment

Imaging Findings

MUCOUS RETENTION CYSTS: MRCs (Figure S45-1) are incredibly common and are frequently noted in patients with a history of chronic sinusitis as a sequela of the infection. They represent obstructed secretions of minor salivary seromucinous glands. Often they are of fluid density and have no to only trace peripheral enhancement. Some authorities believe that they cannot be differentiated on imaging from polyps; however, they are distinguished in many cases by their complete absence of mass effect, their smooth margins, and their scant enhancement. When the margins are wavier, when ostia or bony walls are enlarged, and when the enhancement pattern is crenated, it is a polyp. One should make sure that such lesions are not mucoceles, which usually fill a sinus with nonenhancing tissue.

POLYPS: Polyps result from mucous membrane hyperplasia, have a wavier appearance, and may be associated with atopy/allergic symptoms. Polyps may have different densities and intensities than MRCs, which are virtually always fluid in density/intensity. MRCs are considered asymptomatic. Polyps are more likely to obstruct ostia and to populate both the nasal and the sinus cavities, and they may lead to symptoms. MRCs are four to five times more common than polyps.

Reference

Coleman H, Meer S, Altini M, Reyneke J, Becker P. Maxillary sinus pathology in 119 patients—a histopathologic study. *SADJ*. 2005; 60(4):140, 142-145.

Cross-Reference

Neuroradiology: The Requisites, 3rd ed, 433, 449.

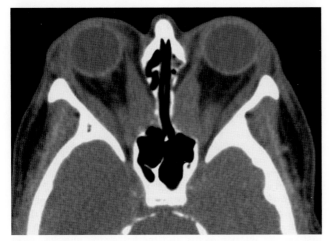

Figure 46-1

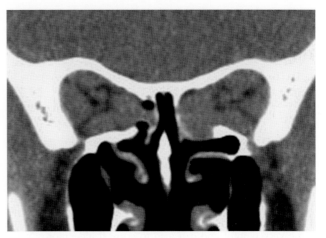

Figure 46-2

HISTORY: A 43-year-old woman has long-standing bilateral proptosis.

1. Which of the following should be included in the differential diagnosis? (Choose all that apply.)
   A. Silent sinus syndrome
   B. Sinusitis and myositis
   C. Bilateral medial orbital wall fractures
   D. Thyroid orbitopathy

2. What percentage of patients with thyroid orbitopathy are euthyroid?
   A. 0% to 10%
   B. 11% to 20%
   C. 21% to 30%
   D. >30%

3. Which symptom usually necessitates surgery for thyroid eye disease?
   A. Exposure keratitis
   B. Diplopia
   C. Dry eyes
   D. Optic neuropathy

4. What is the current recommended surgery for thyroid orbitopathy?
   A. Steroids
   B. Eyelid split and reconstruction
   C. Orbital floor decompression
   D. Endoscopic medial orbital wall decompression

See Supplemental Figures section for additional figures and legends for this case.

CASE 46

Thyroid Eye Disease

1. **D.** The presence of bilateral extraocular muscle enlargement in a patient with proptosis suggests thyroid eye disease. Besides some glycogen deposition diseases, nothing should look like this in the absence of inflammation.

2. **B.** Most patients with thyroid eye disease are hyperthyroid, but some patients are euthyroid or hypothyroid. Some affected patients have been treated for hyperthyroidism and may receive thyroid replacement therapy for hypothyroidism.

3. **A.** The proptosis causes exposure of the cornea. This can be very painful and can lead to corneal ulceration.

4. **D.** Endoscopic treatment of thyroid eye disease has become the preferred method of orbital decompression for thyroid eye disease. From the sinonasal approach, both the orbital floor and the medial orbits can be fractured to relieve the pressure on the orbital apex. (This patient has been decompressed in this fashion.)

Comment

Symptoms of Eye Disease

Thyroid orbitopathy, thyroid eye disease, Graves ophthalmopathy, Graves orbitopathy, thyroid ophthalmopathy, dysthyroid eye disease, and *Basedow disease* refer to the pathologic process in the eye that is associated with thyroid dysfunction. The acute phase is characterized by inflammation and edema of the extraocular muscles with lymphocytic infiltration. There is often injection of the fat as well. The muscular enlargement (Figures S46-1 and S46-2) causes proptosis with associated eyelid retraction. The eyelid retraction leads to exposure of the cornea and the irritation and abrasions that can occur on the surface of the eye. The eyes are dry and painful. In addition, affected patients may have diplopia.

Imaging Findings

In the worst-case scenario, the optic nerve is compressed by the large muscles at the orbital apex. In Figures 46-1 and 46-2, fat remains visible around the optic nerve, but this patient has already been treated with orbital decompression (infracturing) of the medial walls to provide the space for the medial rectus muscle to come off of the optic nerves. The enlarged muscles paradoxically may lead to restriction of eye motion. On imaging, the effects typically seen are first on the inferior rectus and medial rectus muscles, most commonly followed by superior rectus, lateral rectus, and superior oblique muscles. Affected patients have proptosis, edema of the retrobulbar fat, displacement of the lacrimal glands out of the orbit, swelling of the eyelids, and proliferation of the orbital fat (both intraconal and extraconal). The muscular tendons are spared, whereas the bellies of the muscles are markedly expanded. On magnetic resonance imaging, the muscles appear edematous and enhance profusely.

Reference

Kirsch E, Hammer B, von Arx G. Graves' orbitopathy: current imaging procedures. *Swiss Med Wkly.* 2009;139(43-44):618-623.

Cross-Reference

Neuroradiology: The Requisites, 3rd ed, 333b, 342-343.

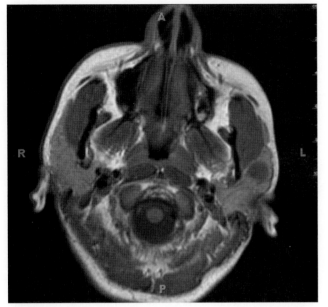

Figure 47-1

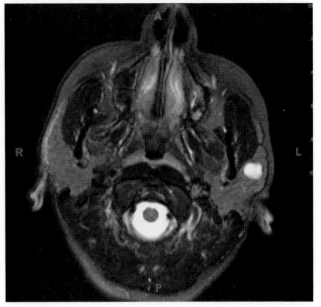

Figure 47-2

HISTORY: A 34-year-old woman was being evaluated for a headache.

1. Which of the following should be included in the differential diagnosis? (Choose all that apply.)
   A. Warthin tumor
   B. Pleomorphic adenoma
   C. Lymph node
   D. Low-grade mucoepidermoid carcinoma

2. What percentage of pleomorphic adenomas dedifferentiate into carcinoma?
   A. 0% to 25%
   B. 26% to 50%
   C. 51% to 75%
   D. >75%

3. What is the typical appearance of a pleomorphic adenoma on dynamic enhancement?
   A. Early rapid wash-in and rapid wash-out
   B. Early rapid wash-in and delayed wash-out
   C. Gradual increase over time, plateau, and maintenance of the plateau
   D. Late persistent enhancement

4. What percentage of parotid tumors are pleomorphic adenomas?
   A. 20% to 40%
   B. 41% to 60%
   C. 61% to 80%
   D. >80%

See Supplemental Figures section for additional figures and legends for this case.

Pleomorphic Adenoma of the Parotid Gland

1. **B, C, and D.** Warthin tumors rarely occur in patients this young. They have a predilection for the tail of the parotid gland.

2. **A.** Carcinoma ex pleomorphic adenoma occurs in only a small percentage of tumors because the masses are usually removed electively. However, the natural history of the tumor, if it is left untreated, is malignant degeneration in 25% of cases in 20 years.

3. **C.** Enhancement increases gradually over time, plateaus, and then is sustained on delayed images with pleomorphic adenomas.

4. **C.** According to the 80% rule, 80% of parotid masses are benign, and that 80% of those are pleomorphic adenomas; thus pleomorphic adenomas represent 64% of tumors.

Comment

Imaging Findings

The most common benign tumor of the salivary glands, the pleomorphic adenoma, has very high signal intensity on T2-weighted images (Figures S47-1 and S47-2). Benign cysts (mucous retention cyst, lymphoepithelial cyst, first branchial cleft cyst, ranula, sialocele, and pseudocyst) may also appear hyperintense on T2-weighted image. Gadolinium is employed to distinguish a pleomorphic adenoma from a cyst: Cysts do not enhance, or if they do, it is only on their periphery, whereas pleomorphic adenomas enhance throughout and thus appear solid.

Incidence of Malignant Salivary Gland Tumors

The smaller the salivary gland, the higher the rate of malignancy in salivary gland tumors. The malignancy rate of salivary gland tumors is 20% to 25% in the parotid gland, 40% to 50% in the submandibular gland, and 50% to 81% in the sublingual glands and minor salivary glands.

Implications of Parotid Pleomorphic Adenoma

Pleomorphic adenomas, also known as *benign mixed tumors,* occur most commonly in middle-aged women. They are the most common parotid mass, representing approximately 65% to 70% of parotid masses and approximately 80% of the benign ones. Of all pleomorphic adenomas, 80% occur in the superficial lobe. Pleomorphic adenomas are the most common benign tumors in the submandibular gland, sublingual gland, and minor salivary glands as well.

In surgical treatment of a pleomorphic adenoma, the danger is the potential for seeding of the operative bed, which would lead to multifocal pleomorphic adenoma or malignant degeneration into an adenocarcinoma. Thus these tumors are treated with wide local excision, with adequate attention to facial nerve preservation.

Reference

Yabuuchi H, Fukuya T, Tajima T, Hachitanda Y, Tomita K, Koga M. Salivary gland tumors: diagnostic value of gadolinium enhanced dynamic MR imaging with histopathologic correlation. *Radiology.* 2003;226(2):345-354.

Cross-Reference

Neuroradiology: The Requisites, 3rd ed, 456-457, 482-484, 486-487, 494.

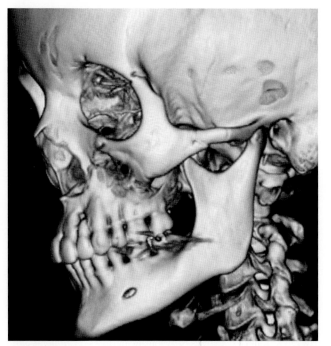

Figure 48-1

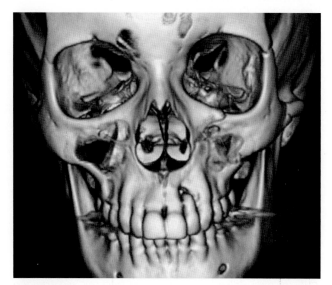

Figure 48-2

HISTORY: A patient suffered facial fractures in an altercation in East Baltimore. Figures 48-1 and 48-2 are three-dimensional reconstructions of computed tomographic scans of facial bones.

1. What type of fracture is shown here?
   A. Trimalar fracture
   B. Fracture of the zygomaticomaxillary complex (ZMC)
   C. LeFort III fracture
   D. Tripod fracture

2. What bone is not included in the ZMC?
   A. Maxilla bone
   B. Zygomaticofrontal suture
   C. Orbital floor
   D. Pterygoid plate

3. What foramen is typically involved in ZMC fractures?
   A. Foramen cecum
   B. Foramen rotundum
   C. Infraorbital foramen
   D. Superior orbital fissure

4. Which part of the zygoma is most frequently fractured?
   A. Zygomaticomaxillary suture
   B. Zygomatic arch
   C. Zygomaticofrontal suture
   D. Sphenozygomatic suture

See Supplemental Figures section for additional figures and legends for this case.

CASE 48

Zygomaticomaxillary Complex Fracture

1. **A, B, and D.** *Zygomaticomaxillary complex fracture* is the formal name for the facial trauma described in this case. *Trimalar fracture* and *tripod fracture* are other names for this type of fracture.

2. **D.** Pterygoid plate fractures are characteristic of the LeFort-type fractures. The other bones are part of the ZMC.

3. **C.** Because of the orbital floor/rim fracture, the infraorbital foramen is involved in ZMC fractures. This often leads to hypesthesia.

4. **B.** The zygomatic arch may be involved in ZMC fractures, but it may also be fractured by itself. Direct blows may cause inward buckling of the zygomatic arch.

Comment

Fracture Locations

ZMC fractures—also known as *tripod fractures* and *trimalar fractures*—are very common (Figures S48-1 and S48-2). Among facial bone fractures, their frequency is less common than nasal bone and orbital floor fractures. As opposed to a blow from frontally at the nose or orbit, these are more commonly roundhouse punches to the side of the face over the zygomatic arch. The structures fractured include the superior attachment to the frontal bone (zygomaticofrontal suture), the medial attachment to the maxilla (zygomaticomaxillary suture), the lateral attachment to the temporal bone (zygomaticotemporal suture), and the deep attachment to the greater wing of the sphenoid bone (zygomaticosphenoidal suture). The zygomaticomaxillary and zygomaticosphenoidal sutures are usually considered a single unit.

Incidence of Zygomatic Fractures

Of zygomatic fractures in toto, ZMC fractures account for 50.7%, zygomaticomaxillary monopod fractures for 25.8%, and isolated fracture of the zygomatic arch for 20.9%. Most fractures necessitate open reduction except for isolated zygomatic arch fractures that do not break the skin. The most common complications after treatment are hypesthesia (56.8%), diplopia (17.0%), and decreased range of motion of the mandible/maxilla (12.5%). The hypesthesia and paresthesia result from involvement of the infraorbital foramen and are in the distribution of cranial nerve branch V_2 with these fractures.

Reference

Hwang K, Kim DH. Analysis of zygomatic fractures. *J Craniofac Surg.* 2011;22(4):1416-1421.

Cross-Reference

Neuroradiology: The Requisites, 3rd ed, 189.

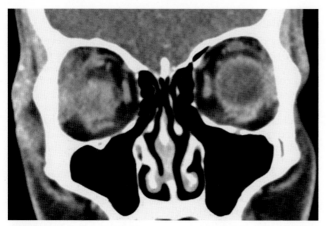

Figure 49-1

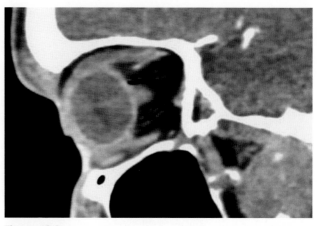

Figure 49-2

HISTORY: A patient has a red eye with swelling and epiphora.

1. Which of the following should be included in the differential diagnosis? (Choose all that apply.)
   A. Periorbital cellulitis
   B. Orbital cellulitis
   C. Orbital phlegmon
   D. Orbital abscess

2. What is the most common source of orbital cellulitis?
   A. Trauma/puncture wounds
   B. Styes/dacryocystitis
   C. Sinusitis
   D. Meningitis

3. How does sinusitis usually lead to orbital cellulitis?
   A. Via retrograde extension into veins
   B. Via blowing the nose and particle debris on cornea
   C. Via meningitis
   D. Via direct spread through thin bone

4. What does "tenting" of the globe imply with an infection?
   A. Axial myopia
   B. Stretching of the optic nerve under pressure, leading to ischemic risk
   C. Abscess
   D. Impending retinal detachment

See Supplemental Figures section for additional figures and legends for this case.

CASE 49

Orbital Cellulitis

1. **B.** The presence of orbital fat injection and muscular thickening, combined with the patient's symptoms, suggests orbital cellulitis.

2. **C.** Many infections of the globe result from irritation by contact lenses, superficial irritation, and corneal lacerations. Orbital cellulitis, however, usually results from spread of sinusitis.

3. **D.** The lamina papyracea, a layer of paper-thin bone, is usually porous enough that it is the route of infection spread from the sinuses to the orbits, which results in orbital sinusitis and/or periosteal abscesses.

4. **B.** Tenting of the globe causes the optic nerve to stretch and become imperiled. This condition is sometimes called *inflammatory staphyloma.*

Comment

Complications of Orbital Cellulitis

Causes of orbital cellulitis include sinusitis (67%), trauma with penetrating injuries (25%), dacryocystitis, and postsurgical and dermatologic infections. The danger of orbital cellulitis is that it can spread to the globe, optic nerve, cavernous sinus, meninges, and brain, which would lead to vascular compromise, venous thrombosis, blindness, meningitis, epidural or cerebral abscess, thrombophlebitis, and phthisis bulbi. Drainage of the sinus or of superiosteal, epidural, or intraconal abscess may be required. Staphylococci and streptococci are the microorganisms most commonly cultured.

Periorbital Versus Orbital Cellulitis

Stranding of the intraconal fat in a patient with a fever and a proptotic, painful eye should prompt evaluation by the clinician. Although the condition may be merely edema in the fat from congestion, it must be treated with aggressive antibiotics and drainage if necessary. Periorbital or preseptal cellulitis is much more common than postseptal orbital cellulitis and is less disconcerting than when the orbital septum has been violated (Figures S49-1, S49-2, and S49-3). The orbital septum is a great barrier to the spread of infections to the orbital contents because it is tough, fibrous tissue that attaches to the palpebral tissues along the tarsal plates as a continuation of the periorbita.

Orbital Cellulitis and Fungi

Because the periorbita is such a good barrier to disease, subperiosteal abscesses may occur without conal or intraconal spread. Computed tomography is ideal for visualizing the sinuses, the bone, the areas of dehiscence, and the potential dangers of surgery. One of the more virulent infections is fulminant mucormycosis, which invariably necessitates orbital exenteration for cure. Otherwise, intracranial spread of mycotic infections may render the patients neurologically impaired. Spread appears to occur along blood vessels (arteries or veins) from the cavernous sinus. Emboli, vasculitis, and aneurysms may be deadly complications.

Reference

LeBedis CA, Sakai O. Nontraumatic orbital conditions: diagnosis with CT and MR imaging in the emergent setting. *Radiographics.* 2008; 28:1741-1753.

Cross-Reference

Neuroradiology: The Requisites, 3rd ed, 339-341.

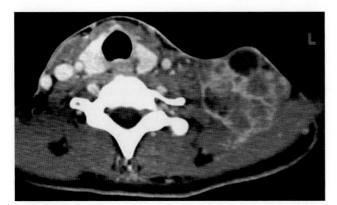

Figure 50-1

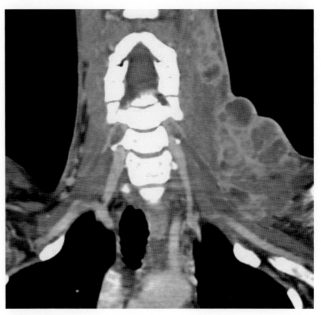

Figure 50-2

HISTORY: A patient presented with a firm, fixed left-sided neck swelling with skin thickening.

1. Which of the following should be included in the differential diagnosis? (Choose all that apply.)
   A. Metastatic breast cancer
   B. Metastatic lung cancer
   C. Nasopharyngeal carcinoma
   D. Mononucleosis

2. What structure is at risk from these lymph nodes?
   A. Thyroglossal duct
   B. Foramen cecum
   C. Brachial plexus
   D. Fossa of Hullenhammer

3. Which neurogenic tumor most commonly affects the brachial plexus?
   A. Schwannoma
   B. Neurofibroma
   C. Neuroma
   D. Malignant peripheral nerve sheath tumor

4. Between which muscles does the brachial plexus pass?
   A. Sternocleidomastoid and anterior scalene
   B. Middle scalene and anterior scalene
   C. Middle scalene and posterior scalene
   D. Anterior scalene and levator scapulae

See Supplemental Figures section for additional figures and legends for this case.

CASE 50

Malignant Adenopathy Infiltrating Brachial Plexus

1. **A, B, and C.** Nodes may develop in the supraclavicular fossa from metastatic breast cancer and metastatic lung cancer. Supraclavicular adenopathy may also be present with nasopharyngeal carcinoma, which would be graded N3. These nodes are unilateral and necrotic; therefore, mononucleosis is unlikely.

2. **C.** The brachial plexus is being invaded by the nodes. The thyroglossal duct is not in proximity. The foramen cecum is at the base of the tongue. There is no such thing as the fossa of Hullenhammer.

3. **B.** Neurofibroma is the most common neurogenic tumor of the brachial plexus. Schwannoma is the second most common, and malignant peripheral nerve sheath tumor is third most common. Neuroma is not histologically a tumor (e.g., Morton neuroma).

4. **B.** The brachial plexus passes between the middle scalene and anterior scalene muscles.

Comment

Associations with Malignant Lymphadenopathy

Malignant lymphadenopathy is the most common cause of malignant involvement of the brachial plexus. The malignancies that affect the brachial plexus include breast and lung lymph nodes, but lung cancers such as Pancoast varieties can directly spread upward to infiltrate the brachial plexus from the lung apex. Lymphoma also may lead to a brachial plexopathy from supraclavicular nodal disease, such as Hodgkin or non-Hodgkin lymphoma.

Imaging Findings

Primary malignancies of the brachial plexus are uncommon. The most frequent are malignant peripheral nerve sheath tumors, possibly in association with neurofibromatosis type I. Sarcomas may also lead to infiltration of the brachial plexus. The anterior scalene muscle (Figure S50-1) is the anterior border of the passageway of portions of the brachial plexus passing from the cervical nerve roots. At this level, the trunks are evident. They pass just above and behind the subclavian artery on coronal imaging (Figure S50-2).

Reference

Gosk J, Rutowski R, Reichert P, Rabczyński J. Radiation-induced brachial plexus neuropathy—aetiopathogenesis, risk factors, differential diagnostics, symptoms and treatment. *Folia Neuropathol.* 2007; 45(1):26-30.

Cross-Reference

Neuroradiology: The Requisites, 3rd ed, 504-505.

Fair Game

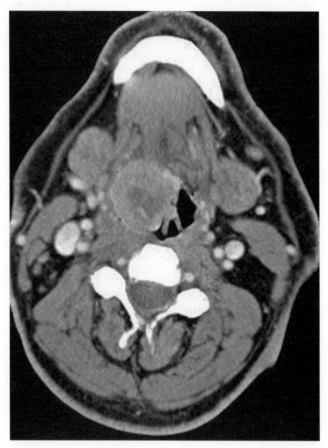

Figure 51-1

HISTORY: A patient has a 2-month history of globus sensation.

1. Which of the following should be included in the differential diagnosis? (Choose all that apply.)
   A. Squamous cell carcinoma
   B. Minor salivary gland cancer
   C. Warthin tumor
   D. Synovial sarcoma

2. In which part of the head and neck is the vallecula located?
   A. Oral cavity
   B. Oropharynx
   C. Hypopharynx
   D. Submental space

3. What structure separates the two sides of the vallecula?
   A. The plica medialis
   B. The pharyngoepiglottic fold
   C. The plica anterialis
   D. The median glossoepiglottic fold

4. Based on the appearance of this cancer in Figure 51-1, what tumor staging is represented?
   A. T1
   B. T2
   C. T3
   D. T4

See Supplemental Figures section for additional figures and legends for this case.

CASE 51

Vallecula Squamous Cell Carcinoma

1. **A and B.** Squamous cell carcinoma is the most common aerodigestive tract tumor. Minor salivary gland cancer may also occur here. Warthin tumor occurs only in and around the parotid gland. Synovial sarcoma is not known to be in this location; it can, however, occur in the hypopharynx.

2. **B.** The vallecula is part of the oropharynx, along with the soft palate, base of tongue, tonsils, and posterior pharyngeal wall.

3. **D.** The median glossoepiglottic fold separates the two sides of the vallecula. The plica medialis does not exist here, and the pharyngoepiglottic fold is more lateral. There is no such structure as a plica anterialis.

4. **A.** T1 staging is indicated in this figure; the cancer is less than 2 cm large. T2 staging implies a size of 2 to 4 cm.

Comment

Treatment Considerations

The issues that are important in considering treatment options for oropharyngeal carcinomas include the following: (1) tumor stage; (2) whether the tumor crosses the midline (which would necessitate a total glossectomy); (3) whether the tumor has invaded mandibular or maxillary bone (which would necessitate flap reconstruction); (4) whether the tumor has invaded the pterygopalatine fossa, which could lead to perineural spread; (5) whether the internal carotid artery is encased, which would render the tumor unresectable; (6) whether the tumor has spread to muscles of mastication; (7) whether the tumor has invaded the skull base; and (8) nodal spread. All of these must be addressed on imaging.

Relevant Anatomy

The anatomic structures included in the oropharynx are the tongue base, soft palate, vallecula, tonsil, and posterolateral pharyngeal wall from the level of the hard palate to the pharyngoepiglottic fold. Below the pharyngoepiglottic fold are the larynx anteriorly and the hypopharynx posteriorly (Figure S51-1).

Imaging Findings

Advanced imaging techniques, such as those involving the apparent diffusion coefficient and perfusion parameters for primary tumors and nodal masses, can potentially differentiate patients who will respond to chemoradiation protocols for advanced cancers from patients who will not respond.

Reference

Kim S, Loevner LA, Quon H, Kilger A, Sherman E, Weinstein G, et al. Prediction of response to chemoradiation therapy in squamous cell carcinomas of the head and neck using dynamic contrast-enhanced MR imaging. *AJNR Am J Neuroradiol.* 2010;31(2):262-268.

Cross-Reference

Neuroradiology: The Requisites, 3rd ed, 388-389, 435-436, 457-468, 470-471, 486, 492, 494.

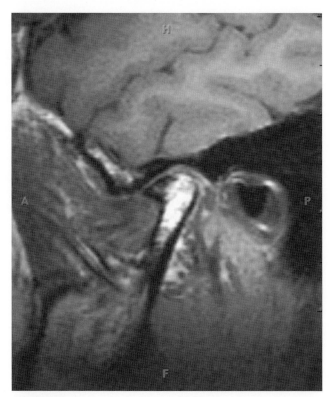

Figure 52-1

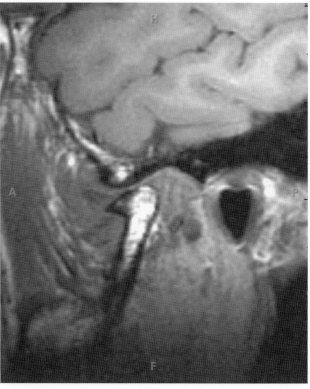

Figure 52-2

HISTORY: A 35-year-old woman complains about long-standing left-sided pain in the temporomandibular joint (TMJ).

1. Which of the following should be included in the differential diagnosis? (Choose all that apply.)
   A. Anterior displacement with recapture
   B. Anterior displacement without recapture
   C. Normal
   D. Posterior meniscus displacement with recapture

2. What does "sideways displacement of a meniscus" refer to?
   A. Medial displacement
   B. Lateral displacement
   C. Medial or lateral displacement
   D. Anterior or posterior meniscus displacement

3. What percentage of the normal symptom-free population have meniscal abnormalities of the TMJ?
   A. <10%
   B. 11% to 20%
   C. 21% to 40%
   D. 41% to 60%

4. What is the biggest technical challenge of evaluating the TMJ on magnetic resonance imaging (MRI)?
   A. Imaging the correct plane of the mandible
   B. Optimizing the contrast
   C. The timing of the enhancement
   D. Getting the patient to open the jaw sufficiently

See Supplemental Figures section for additional figures and legends for this case.

CASE 52

Temporomandibular Joint Disk Disease

1. **B.** The meniscus remains anterior in open- and closed-mouth views. Therefore, there is anterior displacement of the meniscus without recapture.

2. **C.** "Sideways displacement of a meniscus" refers to either medial or lateral displacement. It does not refer to anterior or posterior meniscus displacement.

3. **C.** Approximately 30% of normal symptom-free people have meniscal abnormalities of the TMJ. These abnormalities usually reflect anterior displacement with recapture.

4. **D.** For patients with this condition, opening the jaw sometimes hurts, and the patient cannot keep it open the whole scanning time. One must look at the degree of mandibular condyle displacement to determine whether the opening has been adequate.

Comment

Difficulties with Imaging the Temporomandibular Joint

MRI of the TMJ is fraught with difficulty. Affected patients are often in discomfort. They move a lot. They do not want to open the mouth widely because it elicits discomfort. Once the mouth is open, it is hard to keep open for the 3 to 4 minutes of scan times, and so a bite block must often be used, but that can produce nonphysiologic artifact in images. The plane of section is difficult to achieve in sagittal and coronal views, especially because the right and left TMJs are oriented differently, and yet both are to be scanned at the same time. Furthermore, when the meniscus is anteriorly located, technicians must know to scan not through the joint alone but also in front of the joint to search for a sideways (medial-lateral) displacement of the meniscus (Figures S52-1 and S52-2).

Menisci Displacement

Most menisci become displaced anteriorly, anteromedially, or anterolaterally. They are rarely displaced only in a medial-to-lateral direction. They are not displaced posteriorly because the issue is laxity of the bilaminar zone, which allows the meniscus to slip anteriorly. When the meniscus pops back into place on opening of the jaw, it causes a clicking sound or feeling and, if it goes into the normal location on opening, the condition is termed *anterior displacement with recapture*. In the case described here, however, the meniscus remains anteriorly located, and thus the condition is termed *anterior displacement without recapture*. This is why the open- and closed-mouth views are imaged. The clicking may occur as the meniscus pops forwards anteriorly on closing of the mouth as well.

Associations with Temporomandibular Joint Disease

TMJ disease occurs in young women in their menstruating years. Thus most authorities believe it is hormonally mediated, potentially from the effect of estrogen on the ligamentous laxity of the connective tissue of the bilaminar zone that attaches to the back of the meniscus.

Cross-Reference

Neuroradiology: The Requisites, 3rd ed, 488-489, 490-491.

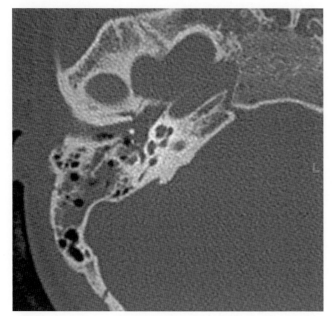
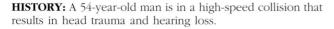

Figure 53-1

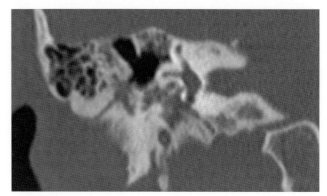

Figure 53-2

HISTORY: A 54-year-old man is in a high-speed collision that results in head trauma and hearing loss.

1. Which of the following is probably the cause of conductive hearing loss in this patient? (Choose all that apply.)
   A. Malleus fracture
   B. Incudomalleolar dislocation
   C. Middle ear hemotympanum
   D. Incudostapedial dislocation
   E. Fracture through the cochlea

2. Fractures along the plane of the petrous apex often extend into which of the following structures?
   A. The external auditory canal
   B. The jugular foramen
   C. The carotid canal
   D. The internal auditory canal

3. What is Battle's sign?
   A. Bloodshot eyes
   B. "Shiners" under the eyelids
   C. Ecchymoses at the mastoid tip
   D. Blood in the external auditory canal

4. Which of the following is *not* a complication of temporal bone fracture?
   A. Meningitis
   B. Facial nerve palsy
   C. Perilymphatic fistula
   D. Cholesterol granuloma

See Supplemental Figures section for additional figures and legends for this case.

CASE 53

Temporal Bone Fracture

1. **C.** Fluid of any kind in the middle ear can cause conductive hearing loss. Incudomalleolar and incudostapedial dislocation are common dislocations but not the most common cause of hearing loss. Malleus fracture and fracture through the cochlea are rare.

2. **C.** Fractures in the plane of the petrous apex may extend along the carotid canal and then into the sphenoid sinus.

3. **C.** Ecchymoses at the mastoid tip may be associated with squamosal temporal bone fracture. Blood in the external auditory canal may be associated with any temporal bone fracture. "Shiners" under the eyelids are associated with orbital and skull base fractures.

4. **D.** Cholesterol granuloma is not considered a complication of temporal bone fracture. Meningitis can occur with tegmen tympani disruption. Facial nerve palsy can result when the tympanic portion of the facial nerve is injured with oblique or horizontal temporal bone fractures. Perilymphatic fistula into the labyrinth can also be caused by temporal bone fracture.

Comment

Classification of Temporal Bone Fractures

The classification of temporal bone fractures has undergone multiple revisions over time. Initially, the differentiation was between horizontal and vertical fractures according to the plane of the tegmen tympani. Physicians later realized that most fractures occurred in an oblique plane and that the classical vertical-versus-horizontal separation was relatively artificial. The current classification differentiates between fractures that involve the labyrinthine structures and those that do not. In describing temporal bone fractures, no matter what the classification, it is important to describe whether each of the following is present:
- Ossicular fracture
- Ossicular dislocation
- Facial nerve transection (canal intact?)
- Labyrinthine fracture
- Tegmen tympani disruption
- Carotid canal involvement
- Blood in the external auditory canal and/or middle ear

Facial Nerve Trauma

Facial nerve trauma occurs more commonly with classical horizontal (longitudinal) fractures and oblique fractures than with vertical (transverse) fractures (Figures S53-1 and S53-2). When facial nerve palsy occurs after trauma, decompression may be required; it should be performed between 2 weeks and 2 months after the injury. The classification of facial nerve injury is the House-Brackmann grading system:

Grade	Characteristics
I. Normal	Normal facial function in all areas
II. Mild dysfunction	**Gross** Slight weakness noticeable on close inspection Possible presence of slight synkinesis At rest, normal symmetry and tone **Motion** Forehead: moderate-to-good function Eye: complete closure with minimal effort Mouth: slight asymmetry
III. Moderate dysfunction	**Gross** Obvious but not disfiguring difference between the two sides Noticeable but not severe synkinesis, contracture, or hemifacial spasm At rest, normal symmetry and tone **Motion** Forehead: slight-to-moderate movement Eye: complete closure with effort Mouth: slightly weak with maximum effort
IV. Moderately severe dysfunction	**Gross** Obvious weakness and/or disfiguring asymmetry At rest, normal symmetry and tone **Motion** Forehead: none Eye: incomplete closure Mouth: asymmetric with maximum effort
V. Severe dysfunction	**Gross** Only barely perceptible motion At rest, asymmetry **Motion** Forehead: none Eye: incomplete closure Mouth: slight movement
VI. Total paralysis	No movement

House, J.W., Brackmann, D.E. Facial nerve grading system. *Otolaryngol Head Neck Surg.* 1985;93(2):146-147.

Reference

Ulug T, Arif Ulubil S. Management of facial paralysis in temporal bone fractures: a prospective study analyzing 11 operated fractures. *Am J Otolaryngol.* 2005;26(4):230-238.

Cross-Reference

Neuroradiology: The Requisites, 3rd ed, 385-416, 596.

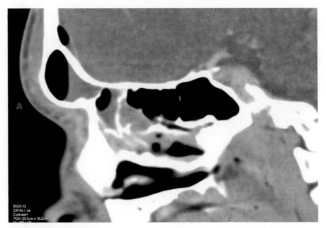

Figure 54-1

HISTORY: A young adult presents with severe head pain and fever.

1. What would be appropriate for the differential diagnosis in this setting? (Choose all that apply.)
   A. Fracture and pneumocephalus from breech of frontal sinus
   B. Polyposis
   C. Sinusitis with epidural abscess
   D. Postoperative cerebrospinal fluid leak
   E. Carcinoma

2. Fracture of which structure most commonly leads to pneumocephalus?
   A. Orbit
   B. Nasal bone
   C. Ethmoid bone
   D. Frontal bone
   E. Mastoid portion of the temporal bone

3. What is Pott's puffy tumor?
   A. A tumor-like paraspinal mass resulting from tuberculous spondylitis
   B. Fibrous dysplasia of the mandibles that leads to puffy cheeks
   C. Soft tissue inflammation in the frontal sinuses, caused by infectious breech of the wall
   D. Sinusitis with epidural abscesses
   E. Sinusitis with an intraparenchymal brain mass

4. In what location is the most common sinusitis-induced abscess?
   A. Intracranial
   B. Retrobulbar orbital
   C. Cheek
   D. Periosteal orbital
   E. Periapical

See Supplemental Figures section for additional figures and legends for this case.

CASE 54

Epidural Abscess from Sinusitis

1. **A and C.** Sinusitis with epidural abscess is apparent in the image. Fracture and pneumocephalus from breech of frontal sinus may be visualized in the differential diagnosis, but contrast medium would generally not be given. No polyps, postoperative changes, or masses are seen in Figure S54-1.

2. **E.** Violation of the air cells within the mastoid portion of the temporal bone often leads to pneumocephalus. Of all cases of pneumocephalus, most result from fractures of that site.

3. **C.** Pott's puffy tumor is soft tissue inflammation superficial to the frontal sinuses that results from infectious breech of the wall. Tuberculous spondylitis is known as *Pott disease*. Fibrous dysplasia of the mandibles leads to puffy cheeks, also known as *cherubism*. Sinusitis with epidural abscesses has no eponym.

4. **D.** Subperiosteal orbital abscess results from ethmoid sinusitis. Retrobulbar orbital abscess is less common than periosteal orbital abscess, and intracranial abscess is less common than any orbital abscess. Periapical abscess results from odontogenic infection and is not often associated with sinusitis.

Comment

Complications of Sinusitis

Intracranial complications of sinusitis can include meningitis, hydrocephalus, parenchymal abscess, subdural empyema, and epidural empyema. In addition, dural sinus and venous thrombosis may result from sinusitis that spreads to the cavernous sinus or the frontal regions. The infection spreads from the frontal sinus to the epidural space via the veins that traverse the valveless diploic space. Streptococcal pathogens are the most common source of epidural abscesses that result from frontal sinusitis.

Treatment of Sinusitis

Treatment of frontal epidural abscesses from sinusitis is usually with intravenous antibiotics and endoscopic sinus surgery to relieve the underlying sinusitis. In rare instances, the collection may be drained via an endoscopic approach from the sinus through the skull base.

Pott's Puffy Tumor

Pott's puffy tumor is a nonneoplastic entity that reflects spread of a sinus inflammatory process into the soft tissues superficial to of the frontal sinus. This is an osteomyelitis of the frontal bone with a subperiosteal abscess that is well circumscribed, inasmuch as it is bordered by the periosteum. Frontal sinusitis and trauma are the most frequent cause of Pott's puffy tumor. It occurs more commonly in young adults than in elderly adults, in part because of the permeability of vascular channels through the frontal sinus in adolescents and young adults. The original description of Pott's puffy tumor was written in 1760 by Sir Percivall Pott, a surgeon in London who thought that this was a tumor, not an infection, in "Observations on the Nature and Consequences of Wounds and Contusions of the Head, Fractures of the Skull."

Reference

Kombogiorgas D, Solanki GA. The Pott puffy tumor revisited: neurosurgical implications of this unforgotten entity. Case report and review of the literature. *J Neurosurg.* 2006;105(2 Suppl): 143-149.

Cross-Reference

Neuroradiology: The Requisites, 3rd ed, 192, 195f, 543-546.

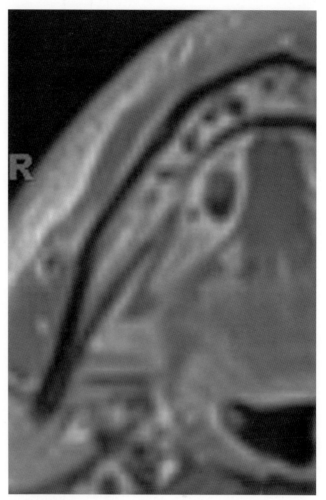

Figure 55-2

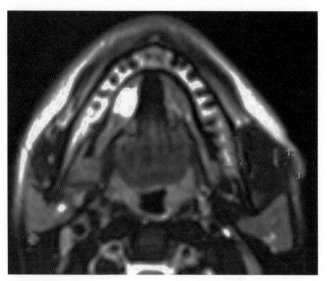

Figure 55-1

HISTORY: A young patient complains of feeling a mass on the right side of the floor of mouth with his tongue.

1. Which of the following should be included in the differential diagnosis? (Choose all that apply.)
   A. Squamous cell carcinoma
   B. Lymphoma
   C. Adenoid cystic carcinoma
   D. Ranula

2. What is the most common primary malignancy of the sublingual gland?
   A. Squamous cell carcinoma
   B. Lymphoma
   C. Adenoid cystic carcinoma
   D. Adenocarcinoma

3. What type of ranula is this?
   A. Submandibular
   B. Submental
   C. Plunging (also called *diving*)
   D. Simple

4. Why is the distinction between a simple and plunging ranula important?
   A. Simple ranulas are treated medically, whereas plunging ranulas are treated surgically.
   B. Simple ranulas have no malignant potential, but plunging ranulas may degenerate into carcinoma.
   C. Simple ranulas are approached intraorally, whereas plunging ranulas are approached transcervically.
   D. Simple ranulas are marsupialized, whereas plunging ranulas are lanced.

See Supplemental Figures section for additional figures and legends for this case.

CASE 55

Ranula

1. **D.** Ranula appears as very bright fluid on T2-weighted images and does not enhance. Squamous cell carcinoma, Lymphoma, and adenoid cystic carcinoma would be solid and usually enhance.

2. **C.** Adenoid cystic carcinoma is the most common primary mass in the minor salivary gland. Squamous cell carcinoma and lymphoma are not primary tumors of the salivary gland. Adenocarcinoma is not common.

3. **D.** This is a simple ranula. It remains in the floor of the mouth, not in submandibular or submental locations. Plunging (diving) ranulas perforate the mylohyoid aperture.

4. **C.** Simple ranulas are approached intraorally, whereas plunging ranulas are approached transcervically. Both are surgical lesions and resected. There is no cancer risk.

Comment

Characteristics of Ranulas

Ranulas may arise from the sublingual gland or minor salivary glands. Some authorities refer to them as _mucous escape cysts,_ whereas others view them as mucous retention cysts; in either case they arise in salivary gland tissue of the sublingual space. They are referred to as _simple ranulas_ (Figures S55-1 and S55-2) when they are small, are in the floor of the mouth, and do not perforate through the mylohyoid muscle to enter the submandibular neck region. Plunging (diving) ranulas usually develop in an area of weakness along the posterior margin of the mylohyoid muscle, where they can then descend into the neck. The distinction between simple and plunging ranulas is thus not trivial.

Treating Ranulas

Simple ranulas are approached surgically by lifting of the tongue and removal or drainage of the ranula via an intraoral approach. Plunging ranulas are best approached by an incision in the neck and removing the cyst from below. The lesions are usually painless. They are palpated as a bulge in the floor of the mouth or below the jaw. The term _ranula_ is derived from _rana,_ Latin for "frog," because of the way a plunging ranula can make the upper anterior neck look like a frog's throat. One should be familiar with the eponyms involving ductal anatomy of the floor of the mouth. There are 8 to 20 ducts of Rivinus that drain the sublingual gland. The Bartholin duct is the largest of these sublingual ducts and opens to the submandibular gland duct (the Wharton duct) near its distal segment on either side of the frenulum in the floor of the mouth.

Reference

La'Porte SJ, Juttla JK, Lingam RK. Imaging the floor of the mouth and the sublingual space. _Radiographics._ 2011;31(5):1215-1230.

Cross-Reference

Neuroradiology: The Requisites, 3rd ed, 453, 482.

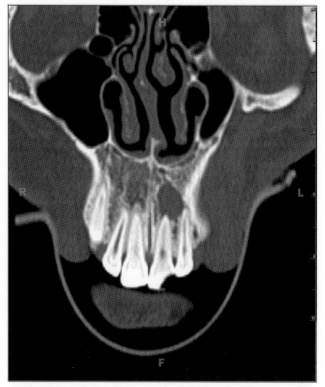

Figure 56-1

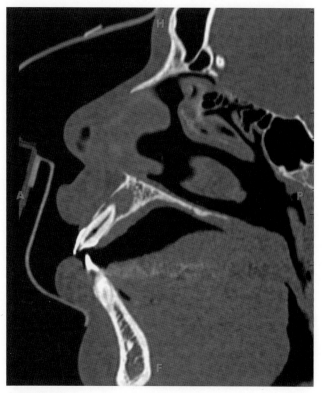

Figure 56-2

HISTORY: A patient has facial trauma with anterior facial pain.

1. Which of the following should be included in the differential diagnosis? (Choose all that apply.)
   A. Dentigerous cyst
   B. Odontogenic keratocyst
   C. Incisive canal cyst
   D. Radicular cyst

2. If a cyst persists after a radicular cyst has been removed, what is it called?
   A. Recurrent cyst
   B. Residual cyst
   C. Reradicular cyst
   D. Retraction cyst

3. What cranial nerve supplies the maxillary incisor teeth sensory function?
   A. V_3
   B. V_2
   C. V_1
   D. VII

4. Radicular cysts affect the maxilla more than the mandible by what ratio?
   A. 2:1
   B. 3:1
   C. 4:1
   D. They actually affect the mandible more than the maxilla.

See Supplemental Figures section for additional figures and legends for this case.

CASE 56

Radicular Cyst

1. **D.** A radicular cyst is present in association with a carious tooth. It would not be a dentigerous cyst because there is no unerupted tooth; nor would it be an odontogenic keratocyst because the tooth is nonvital. An incisive canal cyst would be more medial in location and is unassociated with a carious tooth.

2. **B.** The cyst remaining after a radicular cyst has been removed is called a *residual cyst.*

3. **B.** The second (maxillary nerve) division of the trigeminal nerve (V_2) cranial nerve supplies sensory function to the maxillary incisor teeth through the branches of the greater and lesser palatine nerves.

4. **B.** Radicular cysts affect the maxilla three times more often than the mandible.

Comment

Characteristics of Radicular Cysts

Radicular cysts—also called *periapical cysts* and *apical periodontal cysts*—are the byproduct of periapical dental caries in which a tooth has become nonvital. They occur three times more commonly in the maxilla (with a predilection for incisors and canine teeth) than in the mandible (Figures S56-1 and S56-2), and men are affected more than women. The cysts often enlarge with time and may cause symptoms after having broken through the bone, as in this case. The infection develops from the pulp chamber of the root canal and is often painful. Inflammatory cells and cholesterol clefts are seen histopathologically in the cyst, which is lined by stratified squamous epithelium.

Treating Radicular Cysts

When it has reached an advanced stage, the radicular cyst must be treated surgically. In the early stage, eradication of the infection and root canal surgery with drainage may be enough, but by the time the cyst is expansile and the pressure within it has increased, it must be removed. If some cyst remains behind or regrows, it is called a *residual cyst* and may be removed. The differential diagnosis includes periapical granulomas. Those lesions may enhance more solidly than periapical cysts.

Reference

Scholl RJ, Kellett HM, Neumann DP, Lurie AG. Cysts and cystic lesions of the mandible: clinical and radiologic-histopathologic review, *Radiographics.* 1999;19:1107-1124.

Cross-Reference

Neuroradiology: The Requisites, 3rd ed, 450-451.

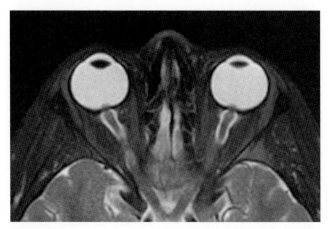

Figure 57-1

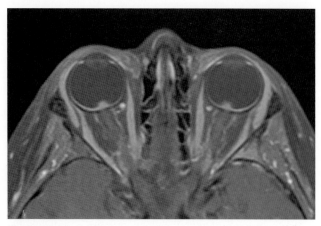

Figure 57-2

HISTORY: An obese patient presents with severe headache, vomiting, and blurred vision.

1. Which of the following should be included in the differential diagnosis? (Choose all that apply.)
   A. Increased intracranial pressure (ICP)
   B. Idiopathic intracranial hypertension (IIH)
   C. Optic neuritis
   D. Pseudotumor cerebri

2. What is the major potential danger of papilledema?
   A. Retinal hemorrhage
   B. Choroidal detachment
   C. Cerebrospinal fluid (CSF) leakage
   D. Ischemic optic neuropathy

3. Which are the findings on magnetic resonance imaging (MRI) of papilledema?
   A. Enlarged optic nerve sheath complex, flattening of the optic nerve insertion on the globe, protrusion of the papilla into the globe, and tortuosity of the nerve
   B. Enlarged optic nerve sheath complex, optic nerve swelling, protrusion of the papilla into the globe, and tortuosity of the nerve
   C. Enlarged optic nerve sheath complex, optic nerve swelling, protrusion of the papilla into the globe, and increased optic nerve signal intensity
   D. Enlarged optic nerve sheath complex, proptosis, protrusion of the papilla into the globe, and tortuosity of the nerve

4. Long-term effects of papilledema do *not* include which of the following?
   A. Optic nerve atrophy
   B. Optic nerve ischemic injury
   C. Cataract formation
   D. Enlargement of the sheath

See Supplemental Figures section for additional figures and legends for this case.

CASE 57

Papilledema

1. **A, B, and D.** Increased ICP and IIH (also known as *pseudotumor cerebri*) cause papilledema. In optic neuritis, the optic nerve itself usually appears bright on T2-weighted images.

2. **D.** Ischemic optic neuropathy can occur as a result of the pressure on the vasculature of the optic nerve. Choroidal detachment and CSF leakage are not associated with papilledema. Retinal hemorrhage is a rare phenomenon.

3. **A.** Enlarged optic nerve sheath complex, flattening of the optic nerve insertion on the globe, protrusion of the papilla into the globe, and tortuosity of the nerve all appear on MRI. The optic nerve might not swell or produce a bright signal, and proptosis is not a feature.

4. **C.** Cataract formation is unrelated to papilledema. Optic nerve atrophy occurs as a chronic condition. Optic nerve ischemic injury can result from diminished vascular flow. The sheath is often enlarged in papilledema.

Comment

Imaging Findings

The patient demonstrates enlarged optic nerve sheath complexes, flattening of the optic nerve insertion on the globe, protrusion of the papilla into the globe (Figure S57-1), tortuosity of the nerve, and enhancement of the papilla (Figure S57-2). The finding of papilledema on MRI of the brain may indicate the presence of IIH, a disease that can, if untreated, lead to blindness. In addition to papilledema, affected patients often have partially or completely empty sella, flattening of the pituitary gland by CSF, and stenosis of the venous sinus. The sinus stenosis may be a source or result of the elevation in ICP caused by venous outflow obstruction and diminished CSF resorption. In some cases, ICP may be elevated as a result of a mass, hematoma, or obstruction of the CSF flow through the ventricles or arachnoid villi. In such cases, the presence of papilledema might suggest the acuity of such a process and the urgency of treatment.

Complications of Papilledema

Papilledema must be addressed because when pressure around the optic nerve sheath complex is elevated for a long time, blood flow can be reduced. This, in turn, can lead to ischemic injury of the nerve and to blindness. In IIH, CSF drainage via multiple taps and/or medications to reduce CSF production are usually necessary. If the condition is recurrent and difficult to treat, fenestration of optic nerve sheath may eliminate the risk. For mass lesions, neurosurgical intervention to remove the obstruction, craniectomy (in the most severe cases), or ventriculostomy for alternative CSF drainage and to reduce pressure may be required.

Tortuosity of the Optic Nerve

Tortuosity of the optic nerve occurs in relation to the fixation points of the distal and proximal nerves. Tortuosity may be in the horizontal or vertical plane and is a relatively nonspecific finding. The "smear sign" refers to partial volume averaging on an axial image of the nerve with fat as the nerve coils upward or downward in the vertical plane.

Incidence

As an indicator of increased ICP, papilledema seen on MRI is not specific. The findings are often delayed. IIH can occur without papilledema. Enhancement of the prelaminar optic nerve as a sign of elevated ICP and IIH is found in only 30% of cases.

Reference

Passi N, Degnan AJ, Levy LM. MR imaging of papilledema and visual pathways: effects of increased intracranial pressure and pathophysiologic mechanisms. *AJNR Am J Neuroradiol.* 2013;34(5):919-924.

Cross-Reference

Neuroradiology: The Requisites, 3rd ed, 256, 345, 369-370.

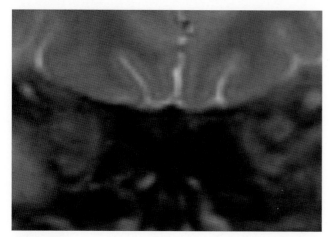

Figure 58-1

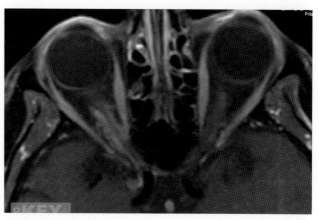

Figure 58-2

HISTORY: A 47-year-old patient has experienced slow. progressive visual blurring over the course of 4 months.

1. Which of the following should be included in the differential diagnosis? (Choose all that apply.)
   A. Optic nerve sheath meningioma
   B. Sarcoidosis
   C. Lymphoma
   D. Subarachnoid seeding from retinoblastoma

2. What is characteristic about optic nerve sheath meningioma and visual loss?
   A. It affects both eyes.
   B. It produces bitemporal hemianopsia.
   C. It affects vision early in the course.
   D. Optic nerve gliomas produce worse visual loss.

3. Which type of meningioma histologically most commonly affects the optic nerve sheath?
   A. Meningothelial
   B. Transitional
   C. Fibroblastic
   D. Malignant aggressive

4. What is the classical sign of optic nerve sheath meningioma?
   A. The molar tooth sign
   B. The tram-track sign
   C. The cap sign
   D. The target sign

See Supplemental Figures section for additional figures and legends for this case.

CASE 58

Optic Nerve Sheath Meningioma

1. **A, B, and C.** Optic nerve sheath meningiomas , sarcoidosis, and lymphoma can manifest as optic nerve sheath enhancement. Subarachnoid seeding from retinoblastoma can look the same, with an enhancing sheath, but would not occur in this age group.

2. **C.** Optic nerve sheath meningiomas affect a patient's vision early in the course with unilateral symptoms.

3. **A.** Meningothelial meningioma histologically affects the optic nerve sheath the most. Transitional meningioma is not as common as meningothelial meningioma. The fibroblastic variety is rare, and malignant aggressive meningioma is very rare.

4. **B.** The tram-track sign is the classical sign of optic nerve sheath meningioma and refers to the enhancing sheath around a nonenhancing nerve. The molar tooth sign is characteristic of Joubert syndrome; the cap sign refers to ependymomas of the spinal cord; and the target sign refers to neurofibromas.

Comment

Incidence of Optic Nerve Meningiomas

Optic nerve meningiomas occur, as do all meningiomas, most commonly in women in their 40s to 60s. Optic nerve meningiomas are lesions that may manifest with striking visual loss early in the course if they arise at the optic canal, where there is less capacity for optic nerve sheath expansion and ischemic injury can subsequently occur. Papilledema and optic nerve atrophy may develop. The lesions occasionally arise not from the optic nerve sheath but from the planum sphenoidale, where they may grow onto both optic nerve sheaths; in that situation, visual loss can be bilateral.

Imaging Findings

The lesions enhance avidly, and thus the differential diagnosis includes any and all entities that infiltrate the dura or subarachnoid space, including metastases and inflammatory lesions (Figures S58-1 and S58-2). Pseudotumor, sarcoid, tuberculosis, fungi, and perioptic neuritis could cause inflammation. Seeding from an ocular melanoma or retinoblastoma is possible, as are leukemia and lymphoma. Optic nerve gliomas are more common than optic nerve sheath meningiomas. The former occur commonly in neurofibromatosis type 1, whereas the latter are more common in neurofibromatosis type 2.

Treatment of Optic Nerve Meningiomas

Treatment currently emphasizes stereotactic radiotherapy. With regard to saving vision, surgical outcomes are poor.

Reference

Kanamalla US. The optic nerve tram-track sign. *Radiology.* 2003;227(3):718-719.

Cross-Reference

Neuroradiology: The Requisites, 3rd ed, 348-349.

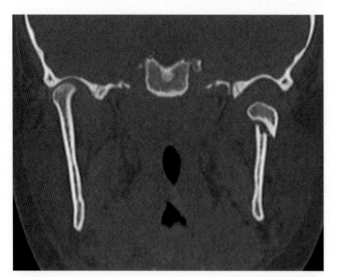

Figure 59-1

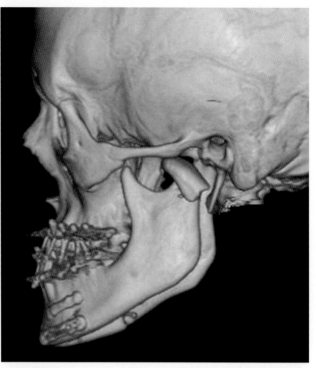

Figure 59-2

HISTORY: A patient presents with jaw pain after having been in an altercation.

1. Which of the following should be included in the differential diagnosis? (Choose all that apply.)
   A. Osteosarcoma
   B. Meniscus dislocation
   C. Traumatic fracture
   D. Pathologic fracture

2. What is the main danger of a mandibular neck fracture?
   A. Rotatory subluxation
   B. Avascular necrosis
   C. Persistent dislocation
   D. Pseudarthrosis

3. What part of the mandible is fractured most commonly?
   A. Body
   B. Angle
   C. Neck
   D. Condyle

4. Which of the following is considered an open fracture?
   A. Fractures that affect the alveolus and teeth
   B. Condylar fracture
   C. Ascending ramus fracture
   D. Neck of mandible fracture

See Supplemental Figures section for additional figures and legends for this case.

CASE 59

Mandible Fracture

1. **C.** The left mandibular neck fracture evident on the coronal two-dimensional image.

2. **B.** The rate of avascular necrosis is highest with mandibular neck fractures, of all mandibular fractures.

3. **A.** The body fractures more commonly than the angle, which is fractured more commonly than the condyle. The neck is not frequently the site of fracture.

4. **A.** By definition, a fracture affecting the teeth and alveolus is analogous to fractures that protrude through the skin and increase the risk of infection, and therefore considered "open."

Comment

Location of Fractures

The mandible, orbital walls, and nasal bones are most commonly fractured in facial trauma. Although one should suspect multiple fractures with any mandibular fracture, nearly 30% of mandibular fractures are isolated, particularly those caused by direct blows. Mandibular condylar fractures and parasymphyseal ones are more commonly multiple than fractures of other portions of the mandible. The left side is affected more commonly than the right, possibly because of a right-handed blow (men have mandibular fractures three to four times more often than do women) and because passengers tend to flinch to the right during a motor vehicle accident. The locations of fractures vary with the cause: parasymphyseal fractures tend to occur with motor vehicle accidents, body fractures with gunshot wounds, and angle fractures with assault.

Displacement of Mandibular Fractures

Displacement of mandibular fractures is dependent on the pull of the muscles of mastication (Figures S59-1 and S59-2). The masseter and temporalis muscles exert upward pull on the angle of the mandible, which distract fractures vertically, whereas the medial and lateral pterygoid muscles distract fractures medially. In addition to fractures, avascular necrosis of the mandible can occur with bisphosphonate therapy, steroid therapy, osteoporosis, and sickle cell disease. Other complications such as technical failure and infections increase with open fractures, delays in surgical reduction, and intravenous drug use.

Reference

Anyanechi CE, Saheeb BD. Mandibular sites prone to fracture: analysis of 174 cases in a Nigerian tertiary hospital. *Ghana Med J.* 2011;45(3):111-114.

Cross-Reference

Neuroradiology: The Requisites, 3rd ed, 187, 188-189, 414-416, 534, 577-578.

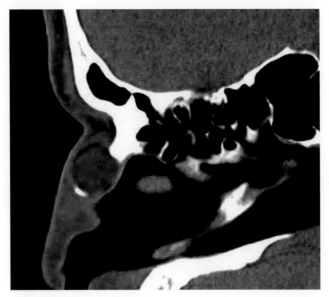

Figure 60-1

HISTORY: An adolescent is not happy with the cosmetic appearance of her nose.

1. Which of the following should be included in the differential diagnosis? (Choose all that apply.)
   A. Lipoma
   B. Nasal glioma
   C. Dermoid
   D. Encephalocele

2. What is the passageway from the sinonasal cavity to the intracranial compartment of a dermal sinus tract?
   A. Anterior neuropore
   B. Foramen cecum
   C. Frontalis ponticulus
   D. Cribriform plate

3. What percentage of nasal dermoids have an intracranial connection?
   A. 0% to 20%
   B. 21% to 40%
   C. 41% to 60%
   D. >60%

4. What percentage of patients with nasal dermoids present with an infection?
   A. 0% to 20%
   B. 21% to 40%
   C. 41% to 60%
   D. >60%

See Supplemental Figures section for additional figures and legends for this case.

CASE 60

Nasal Dermoid

1. **A and C.** The location and density indicate a dermoid. The location is a less likely site for a lipoma, although lipomas contain fat; encephaloceles do not contain fat. The density is not characteristic of nasal glioma.

2. **B.** The foramen cecum is the passageway from the sino-nasal cavity to the intracranial compartment of a dermal sinus tract. The anterior neuropore is an embryologic channel and not located through the nose. There is no such thing as "frontalis ponticulus."

3. **A.** Twelve percent to 18% of nasal dermoids have an intra-cranial connection.

4. **B.** Thirty percent of patients with nasal dermoids present with an infection.

Comment

Imaging Findings

Nasal dermoids typically manifest as a soft tissue mass and/or a tract leading from the nasal bridge or glabella in the midline (Figure S60-1). However, infection may occur, and in some cases, a cheesy off-white material may be expressed from the lesion through the sinus tract. In rare cases, patients may present with an intracranial infection because the pathogens can travel from the dermoid via the dermal sinus tract, through the foramen cecum, to the meninges, which may then result in meningitis.

Incidence of Nasal Dermoids

Boys are affected more commonly than girls, and the average age at discovery is approximately 3 years. Nasal dermoid is the most common midline congenital mass and represents approximately 10% of all head and neck dermoids. Most nasal dermoids are superficial, but 16% affect the nasal cartilage, 12% the cribriform plate, and 10% the nasal bone (like this one).

Reference

Rahbar R, Shah P, Mulliken JB, Robson CD, Perez-Atayde AR, Proctor MR, et al. The presentation and management of nasal dermoid: a 30-year experience. *Arch Otolaryngol Head Neck Surg.* 2003; 129(4):464-471.

Cross-Reference

Neuroradiology: The Requisites, 3rd ed, 422.

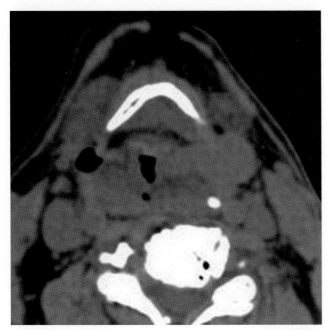

Figure 61-1

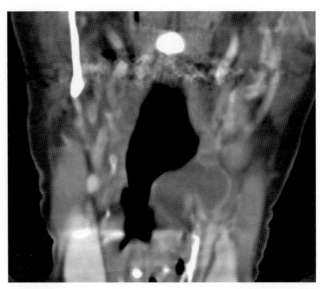

Figure 61-2

HISTORY: A 52-year-old patient with a 35–pack-year smoking history complains of hoarseness.

1. Which of the following should be included in the differential diagnosis? (Choose all that apply.)
   A. Laryngeal cancer
   B. External laryngocele
   C. Mixed laryngocele
   D. Vocal cord paralysis

2. What structure is violated when an internal laryngocele becomes a mixed laryngocele?
   A. The cricothyroid membrane
   B. The cricohyoid membrane
   C. The geniohyoid membrane
   D. The thyrohyoid membrane

3. What is the incidence of cancer in association with a laryngocele?
   A. 0% to 10%
   B. 11% to 20%
   C. 21% to 30%
   D. >30%

4. What is obstructed in a laryngocele?
   A. Minor salivary glands
   B. The piriform sinus
   C. Third branchial arch
   D. The saccule

See Supplemental Figures section for additional figures and legends for this case.

125

CASE 61

Laryngocele

1. **B and C.** An external air-filled laryngocele is present on the right, and a mixed internal and external fluid-filled laryngocele is present on the left. No tumor mass for laryngeal cancer is visible, and there are no findings to indicate vocal cord paralysis.

2. **D.** The thyrohyoid membrane is transgressed when an internal laryngocele becomes a mixed one.

3. **A.** Cancer is associated with 8% of cases of laryngocele. Cancer risk factors of smoking and drinking may change this rate.

4. **D.** The saccule of the laryngeal ventricle is obstructed and then balloons into a laryngocele.

Comment

Imaging Findings

Laryngoceles may be filled with air (as on the right side in this case) or with fluid (as seen on the left side in this case) (Figures S61-1 and S61-2). Laryngoceles may also be external (as seen on the right side in this case), both internal and external (mixed, as seen on the left side of this case), or internal according to whether they perforate the thyrohyoid membrane to breach the space external to the larynx and paraglottic tissues. Laryngoceles result from obstruction at the saccule of the laryngeal ventricle. The radiologist must be very cognizant of a potential mass at the junction of or spanning the levels of the false vocal cord and true vocal cord. Cancers may be the cause of the obstruction in approximately 8% of all cases of laryngocele.

Risks of Laryngoceles

Fluid-filled laryngoceles may be termed *saccular cysts* for the laryngeal saccule. If purulent material fills the laryngocele, it is called a *pyolaryngocele*. People who play wind instruments, glass blowers, and other people who spend much time blowing are at risk for laryngoceles. On the pharyngeal side, pharyngoceles and, of course, Zenker diverticula can develop.

Imaging Options

Computed tomography, because of the thin-section capability and the optimal demonstration of air, is a better study to use for the evaluation of laryngoceles than magnetic resonance imaging. In rare cases, an external fluid-filled laryngocele may simulate a cystic nodal mass or a branchial cleft cyst in the neck at the level of the supraglottis.

Reference

Lancella A, Abbate G, Dosdegani R. Mixed laryngocele: a case report and review of the literature. *Acta Otorhinolaryngol Ital.* 2007;27(5):255-257.

Cross-Reference

Neuroradiology: The Requisites, 3rd ed, 452.

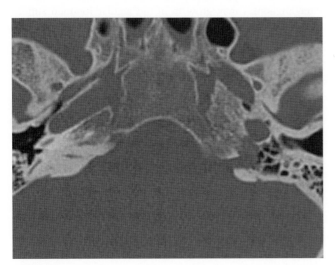

Figure 62-1

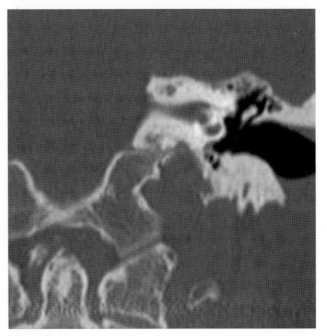

Figure 62-2

HISTORY: A young adult complains of persistent buzzing in the left ear.

1. Which of the following should be included in the differential diagnosis of this lesion? (Check all that apply.)
   A. Carotid body tumor
   B. Pilocytic astrocytoma
   C. Glomus jugulotympanicum
   D. Oligodendroglioma
   E. Multiple myeloma

2. Which cranial nerve passes through the pars nervosa of the jugular foramen?
   A. IX
   B. X
   C. XI
   D. XII
   E. None of the above

3. Of patients with paragangliomas, what percentage have more than one paraganglioma?
   A. 0% to 20%
   B. 21% to 40%
   C. 41% to 60%
   D. 61% to 80%
   E. >80%

4. What structure characteristically is eroded by a glomus jugulare?
   A. Körner septum
   B. Styloid process
   C. Scutum
   D. Pars tuberalis of the jugular foramen
   E. None of the above

See Supplemental Figures section for additional figures and legends for this case.

CASE 62

Glomus Jugulare Tumor

1. **C and E.** Glomus jugulotympanicum could start in the jugular foramen and erode superiorly. Multiple myeloma could lead to a lytic mass in the jugular foramen. A carotid body tumor would be lower in the neck at the carotid bifurcation. Pilocytic astrocytomas do not populate the jugular foramen. Oligodendrogliomas are brain tumors.

2. **A.** IX is the only cranial nerve in the pars nervosa. Cranial nerves X and XI leave via the pars vascularis with the jugular vein, and cranial nerve XII leaves via the hypoglossal canal.

3. **A.** Of patients with paragangliomas, 6% to 8% have more than one.

4. **E.** None of the structures listed is correct; glomus jugulare tumors erode the jugular spine. The Körner septum is seen to be eroded by epidermoids. The styloid process can be eroded by facial nerve masses or nasopharyngeal cancer. The scutum is eroded most frequently by acquired cholesteatoma. There is no such structure as the pars tuberalis of the jugular foramen.

Comment

Characteristics of Glomus Jugulare Tumors

Glomus jugulare tumors characteristically erode the jugular spine of the jugular foramen, the part of the bone that separates the pars nervosa anteromedially from the pars vascularis posterolaterally. The pars vascularis transmits the vagus and spinal accessory nerves (cranial nerves X and XI, respectively). Only the glossopharyngeal nerve (cranial nerve IX) passes through the pars nervosa of the jugular foramen. Paragangliomas may grow from the jugular foramen superiorly to enter the middle ear cavity, where they may manifest as retrotympanic vascular masses (Figures S62-1 and S62-2). A red mass observed behind the eardrum is typically considered an aberrant internal carotid artery or glomus tympanicum; however, as stated, the mass may actually transcend the usual boundaries and be centered in the jugular foramen. Such masses are known as *glomus jugulotympanicum tumors*.

Differential Diagnosis of Glomus Jugulare

Carotid body tumors are the most common of the paragangliomas. Glomus vagale tumors are the tumors most commonly associated with the vagus nerve. Erosive masses in the jugular foramen include metastases, direct spread from nasopharyngeal carcinoma, schwannomas, and paragangliomas. In rare cases, chordomas or myeloma may spread to this location. The schwannomas may be from cranial nerve IX, X, or XI.

Reference

Semaan MT, Megerian CA. Current assessment and management of glomus tumors. *Curr Opin Otolaryngol Head Neck Surg.* 2008; 16(5):420-426.

Cross-Reference

Neuroradiology: The Requisites, 3rd ed, 399-402.

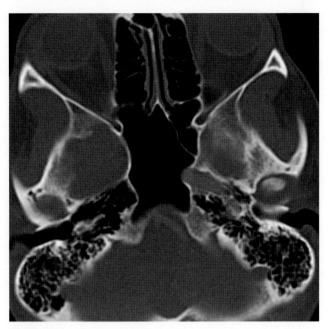

Figure 63-1

HISTORY: A patient is being evaluated for persistent sinusitis.

1. Which of the following should be included in the differential diagnosis? (Choose all that apply.)
   A. Aplasia of the internal carotid artery (ICA)
   B. Aberrant right subclavian artery
   C. Left carotid aneurysm
   D. Aberrant left subclavian artery

2. What dangerous outcome may be associated with an aplastic ICA?
   A. Stroke
   B. Vocal cord paralysis
   C. Moyamoya
   D. Aneurysms

3. What phakomatosis is associated with ICA aplasia?
   A. Tuberous sclerosis
   B. Von Hippel–Lindau disease
   C. Neurofibromatosis type 1
   D. Wyburn-Mason syndrome

4. On which side does ICA aplasia occur at a higher rate?
   A. Left
   B. Right
   C. Equal
   D. Bilateral ICA aplasia is more common than unilateral ICA aplasia

See Supplemental Figures section for additional figures and legends for this case.

CASE 63

Aplasia of the Internal Carotid Artery

1. **A.** ICA aplasia is the correct diagnosis because the petrous carotid canal is absent. An aberrant right subclavian artery courses behind the esophagus. Left carotid aneurysm is not evident, and aberrant left subclavian artery, which is very rare, is not visible at the skull base.

2. **D.** Aneurysms are associated with aplastic ICA at a high rate, 25% to 43%, especially aneurysms of the anterior communicating artery. Moyamoya is not common with ICA aplasia, and there is no direct association with stroke or vocal cord paralysis.

3. **C.** Neurofibromatosis type 1 is associated with ICA aplasia, but it is very rare. Tuberous sclerosis, von Hippel–Lindau disease, and Wyburn-Mason syndrome are not associated with ICA aplasia.

4. **A.** Left-sided ICA aplasia is more common than right-sided ICA aplasia (3:1).

Comment

Imaging Findings

Absence of the ICA is best identified from the absence of the petrous carotid canal, evident in this case (Figure S63-1). When the ICA is missing, the flow to the anterior and middle cerebral arteries is often supplied through intact posterior communicating and anterior communicating arteries.

Pathways of Collateral Circulation

Six pathways of collateral circulation in association with absence of an ICA have been reported and classified (Figure S63-2):
- Type A: The ipsilateral anterior cerebral artery passes through the anterior communicating artery, and the ipsilateral middle cerebral artery runs from the posterior circulation through the posterior communicating artery.
- Type B: The ipsilateral anterior cerebral artery and middle cerebral artery are supplied across a patent anterior communicating artery.
- Type C: Agenesis of ICA is bilateral, and supply to the anterior circulation is through the posterior communicating artery.
- Type D: Agenesis of the cervical portion of the ICA is unilateral, and an intercavernous communication to the ipsilateral ICA siphons flow from the contralateral cavernous ICA.
- Type E: Anterior cerebral arteries are supplied by bilateral hypoplastic but patent ICAs, and middle cerebral arteries are supplied by posterior communicating arteries.
- Type F: Collateral flow to the distal ICA is provided via transcranial anastomoses from the external carotid artery branches via the rete mirabile (as in rabbits).

Incidence of Aplasia of the Internal Carotid Artery

This anomaly is believed to occur in fewer than 0.01% of all individuals. If an intracranial carotid artery is not visible on images but the petrous carotid canal is of normal size, the aberration is probably not congenital in origin but an acquired occlusion.

Risks of Aplasia of the Internal Carotid Artery

Aneurysms, which may result from high flow through the remaining vessels and the shear strain associated, are the major risk of this anomaly. Aneurysms of the anterior communicating artery are the most common.

Reference

Lee JH, Oh CW, Lee SH, Han DH. Aplasia of the internal carotid artery. *Acta Neurochir (Wien)*. 2003;145(2):117-125; discussion, *Acta Neurochir (Wien)*. 2003;145(2):125.

Cross-Reference

Neuroradiology: The Requisites, 3rd ed, 494-499.

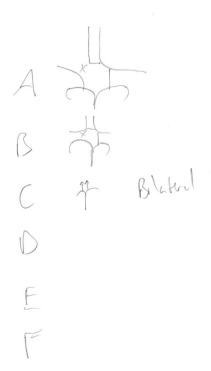

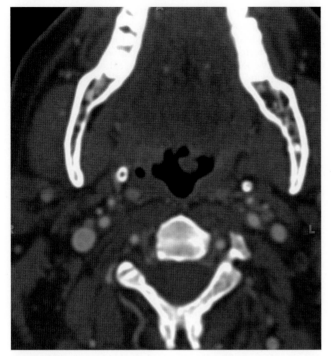

Figure 64-1

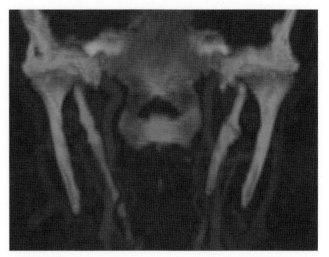

Figure 64-2

HISTORY: An elderly man presents with right ear pain during eating.

1. Which of the following should be included in the differential diagnosis? (Choose all that apply.)
   A. Osteochondroma of the styloid process
   B. Fracture of the styloid process
   C. Myositis ossificans
   D. Eagle syndrome

2. What is the other name for the poststyloid parapharyngeal space?
   A. The retropharyngeal space
   B. The carotid space
   C. The deep lobe of the parotid gland
   D. The longus space

3. What structure does the stylomastoid foramen mark?
   A. The exit of the facial nerve from the skull base
   B. The otic ganglion
   C. Cranial nerve V_3
   D. Cranial nerve V_2

4. What are the two nerves that run along the styloglossus-stylohyoid musculature?
   A. Cranial nerves V_3 (lingual branch) and XII
   B. Cranial nerves IX and XII
   C. Cranial nerves V_2 (buccal branch) and X
   D. Cranial nerve VII, chorda tympani, cranial nerve X, and parasympathetic nerves

See Supplemental Figures section for additional figures and legends for this case.

CASE 64

Eagle Syndrome

1. **D.** Eagle syndrome is a condition involving elongation and calcification of the styloid process, which cause pain on swallowing.

2. **B.** *Carotid space* is the other name for the poststyloid parapharyngeal space because it is posterior to the styloid musculature. The deep lobe of the parotid gland is anterior to the styloid musculature and therefore not "poststyloid."

3. **A.** The facial nerve exits from the skull base and leaves the temporal bone via the stylomastoid foramen. The otic ganglion is nearby, but the stylomastoid foramen is not its marker. Cranial nerve V_3 leaves via the foramen ovale, and cranial nerve V_2 leaves via the foramen rotundum.

4. **A.** Cranial nerves V_3 (lingual branch) and XII run along the sublingual space. Cranial nerves IX, X, and V_2 (buccal branch) are not located in this space. Cranial nerve VII, the chorda tympani, cranial nerve X, and the parasympathetic nerves are not associated with those muscles.

Comment

Characteristics of Eagle Syndrome

Eagle syndrome is an unusual entity, and some authorities do not believe that it causes pain on swallowing. It results from prominence with calcification of the stylohyoid ligament in such a way that the styloid process becomes elongated. The elongated styloid process often indents the pharyngeal mucosa when symptomatic (Figures S64-1 and S64-2). Compression of cranial nerve IX (most commonly) or XII and/or the sympathetic nervous plexus along the carotid artery may yield unusual complaints. The syndrome is named for Watt W. Eagle, a Duke University otolaryngologist who published a report of about 200 affected patients in 1937.

Incidence of Eagle Syndrome

The styloid process is elongated in 4% of the population; the length is usually described as more than 3 to 4 cm. However, fewer than 10% of patients with this elongation have symptoms. Treatment is resection of a portion of the elongated styloid process via an intraoral or extraoral approach. Some physicians inject local anesthetic in the ligament beforehand to ensure that this is the source of the otalgia, dysphagia, and/or headaches.

Reference

Costantinides F, Vidoni G, Bodin C, Di Lenarda R. Eagle's syndrome: signs and symptoms. *Cranio.* 2013;31(1):56-60.

Cross-Reference

Neuroradiology: The Requisites, 3rd ed, 441-444.

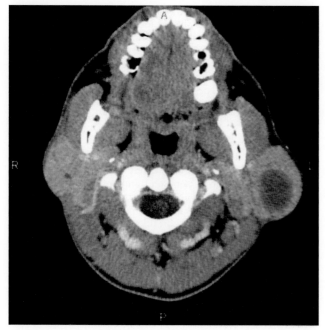

Figure 65-1

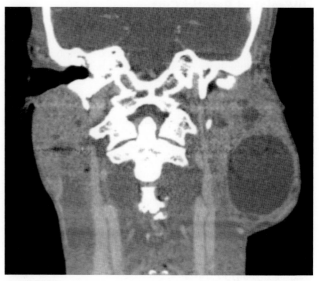

Figure 65-2

HISTORY: A young prostitute has swollen cheeks bilaterally.

1. Which of the following could potentially account for this finding? (Choose all that apply.)
   A. Branchial cleft cyst
   B. Sialocele
   C. Sjögren syndrome
   D. Human immunodeficiency virus (HIV) infection–related lymphoepithelial lesions
   E. None of the above

2. Which branchial cleft cyst is usually associated with the parotid gland?
   A. First
   B. Second
   C. Third
   D. Fourth
   E. Fifth

3. What other parotid masses are associated with HIV infection? (Choose all that apply.)
   A. Lymph nodes
   B. Lymphoma
   C. Metastases from Kaposi sarcoma
   D. All of the above

4. What other parotid masses are associated with Sjögren syndrome? (Choose all that apply.)
   A. Second branchial cleft cysts
   B. Lymphoma
   C. Metastases from Kaposi sarcoma
   D. First branchial cleft cysts

See Supplemental Figures section for additional figures and legends for this case.

CASE 65

HIV-related Parotid Cyst

1. **C and D.** The potential sources of the cysts and nodules in the parotid glands (Figures S65-1 and S65-2) are Sjögren syndrome and HIV infection–related lymphoepithelial lesions. Multiplicity does not suggest branchial cleft cysts or sialoceles.

2. **A.** First branchial cleft cysts are associated with the external auditory canal and the parotid gland.

3. **D.** Benign lymphoepithelial cysts and nodules, lymph nodes, lymphoma, and metastases from Kaposi sarcoma are associated with HIV infection.

4. **B.** Lymph nodes and lymphoma are associated with Sjögren syndrome. Metastases from Kaposi sarcoma and branchial cleft cysts have no association with Sjögren syndrome.

Comment

Causes of Parotid Cysts

Cysts in the parotid gland may have numerous causes; however, entities associated with single cysts are different from those associated with multiple cysts. Solitary cysts may have congenital causes (first branchial cleft cyst), may result from trauma (sialocele), may have inflammatory causes (pseudocyst, mucocele, mucous retention cysts), or may have neoplastic origins (adenoid cystic carcinoma). Of the causes of the multiple cysts in the patient's gland, HIV infection is one of the most common, but in women Sjögren syndrome should be also considered. One should look for rheumatoid changes in the temporomandibular joints or C1-C2 subluxation to suggest Sjögren syndrome on the same study as the parotid gland. Other causes of multiple cysts in the parotid gland include Warthin tumors, which may be a mixture of cystic and solid. Unusual cystic metastases such as those from thyroid papillary carcinoma or some varieties of lymphoma may also be considered.

Implications of Parotid Cysts

HIV-positive patients may present with painful swollen glands. This is usually treated conservatively with anti-inflammatory drugs, but if the pain is persistent and severe, it can also be treated percutaneously with sclerotherapy or low-dose radiation therapy. In most HIV-positive patients, cystic and solid masses are observed in the parotid glands because nodes and lymphoepithelial nodules abound. In addition, one should look for cervical adenopathy and adenoidal hypertrophy, which also may be present. Patients with HIV infection and those with Sjögren syndrome are at higher risk for parotid lymphoma. Kaposi sarcoma may metastasize to the parotid glands as well.

Reference

Rojas R, Di Leo J, Palacios E, Rojas I, Restrepo S. Parotid gland lymphoepithelial cysts in HIV infection. *Ear Nose Throat J.* 2003;82(1):20-22.

Cross-Reference

Neuroradiology: The Requisites, 3rd ed, 476-480, 483-486, 487.

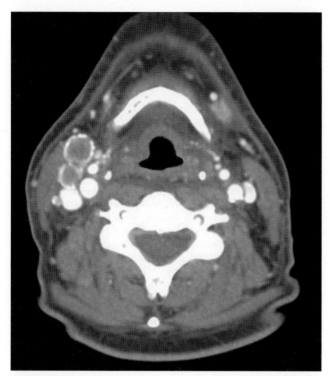

Figure 66-1

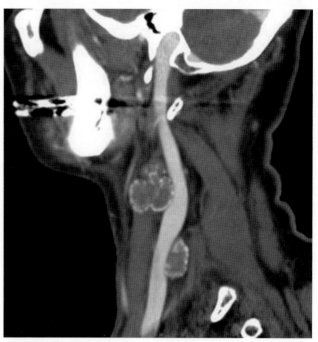

Figure 66-2

HISTORY: An adult presents with long-standing bilateral neck discomfort.

1. Which of the following should be included in the differential diagnosis? (Choose all that apply.)
   A. Calcified nodes from tuberculosis
   B. Calcified nodes from irradiated lymphoma
   C. Calcified nodes from Thorotrast use
   D. Calcified nodes from thyroid cancer

2. Which of the following is *not* a manifestation of thyroid cancer adenopathy?
   A. Calcified nodes
   B. Highly enhancing nodes
   C. Cystic nodes
   D. Hemorrhagic nodes

3. How soon after radiation therapy do lymphoma nodes calcify?
   A. Within 3 months
   B. 3 to 6 months
   C. 6 to 9 months
   D. >9 months

4. What is the level of adenopathy of nodes that are between the hyoid bone and cricoid cartilage but completely behind the jugular vein?
   A. IIA
   B. IIB
   C. III
   D. IIIB
   E. IV

See Supplemental Figures section for additional figures and legends for this case.

CASE 66

Calcified Nodes

1. **A, B, C, and D.** Tuberculosis, irradiated lymphoma, Thorotrast use, and thyroid cancer are all potential causes of calcified nodes. Thorotrast was used as a contrast agent in the 1930s and 1940s.

2. **D.** Hemorrhagic lymph nodes are very uncommon. Thyroid cancer nodes may calcify, may enhance avidly, or may be cystic.

3. **D.** Lymphoma nodes typically calcify 12 months after radiation therapy.

4. **C.** Level III adenopathy consists of lymph nodes that reside between the hyoid bone and cricoid cartilage. Unlike levels I, II, and V nodes, levels III, IV, VI, and VII nodes are not further subdivided into A and B levels.

Comment

Calcified Lymph Node Associations

Calcification of lymph nodes may be secondary to a number of disorders including treated granulomatous infections (e.g., tuberculosis, fungal infections), treated lymphoma, thyroid cancer, silicosis, sarcoidosis, and some mucinous adenocarcinomas. Much of the literature is based on plain radiographs; the onset of calcification in treated lymphoma after radiotherapy is quoted as being 12 months. High-resolution computed tomography may reveal it earlier.

Imaging Findings

Thyroid cancer is unusual in that the nodes associated with it may be calcified, cystic, or hypervascular and may even appear bright on T1-weighted magnetic resonance imaging, presumably because of high colloid content. The other primary tumor that may cause lymph nodes to appear bright on T1-weighted images is melanoma. Thyroid cancer also is unique in that it may lead to retropharyngeal nodes, and many nodes never meet 1-cm size criterion (Figures S66-1 and S66-2).

Nodal Nomenclature

Nodal nomenclature for squamous cell carcinomas in the aerodigestive system is based on location: Level IA nodes are submental; level IB nodes are submandibular; level IIA nodes are in the jugular chain above the hyoid bone and *not* completely behind the jugular vein; level IIB nodes are in the jugular chain above the hyoid and completely behind the jugular vein; level III nodes are in the jugular chain between the hyoid bone and the cricoid cartilage; level IV nodes are in the jugular chain below the cricoid cartilage and down to the clavicle; level VA nodes are completely behind the sternocleidomastoid muscle and above the cricoid cartilage; level VB nodes are completely behind the sternocleidomastoid muscle and below the cricoid cartilage; level VI nodes are anterior visceral; and level VII nodes are anterior mediastinal.

Reference

Gawne-Cain ML, Hansell DM. The pattern and distribution of calcified mediastinal lymph nodes in sarcoidosis and tuberculosis: a CT study. *Clin Radiol.* 1996;51(4):263-267.

Cross-Reference

Neuroradiology: The Requisites, 3rd ed, 470-471, 472.

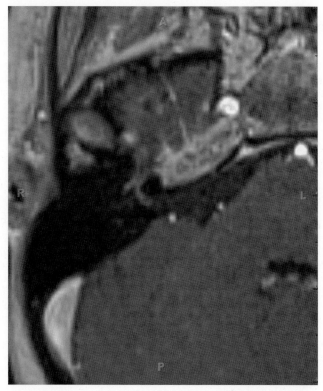

Figure 67-1

HISTORY: A middle-aged woman has a 1-week history of right facial droop.

1. Which of the following should be included in the differential diagnosis? (Choose all that apply.)
   A. Labyrinthitis
   B. Otospongiosis
   C. Lyme disease
   D. Bell palsy

2. Which of the following portions of cranial nerve VII do not normally enhance on magnetic resonance imaging (MRI)?
   A. Preganglionic segment
   B. Geniculate ganglion
   C. Tympanic segment
   D. Intramastoid segment

3. What is the explanation for the classical location of enhancement of cranial nerve VII in Bell palsy?
   A. That portion of the nerve has a more capacious blood-brain barrier.
   B. There is retrograde spread of blood from the gasserian ganglion.
   C. That location has a more vascular bed.
   D. This is the tightest portion of the bony course of the nerve.

4. Which of the following is *not* a frequent cause of cranial nerve VII palsies?
   A. Bell palsy
   B. Malignant parotid tumors
   C. Schwannomas of cranial nerve VII
   D. Vertical temporal bone fractures

See Supplemental Figures section for additional figures and legends for this case.

CASE 67

Bell Palsy

1. **C and D.** Lyme disease and Bell palsy are possible causes of enhancement of cranial nerve VII (the facial nerve). Labyrinthitis and otospongiosis would not be included in the differential diagnosis because there is no enhancement of the facial nerve from these conditions. They may cause labyrinthine enhancement.

2. **A.** The preganglionic segment should not enhance. The geniculate ganglion, the tympanic horizontal segment, and the descending intramastoid segment often enhance.

3. **D.** The enhancement of the facial nerve in Bell palsy is caused by compression at the tightest portion of the bony course of the nerve. The swollen nerve becomes inflamed at the tight opening of the fallopian canal between the fundus of the internal auditory canal and the preganglionic segment. This causes it to enhance on imaging.

4. **C.** It is uncommon for a schwannoma to cause a paralysis. Bell palsy and malignant parotid tumors often cause facial nerve paralysis, and vertical temporal bone fractures often injure the facial nerve, which leads to its paralysis.

Comment

Cause of Bell Palsy

The cause of Bell palsy is still obscure, but it is believed to represent a viral infection of the nerve that leads to palsy, most likely from the herpes simplex virus. Although the infection is usually self-limited, a small percentage of patients develop permanent facial changes. The imaging findings include diffuse or focal enhancement of the facial nerve, which is complicated by the fact that the facial nerve in its geniculate ganglion, tympanic segment, and intramastoid segment may normally show (asymmetric) enhancement (Figure S67-1). The labyrinthine segment and intracanalicular segment do not normally enhance because they do not have the typical venous plexus around the nerve like the other segments. Nonetheless, on 3.0-T MRI, the nerve may be accentuated after gadolinium administration, which may resemble nerve enhancement in these segments. Because the entrance from the intracanalicular segment to the fallopian canal is the tightest orifice through which the nerve must pass, the swollen nerve is said to become even more inflamed at this location; hence the avid enhancement.

Causes of Facial Nerve Enhancement

The numerous other causes of facial nerve enhancement include Lyme disease, sarcoidosis, herpetic infections, carcinomatous meningitis, perineural neoplastic spread, and tuberculosis. If a mass observed in the parotid gland is associated with facial palsy, it should be considered malignant until proven otherwise. It is decidedly rare for pleomorphic adenomas (the most common benign parotid mass) and Warthin tumors (the second most common benign parotid mass) to cause a facial nerve paralysis. Adenoid cystic carcinoma is the malignancy that most commonly causes perineural spread of paralysis up cranial nerve VII.

Reference

Gilden DH. Clinical practice. Bell's palsy. *N Engl J Med.* 2004;351(13): 1323-1331.

Cross-Reference

Neuroradiology: The Requisites, 3rd ed, 404, 413-414.

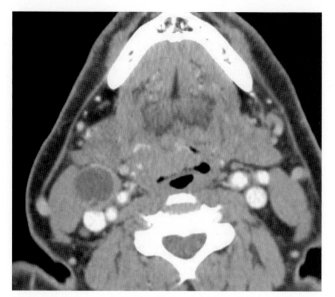

Figure 68-1

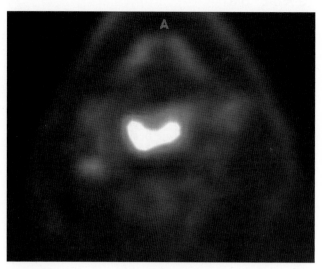

Figure 68-2

HISTORY: A 71-year-old patient has had a globus sensation for months and now has a mass in the right neck.

1. Which of the following should be included in the differential diagnosis? (Choose all that apply.)
   A. Oral cavity cancer
   B. Oropharyngeal cancer
   C. Hypopharyngeal cancer
   D. Supraglottic larynx cancer

2. What benign lesions occur in the floor of the mouth?
   A. Ranulas, dermoids, lymphangiomas, thyroglossal duct cysts, and hemangiomas
   B. Ranulas, Rathke cysts, lymphangiomas, thyroglossal duct cysts, and hemangiomas
   C. Ranulas, dermoids, Tornwaldt cysts, thyroglossal duct cysts, and hemangiomas
   D. Ranulas, dermoids, lymphangiomas, goiters, and hemangiomas

3. What stage tumor of the oropharynx is characterized by invasions of the extrinsic tongue muscles?
   A. T1
   B. T2
   C. T3
   D. T4

4. What is the most common site of oral cavity cancer?
   A. The lip
   B. The floor of the mouth
   C. The oral tongue
   D. The base of the tongue

See Supplemental Figures section for additional figures and legends for this case.

CASE 68

Oropharyngeal Cancer

1. **B.** Because this mass is in the base of the tongue, and because the base of the tongue is considered part of the oropharynx, this manifestation represents oropharyngeal cancer (Figures S68-1 and S68-2).

2. **A.** Ranulas, dermoids, lymphangiomas, thyroglossal duct cysts, and hemangiomas are benign lesions that occur in the floor of the mouth. Rathke cysts occur in the sella/suprasellar region, Tornwaldt cysts occur in the nasopharynx, and goiters occur in the lower neck.

3. **D.** Invasions of the extrinsic tongue muscles in oropharyngeal cancer lead to classification as stage T4A tumor.

4. **A.** The most common site of oral cavity cancer is the lip.

Comment

Treatment of Oropharyngeal Cancer

Head and neck surgeons require 2-cm margins around a visible tumor to ensure that they have resected all macroscopic and microscopic disease. However, they may use the periosteum of the mandible and periorbita of the orbit as a margin, even if the tumor is small. The risk of lymph node metastases, local and nodal recurrences, and death from the tumor is higher when neurovascular structures of the tongue base are invaded by tumor. The lingual nerve, lingual artery, and hypoglossal nerve course in the sublingual space, close to the styloglossus-hyoglossus complex; if the fat is obliterated between the tumor and either this muscle or the enhancing vessels, and if margins of the tumor appear irregular in the sublingual space, the neurovascular sheath has been infiltrated. Even if the tumor is small, the artery and the nerves may be included in the 2-cm margin.

Nodal drainage from the oral cavity cancers includes: level 1 (submandibular and submental) nodes and level 2 (high jugular chains) nodes.

Tumor staging of oropharyngeal cancer is as follows:
- T1: ≤2 cm in size
- T2: >2 cm, ≤4 cm in size
- T3: >4 cm in size or extension to lingual surface of epiglottis
- T4A (moderately advanced): invasion of larynx, cortical bone, deep (extrinsic) muscles, and medial pterygoid muscle
- T4B (very advanced): invasion of masticator space, lateral pterygoid, pterygoid plates, skull base, internal carotid artery, and nasopharynx

Reference

Mukherji SK, Weeks SM, Castillo M, Yankaskas BC, Krishnan LA, Schiro S: Squamous cell carcinomas that arise in the oral cavity and tongue base: can CT help predict perineural or vascular invasion? *Radiology.* 1996;198:157-162.

Cross-Reference

Neuroradiology: The Requisites, 3rd ed, 393.

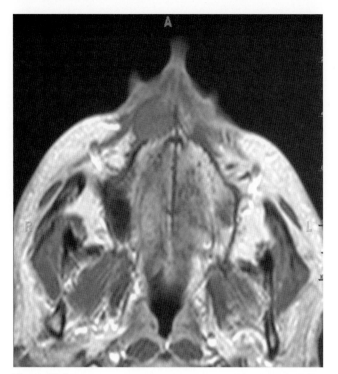

Figure 69-1

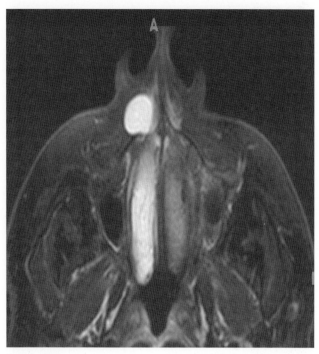

Figure 69-2

HISTORY: A young patient has chronic painless swelling in the right naris.

1. Which cyst should be considered in the differential diagnosis of this lesion? (Choose all that apply.)
   A. Nasolabial cyst
   B. Nasopalatine cyst
   C. Globulomaxillary cyst
   D. Globulolabial cyst

2. Which of the following is not a congenital cyst?
   A. Incisive canal cyst
   B. Nasopalatine cyst
   C. Globulomaxillary cyst
   D. Dentigerous cyst

3. Which cyst is associated with basal cell nevus syndrome?
   A. Radicular cyst
   B. Keratocystic odontogenic tumor
   C. Nasopalatine cyst
   D. Globulomaxillary cyst
   E. Dentigerous cyst

4. What cyst is associated with an unerupted tooth?
   A. Radicular cyst
   B. Keratocystic odontogenic tumor
   C. Nasopalatine cyst
   D. Globulomaxillary cyst
   E. Dentigerous cyst

See Supplemental Figures section for additional figures and legends for this case.

CASE 69

Nasopalatine Cyst

1. **A.** Nasolabial cysts are more superficial, and globulomaxillary cysts are more lateral than appears in this image. There is no such entity as a globulolabial cyst.

2. **D.** A dentigerous cyst is not considered a congenital cyst (present from birth). Incisive canal cysts, nasopalatine cysts, and globulomaxillary cysts are all congenital.

3. **B.** Keratocystic odontogenic tumors are associated with basal cell nevus syndrome. Previously, these were called *odontogenic keratocysts*. Radicular cysts are associated with a carious nonvital tooth. Nasopalatine cysts and globulomaxillary cysts are congenital but not syndromic.

4. **E.** Dentigerous cysts are associated with an unerupted tooth.

Comment

Location of Nasopalatine Cysts

The nasopalatine cyst is also termed the *incisive canal cyst* because it resides in close proximity posterior to the incisors bilaterally. It is the most common noninflammatory cyst in the maxilla, and it may appear bright or dark on T1-weighted images, bright on T2-weighted images (Figures S69-1 and S69-2), and hypodense on computed tomographic scans. Such cysts are usually discovered as incidental findings, but some grow so large that they cause the upper lip to bulge, some become inflamed, and some cause distortion of the alignment of the maxillary teeth. The nasopalatine cysts are more medial than the globulomaxillary cysts and are on the inside of the mouth, as opposed to the nasoalveolar/nasolabial cysts, which are more superficial.

Classification of Nasopalatine Cysts

Although these cysts were initially thought to be fissural cysts, the World Health Organization has classified them as developmental, epithelial, and nonodontogenic cysts of the maxilla. The incidence peaks between the ages of 50 and 60 years, and men are affected more commonly than are women. Treatment is usually complete removal. There is no malignant potential. The nasopalatine nerve is an offshoot of cranial nerve V_2 (maxillary nerve) and innervates the anterior teeth.

Reference

Escoda Francolí J, Almendros Marqués N, Berini Aytés L, Gay Escoda C. Nasopalatine duct cyst: report of 22 cases and review of the literature. *Med Oral Patol Oral Cir Bucal.* 2008;13(7):E438-E443.

Cross-Reference

Neuroradiology: The Requisites, 3rd ed, 445.

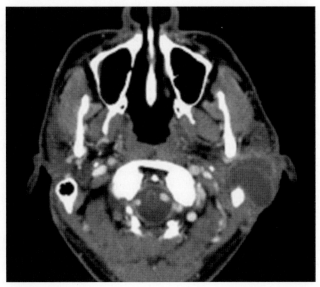

Figure 70-1

HISTORY: A young adult has a painless swelling in the left ear.

1. Which of the following should be included in the differential diagnosis? (Choose all that apply.)
   A. Sialocele
   B. Lymphoepithelial cyst
   C. First branchial cleft cyst (BCC)
   D. Adenoid cystic carcinoma

2. What is the difference between Arnot type I and Arnot type II first BCCs?
   A. Arnot type I cysts communicate with the external auditory canal (EAC), whereas Arnot type II cysts do not.
   B. Arnot type II cysts communicate with the EAC, whereas Arnot type I cysts do not.
   C. Arnot type I cysts are superficial to the sternocleidomastoid muscle, whereas Arnot type II cysts are deep.
   D. Arnot type I cysts communicate with the palatine tonsil, whereas Arnot type II cysts do not.

3. What entity besides human immunodeficiency virus (HIV) infection/acquired immunodeficiency syndrome (AIDS) is associated with lymphoepithelial cysts?
   A. Human papillomavirus–positive carcinomas
   B. Lymphoma
   C. Sialosis
   D. Sjögren syndrome

4. What is the difference between a sialocele and a pseudocyst of the parotid gland?
   A. Sialoceles communicate with the ductal system, whereas pseudocysts do not.
   B. Pseudocysts communicate with the ductal system, whereas sialoceles do not.
   C. Sialoceles communicate with the skin surface, whereas pseudocysts do not.
   D. Pseudocysts communicate with the skin surface, whereas sialoceles do not.

See Supplemental Figures section for additional figures and legends for this case.

CASE 70

First Branchial Cleft Cyst

1. **A, B, and C.** Sialocele is a cystic lesion that appears often after trauma and can look like the lesion shown in Figure S70-1. Lymphoepithelial cysts are often seen with nodules and are multiple in patients infected with human immunodeficiency virus (HIV). First BCCs often occur in the parotid gland. Adenoid cystic carcinoma lesions are usually not truly cystic and would not be included in the differential diagnosis.

2. **B.** Arnot type II first BCCs communicate with the EAC—there is a fistula to the EAC—whereas Arnot type I first BCCs do not.

3. **D.** Sjögren syndrome is associated with lymphoepithelial cysts and is also characterized by benign lymphoepithelial lesions. There is no association between lymphoepithelial cysts—or, moreover, parotid cysts—and human papillomavirus–positive carcinomas or sialosis. Lymphoma can occur with lymphoepithelial cysts in patients with HIV(+) and/or Sjögren syndrome.

4. **A.** Sialoceles communicate with the ductal system, whereas pseudocysts do not.

Comment

Characteristics of First Branchial Cleft Cysts

First BCCs are the second most common BCCs after second BCCs. They are intimately associated with the external ear and parotid gland and arise superior to the typical location of second BCCs, which most commonly lie at the level of the submandibular gland. Depending on whether they communicate with the EAC, first BCCs are classified as Arnot type I (no communication) or type II (communication). The course of the cysts is benign, but they may become infected.

Types of Parotid Cysts

Sialoceles are usually a result of blunt or penetrating trauma. They represent a pool of saliva that still communicated with the parent duct. They most commonly occur in the parotid gland. Pseudocysts are usually postinflammatory, resulting from rupture of the glandular architecture, but they may also result from trauma. They represent a collection that no longer communicates with the normal ductal system. Sjögren syndrome, like HIV infection/AIDS, may be characterized by bilateral and multiple cysts and nodules in the parotid glands. These lesions are commonly referred to as *benign lymphoepithelial lesions* in acknowledgment that they may be cysts or lymphoid aggregates. Sjögren syndrome is also noteworthy for the possibility of lymphoma in the parotid gland; thus any dominant solid mass in the parotid gland of a patient with Sjögren syndrome should be aspirated/biopsied.

Reference

Goff CJ, Allred C, Glade RS. Current management of congenital branchial cleft cysts, sinuses, and fistulae. *Curr Opin Otolaryngol Head Neck Surg.* 2012;20(6):533-539.

Cross-Reference

Neuroradiology: The Requisites, 3rd ed, 445, 487, 495.

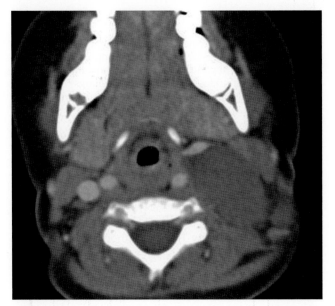

Figure 71-1

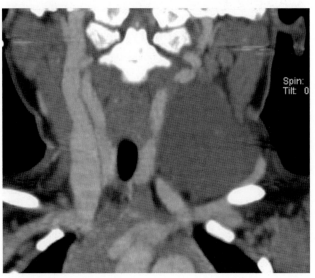

Figure 71-2

HISTORY: A 17-year-old boy presents with neck swelling on the left side.

1. Which of the following should be included in the differential diagnosis? (Choose all that apply.)
   A. Branchial cleft cyst
   B. Cystic nodal mass
   C. Jugular lymphatic sac
   D. Tornwaldt cyst

2. Which primary tumor is the most rarely associated with cystic lymph nodes?
   A. Papillary carcinoma of the thyroid
   B. Human papillomavirus (HPV)–positive squamous cell carcinoma
   C. HPV-negative squamous cell carcinoma
   D. Melanoma

3. What size node constitutes N2 disease with thyroid cancer?
   A. 3 cm
   B. 6 cm
   C. Bilateral nodes
   D. There is no N2 classification for thyroid cancer

4. If an HPV-positive squamous cell carcinoma is found in aspirate from a neck node, where is the primary tumor typically found?
   A. Oropharynx
   B. Hypopharynx
   C. Thyroid gland
   D. Esophagus

See Supplemental Figures section for additional figures and legends for this case.

CASE 71

Cystic Node from Papillary Carcinoma

1. **A, B, and C.** All of these could be cystic lesions in the neck of a young patient. The Tornwaldt cyst, however, is found in the nasopharynx.

2. **D.** Melanoma is the least likely to be associated with cystic lymph nodes. Papillary carcinoma of the thyroid and HPV-positive squamous cell carcinoma are the most likely. HPV-negative squamous cell carcinoma is not as commonly associated with cystic nodes but it is particularly associated with tonsil primary tumors.

3. **D.** There is no N2 classification for thyroid cancer. The node classifications for this type of cancer include only N0, N1a, and N1b. Furthermore, size does not matter in the classification of thyroid cancer, as opposed squamous cell carcinoma elsewhere.

4. **A.** If an HPV-positive node of squamous cell carcinoma is found in neck aspirate, the primary tumor is typically located in the oropharynx.

Comment

Classic Neoplastic Causes of Cystic Lymph Nodes

Cystic lymph nodes are characteristic of two primary tumors: papillary carcinoma of the thyroid and HPV-positive squamous cell carcinoma. In this case, the image showed a very small thyroid cancer; the node was identified as metastatic in nature and as papillary carcinoma (Figures S71-1 and S71-2), and the cancer was removed. The node is the initial presentation, as in this case, in about 15% of cases of papillary cancers.

Ultrasound Features

Features on ultrasound imaging of cystic papillary cancer nodes include the following:
- Purely cystic nodes in 6.2% of cases
- Cystic nodes in younger patients
- Thick outer wall of nodes in 35% of cases
- Internal nodularity in 43% of cases
- Internal septations in 57% of cases

Nodal Disease

With squamous cell carcinoma, size criteria are used to determine whether a node is benign or malignant. However, in the thyroid gland, tiny thyroid papillary carcinoma metastases can be present in the nodes (as well as in the lungs). The nodal staging is therefore based on location; regional lymph nodes are the central compartment, lateral cervical, and upper mediastinal lymph nodes:
- N0: No regional lymph node metastasis
- N1: Regional lymph node metastasis
- N1a: Metastasis to level VI (pretracheal, paratracheal, and prelaryngeal/Delphian nodes)
- N1b: Metastasis to unilateral, bilateral, or contralateral cervical or retropharyngeal lymph nodes or to superior mediastinal lymph nodes

Classification of Primary Thyroid Tumors

The primary thyroid tumor is staged on the basis of size and extent of invasion into neighboring structures:
- T1: Tumor ≤2 cm in greatest dimension and limited to thyroid
  - T1a: Tumor ≤1 cm and limited to thyroid
  - T1b: Tumor >1 cm but <2 cm and limited to thyroid
- T2: Tumor >2 cm but <4 cm in greatest dimension and limited to thyroid
- T3: Tumor >4 cm in greatest dimension and limited to the thyroid or with minimal extrathyroid extension (extension to sternothyroid muscle or perithyroid soft tissues)
- T4a: Tumor of any size extending beyond the thyroid capsule to invade subcutaneous soft tissues, larynx, trachea, esophagus, or recurrent laryngeal nerve or anaplastic carcinoma, surgically resectable
- T4b: Tumor invading prevertebral fascia or encasing carotid artery or mediastinal vessels, or anaplastic carcinoma, unresectable

Reference

Wunderbaldinger P, Harisinghani MG, Hahn PF, Daniels GH, Turetschek K, Simeone J, et al. Cystic lymph node metastases in papillary thyroid carcinoma. *AJR Am J Roentgenol*. 2002;178(3):693-697.

Cross-Reference

Neuroradiology: The Requisites, 3rd ed, 508-509.

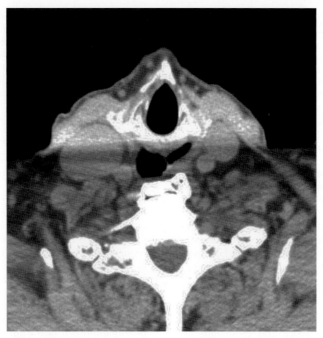

Figure 72-1

HISTORY: The patient is having pain on swallowing and once coughed up a partially eaten cookie.

1. What should the differential diagnosis include? (Check all that apply.)
   A. Laryngocele
   B. Zenker diverticulum
   C. Pharyngocele
   D. Saccular cysts

2. In which direction do most Zenker diverticula point?
   A. Anterior
   B. Superior
   C. Left
   D. Right
   E. None of the above

3. With what condition is Zenker diverticulum associated?
   A. Plummer-Vinson syndrome
   B. Barrett esophagus
   C. Achalasia
   D. Hiccups
   E. None of the above

4. Risk factors for upper esophageal carcinoma do *not* include which of the following?
   A. Plummer-Vinson syndrome
   B. Barrett esophagus
   C. Achalasia
   D. Hiccups
   E. None of the above

See Supplemental Figures section for additional figures and legends for this case.

CASE 72

Zenker Diverticulum

1. **B and C.** These entities are outpouchings of the digestive tube; if the outpouching is from the pharynx, the lesion may be a pharyngocele, whereas if the outpouching is from the upper esophageal segment, it is a Zenker diverticulum.

2. **D.** Most Zenker diverticula point to the right.

3. **E.** There is no association between Zenker diverticulum and Plummer-Vinson syndrome, Barrett esophagus, achalasia, or hiccups.

4. **D.** There is no association between risk factors for upper esophageal carcinoma and hiccups. Plummer-Vinson syndrome, Barrett esophagus, and achalasia are risk factors for upper esophageal carcinoma.

Comment

Types of Small Air Collections

Small air collections along the trachea and esophagus are fairly common, and most are probably normal variants, the effects of a collapsed airway or alimentary canal rather than true diverticula. Those that occur in association with the larynx are called *laryngoceles*. They may be internal (not perforating through the thyrohyoid membrane), external (extending via a stalk through the thyrohyoid membrane and manifesting outside the airway confines), or mixed. Those that are superinfected are called *pyolaryngoceles* because they often fill with purulent fluid. In the presence of a laryngocele, one must consider the possibility of an obstructing lesion at the saccule/appendix of the laryngeal ventricle as a potential source. In general, laryngoceles are more common in people who play brass instruments, glass blowers, and people who abuse their voices.

Location of Pharyngoceles

Pharyngoceles have a predilection for a weak area between the superior and middle pharyngeal constrictor muscles, This is at or just below the level of the palatine tonsils. The second weak area for pharyngoceles to develop is between the middle and inferior constrictor muscles at the base of the piriform sinus. They too may be internal, external, and mixed. Distinguishing between laryngoceles and pharyngoceles is sometimes difficult, especially with the external varieties, in which the "connection" may be petite or obscured. Both are more common in men than in women and in adults in middle age.

Zenker Diverticulum versus Killian Jamieson Diverticulum

Zenker diverticulum is also termed a *pharyngoesophageal diverticulum*. It usually occurs in close association with the cricopharyngeus muscle and is more common in elderly women and in patients with achalasia or other types of esophageal motility dysfunction in which the intrapharyngeal/esophageal pressure increases. It is a source of dysphagia and regurgitation of undigested foodstuffs. Aspiration pneumonia is the most serious complication. The Zenker diverticulum typically arises from the posterior wall of the pharyngoesophageal segment in a midline area of weakness just above the cricopharyngeus (i.e., Killian dehiscence) and points to the right (Figure S72-1). To add to the confusion, Killian-Jamieson diverticulum is a rare form of pharyngoesophageal diverticulum of the cervical esophagus that protrudes through a muscular gap (the Killian-Jamieson space) in the anterolateral wall of the cervical esophagus inferior to the cricopharyngeus. Most Killian-Jamieson diverticula are either left-sided or bilateral. A single right-sided Killian-Jamieson diverticulum is rare. These diverticula may contain air, fluid, and debris. Tracheal diverticula are usually asymptomatic and observed as a right-sided paratracheal air-containing pouch. High-resolution computed tomography often shows a connection between the tracheal lumen and the diverticulum.

Reference

Prisman E, Genden EM. Zenker diverticulum. *Otolaryngol Clin North Am.* 2013;46(6):1101-1111.

Cross-Reference

Neuroradiology: The Requisites, 3rd ed, 453.

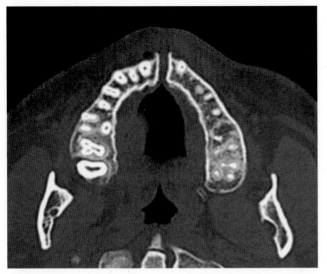

Figure 73-1

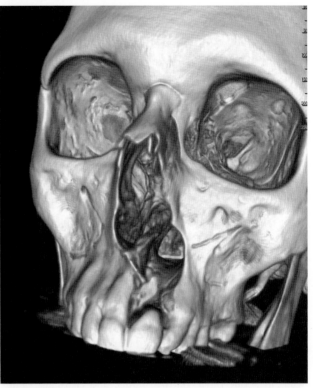

Figure 73-2

HISTORY: The patient has had a lifetime lisp.

1. What is the likely cause of the abnormality shown? (Check all that apply.)
   A. Trauma
   B. Neoplasm
   C. Congenital condition
   D. Vascular band
   E. None of the above

2. The hard palate normally fuses between which weeks of gestation?
   A. 0 and 10 weeks
   B. 10 and 20 weeks
   C. 20 and 30 weeks
   D. 30 and 40 weeks

3. Which develops first in gestation: the lips or palate?
   A. Lips
   B. Palate
   C. Same time
   D. None of the above

4. Which of the following are associated with cleft lips and/or palates? (Check all that apply.)
   A. Basal encephaloceles
   B. Callosal anomalies
   C. Optic nerve dysplasias
   D. All of the above

See Supplemental Figures section for additional figures and legends for this case.

CASE 73

Cleft Palate

1. **C.** The abnormality shown in Figures S73-1 and S73-2, a cleft palate, is congenital. It is too widely spaced to have resulted from trauma. No mass or vessel is present, and so it is not a neoplasm or vascular band.

2. **B.** The hard palate normally fuses during the twelfth week of gestation.

3. **A.** The lips develop first in gestation, at week 7. The palates develop at week 12.

4. **D.** All of the above. Basal encephaloceles, callosal anomalies, and optic nerve dysplasias are associated with cleft lips and/or palates.

Comment

Lip and Palate Formation

The lips form by the seventh week of gestation and the palate by the twelfth week of gestation. Multiple genes are involved in the regulation of this process, including the *FOXE1* gene, which is found on chromosome 9, and the *TBX22* gene, located on the X chromosome. Cleft palates occur in about 1 per 700 live births, and cleavages of the lip and soft palate are frequently concomitant. Affected children have problems with swallowing and nasal speech; however, the condition can be readily corrected surgically in childhood.

Incidence of Cleft Deformities

Of all cases of cleft deformities, 50% involve combined cleft lip and palate (unilateral clefts are three times more common than bilateral clefts), 20% are isolated cleft lips (unilateral clefts are nine times more common), and 30% are isolated cleft palate. Native Americans and Asians have a higher rate of cleft deformities than do white populations. Several syndromes are also associated with cleft lips and palates, including Loeys-Dietz syndrome, van der Woude syndrome, and Stickler syndrome. Maternal smoking and alcohol use also raise the risk of these deformities in their fetuses.

Treatment of Cleft Deformities

One of the issues with cleft palates is the association with intracranial anomalies, which include cephaloceles, optic nerve dysplasias, and callosal dysgenesis. Hypertelorism may coexist. Although treatment usually occurs in early childhood, bone grafting may be necessary in late childhood to address closure issues. The appearance of the maxilla and facial bones after treatment usually shows asymmetries, including deviation, narrowing, and descent of the nasal aperture; deviation of the nasal septum; and deviation of anterior nasal spine away from the cleft. Remnants of the cleft are more common posteriorly than anteriorly.

Reference

Kolbenstvedt A, Aaløkken TM, Arctander K, Johannessen S. CT appearances of unilateral cleft palate 20 years after bone graft surgery. *Acta Radiol.* 2002;43(6):567-570.

Cross-Reference

Neuroradiology: The Requisites, 3rd ed, 442.

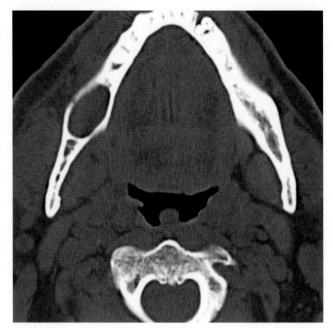

Figure 74-1

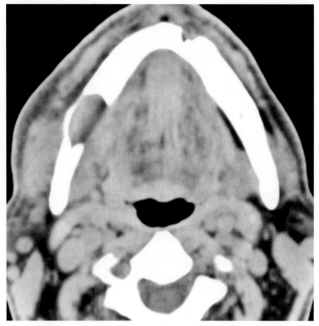

Figure 74-2

HISTORY: A 30-year-old patient is experiencing right-sided jaw pain.

1. Which of the following are the possible causes of the bone lesion in this patient in view of the history provided? (Choose all that apply.)
   A. Unicameral bone cyst
   B. Metastasis
   C. Osteonecrosis from bisphosphonate administration
   D. Radicular cyst
   E. Keratocystic odontogenic tumor (KOT)

2. The long axis of which cyst is usually parallel to the long axis of the mandible?
   A. Residual cyst
   B. Dentigerous cyst
   C. Nasopalatine cyst
   D. Radicular cyst
   E. KOT

3. What syndrome is associated with KOTs?
   A. Gardner
   B. Gradenigo
   C. Gorham
   D. Gorlin

4. Which of the following cysts are more commonly unilocular than multilocular? (Choose all that apply.)
   A. Unicameral bone cyst
   B. Dentigerous cyst
   C. Nasopalatine cyst
   D. Radicular cyst
   E. All of the above

See Supplemental Figures section for additional figures and legends for this case.

CASE 74

Keratocystic Odontogenic Tumor

1. **A and E.** Unicameral bone cyst and KOT are the possible causes of the bone lesion in this patient given the shape and orientation and borders.

2. **E.** The long axis of a KOT is parallel to the long axis of the mandible. The dentigerous cyst and radicular cyst are more vertically oriented to the mandible. The nasopalatine cyst occurs in the maxilla, not in the mandible.

3. **D.** Gorlin syndrome is associated with KOTs. Gardner syndrome is associated with osteomas; Gradenigo syndrome, with petrous apicitis; and Gorham syndrome, with vanishing bone or osteolysis.

4. **E.** Unicameral bone, dentigerous, nasopalatine, and radicular cysts are more commonly unilocular than multilocular.

Comment

Classification of Keratocystic Odontogenic Tumors

Because of their neoplastic nature—their aggressive behavior, high mitotic activity histologically, and associated mutation of the protein patched homolog 1 *(PTCH1)* gene—the World Health Organization designated odontogenic keratocysts as KOTs (i.e., neoplasms). Thus these lesions are considered tumors rather than cysts, and KOTs now represent nearly one third of all primary odontogenic tumors, surpassing odontomas and ameloblastomas in frequency. Of all other odontogenic cysts, 50% are radicular cysts, 30% are dentigerous cysts, and 15% are residual cysts (radicular cysts after a tooth has been removed).

Orientation of Keratocystic Odontogenic Tumor

KOTs are sometimes distinguished from other odontogenic cysts because they are usually oriented in the long axis of the mandible or maxilla, not the short axis (Figures S74-1, S74-2, and S74-3). It is usually not associated with a carious tooth (radicular/periapical cyst) and may or may not be associated with an undescended unerupted tooth (dentigerous cyst). KOTs are three times more common in the mandible than in the maxilla and usually occur in the premolar-molar regions.

Imaging Findings

On imaging, KOTs have smooth, expanded, scalloped margins. Most KOTs are multilocular, but the presence of a unilocular lesion, as in this case, should not exclude the diagnosis of KOT. On unenhanced computed tomography, they often appear hyperdense because of keratin content. Their solid portions do not enhance, and the lesions can therefore be distinguished from benign ameloblastomas.

Components of Gorlin Syndrome

Patients with Gorlin syndrome—also known as *basal cell nevus syndrome* and *nevoid basal cell carcinoma syndrome*—may have (1) basal cell carcinomas of the skin (90% of cases), (2) falcine and dural calcification, (3) KOTs (75% of cases), (4) bifid or fused ribs, (5) palmar and plantar pits, and (6) first-degree relatives with the disorder. In comparison with the general population, such patients have a higher rate of medulloblastomas. The origin of the disease has been isolated to an autosomal dominant genetic defect of chromosome 9 that leads to mutations of the *PTCH1* gene.

Reference

Avelar RL, Antunes AA, Carvalho RW, Bezerra PG, Oliveira Neto PJ, Andrade ES. Odontogenic cysts: a clinicopathological study of 507 cases. *J Oral Sci.* 2009;51(4):581-586.

Cross-Reference

Neuroradiology: The Requisites, 3rd ed, 450-451.

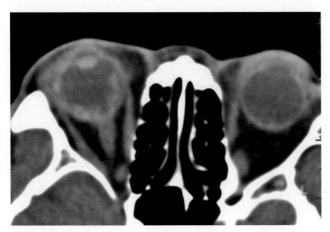

Figure 75-1

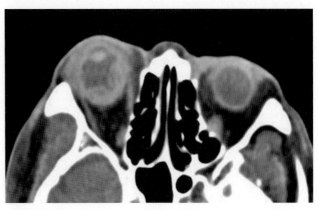

Figure 75-2

HISTORY: A patient who has diabetic retinopathy has post-traumatic visual loss.

1. Which of the following should be included in the differential diagnosis? (Choose all that apply.)
   A. Retinal detachment
   B. Choroidal detachment
   C. Scleral detachment
   D. Anterior hyphema

2. Which of the following is associated with retinal detachments?
   A. Termination at the ora serrata
   B. Cupping at the optic nerve insertion
   C. Retinoblastoma
   D. Scintillations
   E. All of the above

3. Which of the following is true?
   A. Choroidal detachments result from tears of the vortex veins.
   B. Retinal detachments result from tears of the vortex arteries.
   C. Retinal detachments result from tears of the ophthalmic arteries.
   D. Retinal detachments result from tears of the ophthalmic veins.
   E. None of the above.

4. What is the value of scleral banding procedures?
   A. Reapposition of retinal membranes
   B. Dilation and curettage of the membranes
   C. Filling the vitreous humor with material to tamponade the bleed
   D. All of the above

See Supplemental Figures section for additional figures and legends for this case.

CASE 75

Traumatic Retinal Detachment

1. **A.** Retinal detachment is the most likely diagnosis. There is no evidence of anterior chamber blood, choroidal detachment, or scleral hemorrhage.

2. **E.** Termination at the ora serrata, cupping at the optic nerve insertion, retinoblastoma, and scintillations are all associated with retinal detachments.

3. **A.** Tears of the vortex veins may be associated with choroidal detachments. Retinal detachment is not caused by tears of the large ophthalmic vessels of the orbit.

4. **A.** The value of scleral banding procedures is reapposition of retinal membranes.

Comment

Causes of Retinal Detachment

Retinal detachment results from a separation of the sensory epithelium of the retina from the deeper pigmented epithelium with accumulation of fluid. The retinal epithelium ends at the ora serrata, which is positioned at the 10 o'clock and 2 o'clock positions on the globe (Figures S75-1 and S75-2), whereas choroidal detachments extend to the ciliary apparatus further anteriorly. There are numerous potential causes of retinal detachments; however, trauma, axial myopia, diabetes, cytomegalovirus retinitis, and ocular neoplasms are predisposing factors. Often the posterior vitreous humor also is torn,

and vitreous fluid may cause dissection between the retinal epithelial layers.

Implications of Retinal Detachments

If left untreated, retinal detachments lead to total loss of light perception in the eye in more than 50% of cases. Treatment should be prompt to prevent scarring, hypotony, and deconvolution to phthisis bulbi. Reapposition of the sensory and pigmented layers can be achieved by the following methods:

1. Retinopexy, in which adhesions are created through the use of diathermy, cryotherapy, and photocoagulation

2. Scleral buckles or bands with silicone rubber or sponges or with tantalum, which indent the globe

3. Intraocular tamponade with gas, air, or silicone oil bubble

4. Vitrectomy

Surgical Complications

Possible surgical complications include choroidal detachment, especially with scleral buckling, which occurs in one third of cases. It resolves over the course of weeks.

Reference

Lane JI, Watson RE Jr, Witte RJ, McCannel CA. Retinal detachment: imaging of surgical treatments and complications. *Radiographics*. 2003;23(4):983-994.

Cross-Reference

Neuroradiology: The Requisites, 3rd ed, 324.

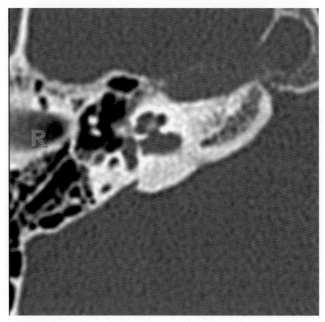

Figure 76-1

HISTORY: A 30-year-old woman is experiencing predominantly conductive hearing loss.

1. Which of the following should be included in the differential diagnosis? (Choose all that apply.)
   A. Labyrinthitis ossificans
   B. Otomastoiditis
   C. Otospongiosis
   D. Otosclerosis

2. Where is the classic location for fenestral otospongiosis?
   A. Aditus ad antrum
   B. Cochleariform process
   C. Fissula ante fenestram
   D. Sinus tympani and pyramidal eminence

3. How does otospongiosis cause conductive hearing loss?
   A. It causes tympanosclerosis.
   B. It causes the stapes to stop moving.
   C. It dislocates the ossicles.
   D. It poisons the organ of Corti.

4. How does otospongiosis cause sensorineural hearing loss?
   A. It causes tympanosclerosis.
   B. It causes the stapes to stop moving.
   C. It poisons the utricle and saccule.
   D. It poisons the organ of Corti.

See Supplemental Figures section for additional figures and legends for this case.

CASE 76

Otospongiosis

1. **C and D.** Otospongiosis and otosclerosis are synonymous and should be included in the differential diagnosis. Labyrinthitis ossificans does not cause new bone growth or osteolysis at the stapes footplate. Also, the image in this case does not show middle ear or mastoid opacification.

2. **C.** The fissula ante fenestram is where fenestral otospongiosis occurs. Aditus ad antrum is the channel between the middle ear and mastoid and where otitis media and cholesteatomas travel. The cochleariform process is where the tensor tympani tendon attaches. The sinus tympani and pyramidal eminence are parts of the hypotympanum; pars tensa cholesteatomas may reside there.

3. **B.** Otospongiosis causes conductive hearing loss by causing the stapes to stop moving and by fixing the footplate in place.

4. **D.** Enzymatic degradation of the hair cells of the organ of Corti causes the sensorineural hearing loss. Impingement upon the cochlear walls by the otospongiotic focus, causing a narrowing of the lumen of the cochlea, can also lead to sensorineural hearing loss.

Comment

Complications of Otospongiosis

Otospongiosis is an unusual disorder that can cause conductive, sensorineural, or, most commonly, mixed hearing loss. The conductive loss occurs as a result of the new bone growth at the fissula ante fenestram, which causes the more anterior portion of the footplate of the stapes at the oval window to become fixed (Figure S76-1), which prevents it from vibrating from sounds. On occasion, the whole oval window is occluded by new spongiotic bone growth. Current treatment involves a stapedotomy, in which a small hole in the stapes footplate is made with placement of a small-diameter Teflon wire piston into the vestibule.

The sensorineural hearing loss in otospongiosis results from enzymatic injury to the hair cells of the organ of Corti, hyalinization of the spiral ligament, vascular shunting, or narrowing of the cochlear canals and distortion of the basement membrane. Otospongiosis is bilateral in 80% of cases, but the degree of severity may not be symmetric.

Manifestation of Otospongiosis

The disease may be fenestral, as described previously, or retrofenestral, in which the new bone growth may be apposed to or even encircle the cochlea. The cochlear retrofenestral form may occlude the round window, which renders insertion of a cochlear implant more problematic. Either way, it is an autosomal dominant disorder with higher penetrance in affected female patients than in affected male patients. The differential diagnosis includes otosyphilis, osteogenesis imperfecta, and Paget disease. Because the incidence of otospongiosis peaks in the 20s, osteogenesis imperfecta and Paget disease can be ruled out in this patient.

Reference

Sakai O, Curtin HD, Fujita A, Kakoi H, Kitamura K. Otosclerosis: computed tomography and magnetic resonance findings. *Am J Otolaryngol.* 2000;21:116-118.

Cross-Reference

Neuroradiology: The Requisites, 3rd ed, 408-410.

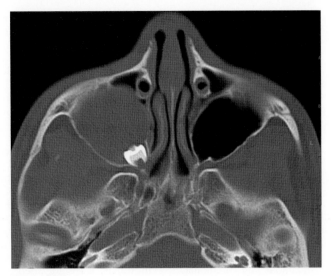

Figure 77-1

HISTORY: A young patient complains of constant right-sided nasal congestion.

1. Which of the following should be included in the differential diagnosis? (Choose all that apply.)
   A. Radicular cyst
   B. Dentigerous cyst
   C. Odontogenic keratocyst
   D. Ameloblastoma

2. What is the new name for odontogenic keratocyst?
   A. "Keratocystic odontocyst"
   B. "Basal cell cyst"
   C. "Keratocystic odontogenic tumor"
   D. "Residual cyst"

3. What is the possible complication of removal of a periapical cyst?
   A. Basal cell carcinoma
   B. Squamous cell carcinoma
   C. Oral antral fistula
   D. Dentigerous cyst

4. What is the typical location of a globulomaxillary cyst?
   A. Between medial incisors
   B. Between medial and lateral incisors
   C. Between lateral incisor and canine tooth
   D. Between molars

See Supplemental Figures section for additional figures and legends for this case.

CASE 77

Dentigerous Cyst

1. **B.** Dentigerous cysts are often associated with an unerupted tooth. Odontogenic keratocyst is usually not associated with an unerupted tooth. No carious tooth is evident, and so the diagnosis would not be a radicular cyst.

2. **C.** The new name for odontogenic keratocyst is "keratocystic odontogenic tumor" (KOT). This is because the World Health Organization believes this to be a low-grade neoplasm.

3. **C.** Oral antral fistula is a possible complication of removal of a periapical cyst. A communication can develop between the oral cavity and the maxillary antrum. There are no known associations between the removal of a periapical cyst and basal cell carcinoma, squamous cell carcinoma, or dentigerous cysts.

4. **C.** The typical location of a globulomaxillary cyst is between the lateral incisor and the canine tooth.

Comment

Dental Cysts

Symptoms in association with an unerupted tooth, as in this case, indicate a dentigerous cyst (also sometimes referred to as a *primordial cyst*). Dentigerous cysts are more common in the mandible than in the maxilla. They are found more commonly in the premolar and molar areas than elsewhere (Figure S77-1).

Odontogenic cysts include such benign congenital cysts as nasopalatine cysts and globulomaxillary cysts. Patients with holoprosencephaly may have a solitary median maxillary central incisor, which may suggest an issue with cleavage.

Keratocystic Odontogenic Tumors

KOTs have been reclassified as neoplasms by the World Health Organization, and the term *keratocystic odontogenic tumor* has replaced the term *odontogenic keratocysts*. KOTs represent nearly one third of all primary odontogenic tumors, surpassing odontomas and ameloblastomas in frequency. According to Johnson and colleagues (2013), 54.6% of odontogenic cysts are radicular cysts, 20.6% are dentigerous cysts, and 11.7% are KOTs. Of odontogenic tumors, 36.9% are ameloblastomas, 14.3% are KOTs, 6.5% are odontogenic myxomas, 4.1% are adenomatoid odontogenic tumors, and 1.6% are ameloblastic fibromas.

Reference

Johnson NR, Gannon OM, Savage NW, Batstone MD. Frequency of odontogenic cysts and tumors: a systematic review. *J Investig Clin Dent.* 2014;5(1):9-14.

Cross-Reference

Neuroradiology: The Requisites, 3rd ed, 450-451.

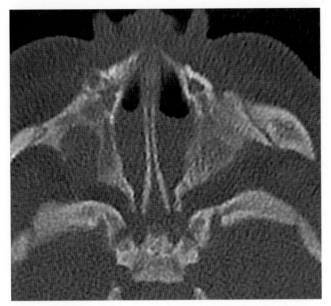

Figure 78-1

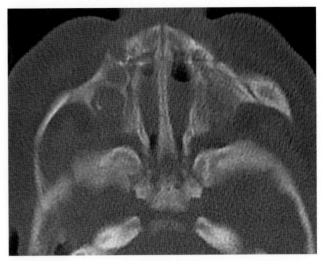

Figure 78-2

HISTORY: The patient is a 4-year-old child with nasal obstruction.

1. On the basis of the images, what should be included in the causes of this child's nasal obstruction? (Choose all that apply.)
   A. Membranous choanal atresia
   B. Bony choanal atresia
   C. Nasal aperture stenosis
   D. Polyps

2. What percentage of choanal atresia is mixed bony-membranous?
   A. <20%
   B. 21% to 40%
   C. 41% to 60%
   D. 61% to 80%
   E. >80%

3. Which syndrome is associated with choanal atresia?
   A. CHARGE
   B. Gorlin
   C. Tuberous sclerosis
   D. VACTERL syndrome

4. What width of the vomer in a child suggests choanal stenosis or atresia?
   A. 2 mm
   B. >3 mm
   C. 4 mm
   D. 5 mm
   E. 6 mm

See Supplemental Figures section for additional figures and legends for this case.

CASE 78

Choanal Atresia

1. **A and B.** Membranous choanal atresia and bony choanal atresia are the probable causes of the nasal obstruction. Soft tissue is obstructing the nasal cavity; this may represent secretions or membranous choanal atresia. Also, there is bony narrowing posteriorly. Probable causes do not include nasal aperture stenosis, inasmuch as the nasal aperture is normal in width, or polyps, inasmuch as there is nothing polypoid in the nose.

2. **D.** Of all cases of choanal atresia, 70% are mixed bony-membranous.

3. **A.** CHARGE is associated with choanal atresia: *c*oloboma, *h*eart disease, choanal *a*tresia, *r*etardation, *g*enital hypoplasia, and *e*ar anomalies. There are no associations between choanal atresia and Gorlin syndrome (nevoid basal cell carcinoma syndrome), tuberous sclerosis, and VACTERL syndrome (*v*ertebral anomalies, *a*nal atresia, *c*ardiac defects, *t*racheoesophageal fistula and/or *e*sophageal atresia, *r*enal anomalies and *l*imb defects).

4. **E.** Vomer width of 6 mm in a child suggests choanal stenosis or atresia. The posteroinferior vomer normally measures less than 2.3 mm in width and should not exceed 5.5 mm in children younger than 8 years.

Comment

Incidence of Bilateral Choanal Atresia

Bilateral choanal atresia may lead to infantile respiratory distress because neonates are obligate nose breathers. The diagnosis is usually made clinically by the inability to pass a nasogastric tube in a newborn with a breathing disorder. Unilateral choanal atresia is twice as common as bilateral choanal atresia, but the diagnosis may, as a result, be delayed. Choanal atresia is also twice as common in girls as in boys, but the overall incidence is 0.82 per 10,000 live births. The cause is failure of perforation of the buccopharyngeal membrane. Low levels of fetal thyroid hormones may be a factor in the development of this disorder.

Imaging Findings

In the past, 90% of cases of choanal atresias were said to be bony. Currently, most cases are thought to be combined membranous and bony (Figures S78-1, S78-2, and S78-3). It is difficult to determine radiologically whether the soft tissue anterior to the bony narrowing is secondary to retained secretions in the nose or to membranous atresia. Suctioning should be performed immediately before scanning to reduce the likelihood that the soft tissue represents mucus, as opposed to membranous choanal atresia. The posterior edge of the vomer is flared and widened in choanal atresia (see Figure S78-2). It should not measure greater than 5.5 mm, but this depends in part on the overall stature of the child.

Reference

Cedin AC, Atallah AN, Andriolo RB, Cruz OL, Pignatari SN. Surgery for congenital choanal atresia. *Cochrane Database Syst Rev.* 2012;(2):CD008993.

Cross-Reference

Neuroradiology: The Requisites, 3rd ed, 421-422.

CASE 79

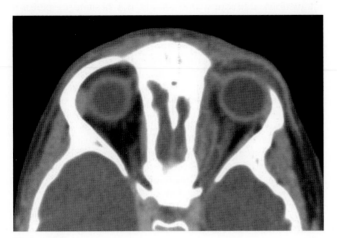

Figure 79-1

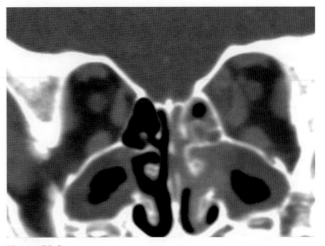

Figure 79-2

HISTORY: A teenager has had fever and left eye pain for 4 days.

1. What should be included in the differential diagnosis on this case? (Choose all that apply.)
   A. Subperiosteal abscess
   B. Sinusitis
   C. Periorbital cellulitis
   D. Orbital cellulitis

2. What is *not* a risk factor for the development of subperiosteal abscesses?
   A. Sinusitis
   B. Pediatric age group
   C. Immunodeficiency
   D. Hypercalcemia

3. What percentage of patients with sinusitis have orbital manifestations?
   A. <5%
   B. 6% to 10%
   C. 11% to 15%
   D. >15%

4. Why is ethmoid sinusitis most commonly associated with orbital complications?
   A. Proximity
   B. Valveless veins
   C. Anterior and posterior ethmoid artery openings to the orbit
   D. Thinness of the lamina papyracea
   E. All of the above

See Supplemental Figures section for additional figures and legends for this case.

CASE 79

Periorbital Subperiosteal Abscess

1. **A, B, C, and D.** Sinusitis, visible on the images, may lead to a subperiosteal abscess and orbital cellulitis. Because of the edema in the retrobulbar fat and the swelling of the superficial soft tissues, periorbital and orbital cellulitis may be present.

2. **D.** Sinusitis and immunodeficiency are risk factors for the development of subperiosteal abscesses. These abscesses are much more common in children than in adults because of the more dehiscent bone. There are no known associations between subperiosteal abscesses and hypercalcemia.

3. **A.** Fewer than 5% of patients with sinusitis have orbital manifestations. The actual percentage is quoted to be approximately 1% to 3%.

4. **E.** Ethmoid sinusitis is most commonly associated with orbital complications because of proximity, valveless veins, openings of the anterior and posterior ethmoid arteries to the orbit, thinness of the lamina papyracea, and propensity for dermal sinus tracts.

Comment

Imaging Findings

On imaging, the subperiosteal abscess of the orbit usually appears as a low-density, well-defined collection along the medial orbit adjacent to ethmoid sinusitis which is the usual source of the infection (Figures S79-1 and S79-2). The walls of these collections often do *not* enhance and yet are mature abscess collections. Treatment should be aggressive, with intravenous antibiotics; one should not hesitate to perform surgical drainage, especially in children who are predisposed to these infections because of the risk to the optic nerve. Despite the excellent barrier function of the periorbita (i.e., the periosteum of the orbital walls), this disease may spread into the retroconal orbit. In about 20% of cases, sinusitis progresses to retrobulbar inflammatory optic neuritis, and its first indication may be stranding of the orbital fat or enlargement and low density of the extraocular muscles. Septic thromboses of veins or small arteries from the progressive infection have a well-known potential to cause necrosis of the nerve. Visual disturbance, culminating in diplopia, may be secondary to the effects on the medial rectus muscle. Visual blurring may also result from optic nerve injury by direct compression by the collection or by an ischemic vasculitic mechanism.

Treatment of Periorbital Subperiosteal Abscess

Loss of visual acuity, nonmedial abscess, intracranial spread, severe mass effect or pain, clinical deterioration, and failure to improve within 48 hours of antibiotic treatment are criteria for surgical treatment. Surgery may be performed via an endoscopic approach. The pathogens may be aerobic (more often streptococcal than staphylococcal) or anaerobic (*Bacteroides* organisms). After drainage, broad-spectrum antibiotic therapy is indicated. In decreasing order of frequency, the orbital complications of sinusitis include preseptal cellulitis, orbital cellulitis, subperiosteal abscess, and orbital abscess.

Reference

Soon VT. Pediatric subperiosteal orbital abscess secondary to acute sinusitis: a 5-year review. *Am J Otolaryngol.* 2011;32(1):62-68.

Cross-Reference

Neuroradiology: The Requisites, 3rd ed, 321.

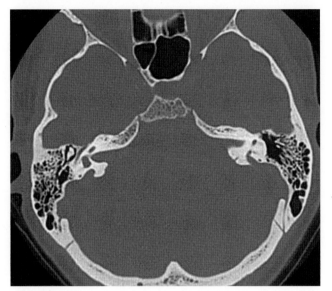

Figure 80-1

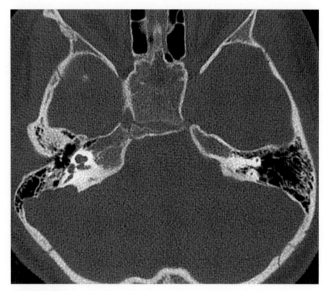

Figure 80-2

HISTORY: A patient has long-standing sensorineural hearing loss.

1. Which of the following should be included in the differential diagnosis? (Choose all that apply.)
   A. Enlarged vestibular aqueduct syndrome
   B. Mondini malformation
   C. Michel deformity
   D. Cock deformity

2. What congenital deformity may be associated with enlarged vestibular aqueduct syndrome?
   A. Mondini malformation
   B. Michel deformity
   C. Cock deformity
   D. VACTERL syndrome

3. Which of the following diameters represents abnormal enlargement of the vestibular aqueduct?
   A. >0.3 mm
   B. >0.5 mm
   C. >0.8 mm
   D. >1.5 mm

4. What is the term currently used for classic Mondini syndrome?
   A. "Incomplete partition type I"
   B. "Incomplete partition type II"
   C. "Incomplete partition type III"
   D. "Pendred syndrome"

See Supplemental Figures section for additional figures and legends for this case.

CASE 80

Enlarged Vestibular Aqueduct Syndrome

1. **A.** Enlarged vestibular aqueduct syndrome should be included in the differential diagnosis. The differential diagnosis would not include Mondini malformation, Michel deformity, or Cock deformity, inasmuch as there is no problem with cochlea spiralization, cochlea and vestibule development, or cochlea and vestibule separation.

2. **A.** Mondini malformation may be associated with enlarged vestibular aqueduct syndrome. These two often coexist. There is no association between enlarged vestibular aqueduct syndrome and Michel deformity, Cock deformity, or VACTERL syndrome (*v*ertebral anomalies, *a*nal atresia, *c*ardiac defects, *t*racheoesophageal fistula and/or *e*sophageal atresia, *r*enal anomalies and *l*imb defects).

3. **D.** An abnormally enlarged vestibular aqueduct has a diameter exceeding 1.5 mm. The affected aqueduct can also be compared with the adjacent semicircular canal caliber. If it is larger, this diagnosis should be considered.

4. **B.** "Incomplete partition type II" is the current, new term used for classic Mondini syndrome. Incomplete partition type I is the term for cystic cochleovestibular malformation. Incomplete partition type III is a rare condition in which the modiolus is not formed and the cochlea is in an abnormally medial location. Pendred syndrome is a genetic disorder with bilateral sensorineural hearing loss and goiter, which may result from bilateral enlarged vestibular aqueduct syndrome.

Comment

Causes of Congenital Sensorineural Hearing Loss

The enlarged vestibular aqueduct syndrome is one of the most common causes of congenital sensorineural hearing loss. It is manifested as enlargement of the bony canal of the vestibular aqueduct on computed tomography (CT) or enlargement of the endolymphatic sac, visualized directly on magnetic resonance imaging (MRI). This disorder may be associated with a Mondini malformation (see Figure S80-2). Among the many causes of neonatal hearing loss are congenital TORCH infections (*t*oxoplasmosis, *o*ther infections, *r*ubella, *c*ytomegalovirus, and *h*erpes simplex virus), medication effects, trauma, and hypoxic ischemic injuries. Other causes include congenital disorders such as external auditory canal atresia.

Enlargement of the Vestibular Aqueduct

The size of the vestibular aqueduct is easy to determine on high-resolution CT (Figures S80-1, S80-2, and S80-3). When the midpoint diameter of the vestibular aqueduct is greater than 1.5 mm according to Valvassori criteria or larger than the width of the posterior semicircular canal, it is classified as abnormally enlarged. According to Cincinnati criteria, however, 1 mm on CT is a more appropriate cutoff. The disorder is bilateral in approximately half of cases.

On MRI the endolymphatic sac is actually visible (Figures S80-4 and S80-5) as intensity of cerebrospinal fluid along the posterolateral temporal bone, paralleling the petrous angle.

Other Forms of Hearing Loss

Michel deformity is complete labyrinthine aplasia. Mondini malformation is a form of incomplete partition (type II); a cystic cochleovestibular malformation is another form of incomplete partition (type I; previously referred to as a *Cock deformity*). Incomplete partition type III, which is very uncommon, consists of absence of the modiolus with a cochlea that lies along the lateral border of the internal auditory canal. Patients with Pendred syndrome may have bilateral sensorineural hearing loss as a result of bilateral enlargement of the vestibular aqueducts. They may also be hypothyroid and have a goiter. Pendred syndrome is associated with mutations in the *SLC26A4* gene. No treatments have been uniformly successful. Cochlear implantation has had only limited success.

Reference

Huang BY, Zdanski C, Castillo M. Pediatric sensorineural hearing loss, part 1: practical aspects for neuroradiologists. *AJNR Am J Neuroradiol.* 2012;33(2):211-217.

Cross-Reference

Neuroradiology: The Requisites, 3rd ed, 414.

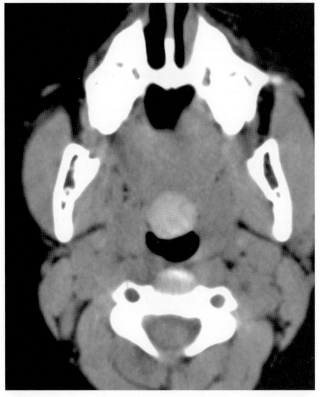

Figure 81-1

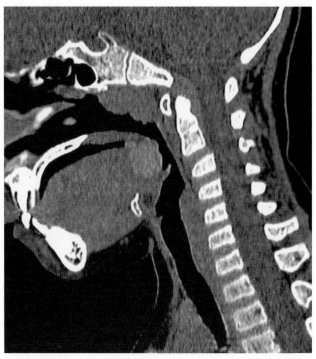

Figure 81-2

HISTORY: A child has a globus sensation.

1. Which of the following should be included in the differential diagnosis? (Choose all that apply.)
   A. Lingual thyroid gland
   B. Thyroglossal duct cyst
   C. Lymphoma
   D. Hemangioma
   E. None of the above

2. In what percentage of people with lingual thyroid tissue is that tissue the only thyroid tissue in the body?
   A. 0% to 25%
   B. 26% to 50%
   C. 51% to 75%
   D. >75%

3. Thyroid cancer is more common in people with lingual thyroid tissue than in those with which of the following?
   A. Thyroglossal duct cysts
   B. Native thyroid tissue
   C. Multinodular goiters
   D. Multiple endocrine neoplasia II

4. Of the sites listed, which is the most common for struma thyroidea?
   A. Oral cavity
   B. Oropharynx
   C. Omphalus
   D. Ovary
   E. Omentum

See Supplemental Figures section for additional figures and legends for this case.

CASE 81

Lingual Thyroid Gland

1. **A.** The gland is not cystic and is too hyperdense to be thyroglossal duct cyst or lymphoma. In a child like this, a hemangioma can occur in this location and be dense, but not this dense!

2. **D.** The lingual thyroid tissue is the only thyroid tissue in the body in 80% of cases.

3. **A.** The rate of cancer in thyroglossal duct cysts is exceedingly low because affected patients rarely have functioning thyroid tissue. The rate of cancer in lingual thyroids is like that in any thyroid tissue. Patients with multiple endocrine neoplasia II have a higher rate of pheochromocytoma and medullary thyroid carcinoma.

4. **D.** The most common site for struma thyroidea is the ovary. Its occurrence in the other sites is very rare.

Comment

Presentation of the Lingual Thyroid Gland

A lingual thyroid gland may manifest as a globus sensation in an adolescent child when it enlarges as a result of the hormonal surges associated with pubescence. Females are affected more commonly than males by a 7:1 ratio. The mass sensation prompts imaging and, it is hoped, a correct diagnosis, inasmuch as few lesions in this location are hyperdense on an unenhanced scan (Figures S81-1 and S81-2). Unfortunately, an enhanced scan can cause confusion because avid enhancement in this location could also be attributed to hemangiomas and lymphomas, which can also present in adolescents.

Thyroid Function and Thyroid Lesions

In 80% of cases of lingual thyroid gland, the gland is the only thyroid tissue in the body. Nuclear medicine scanning is performed to see whether there is thyroid tissue elsewhere that can take over thyroid hormone production if the lingual thyroid is removed. Thyroid cancers can occur in lingual thyroid tissue. The thyroid tissue in thyroglossal duct cysts is only rarely functional; thus the rate of cancer with these cysts is much lower. Thyroglossal duct cysts are unusual in this location; most occur below the hyoid bone, and if they occur in the tongue, they are usually much further inferior. Most patients with a lingual thyroid gland are either euthyroid or hypothyroid. They should be treated with supplements only until they resume a euthyroid state.

Reference

Gupta M, Motwani G. Lingual thyroid. *Ear Nose Throat J*. 2009;88(6):E1.

Cross-Reference

Neuroradiology: The Requisites, 3rd ed, 445.

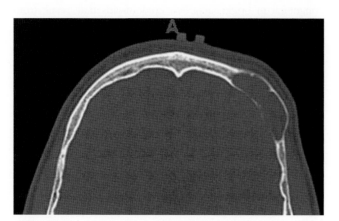

Figure 82-1

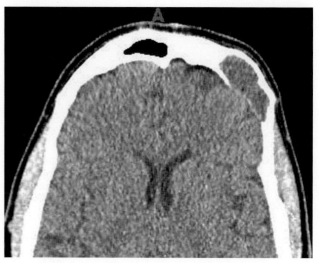

Figure 82-2

HISTORY: A middle-aged patient notices a focal area of skull irregularity when combing his hair.

1. Which of the following should be considered in the differential diagnosis? (Check all that apply.)
   A. Metastasis
   B. Paget disease
   C. Eosinophilic granuloma
   D. Hemangioma
   E. Epidermoid

2. Punched-out lesions of the skull are characteristic of each listed lesion except which one?
   A. Myeloma
   B. Tuberculosis
   C. Epidermoid
   D. Eosinophilic granuloma
   E. None of the above

3. Which of the following is associated with epidermoids of bone?
   A. Gardner syndrome
   B. Klippel-Feil syndrome
   C. McCune-Albright syndrome
   D. Klippel-Trenaunay-Weber syndrome
   E. None of the above

4. What percentage of epidermoids are intradural versus extradural?
   A. 75% intradural, 25% extradural
   B. 50% intradural, 50% extradural
   C. 75% extradural, 25% intradural
   D. 5% intradural, 95% extradural

See Supplemental Figures section for additional figures and legends for this case.

CASE 82

Epidermoid

1. **E.** Metastasis rarely expands and thins the bone. Paget disease is usually blastic, and bony margins are rarely thinned even when the disease is in the lytic phase. In eosinophilic granuloma, the bone usually has beveled edges. Hemangioma is bubbly, not lytic.

2. **C.** Myeloma, tuberculosis, and eosinophilic granuloma manifest with punched-out lesions of the skull. Epidermoid lesions are lytic and more expansile but not punched out.

3. **E.** Epidermoids do not have any known associations with syndromes. Gardner syndrome is associated with osteomas; Klippel-Feil syndrome, with craniovertebral anomalies; McCune-Albright syndrome, with fibrous dysplasia; and Klippel-Trenaunay-Weber syndrome, with venous vascular malformations.

4. **A.** Of all epidermoids, 75% are intradural (25% are extradural).

Comment

Appearance of Epidermoids of the Calvaria

Epidermoids of the calvaria are among the 25% of extradural epidermoids. They usually manifest in young adults, most commonly as a localized lump in the skull and detected by the patient. They are lytic lesions that thin the bone and have sclerotic margins, as opposed to lesions such as eosinophilic granuloma that have punched-out margins. They are defined usually as intradiploic lesions of the skull, centered within the calvarial margins and expanding in both directions (Figures S82-1 and S82-2). Whereas most lesions are thought to be congenital in origin, acquired epidermoids may result from trauma or iatrogenic causes in which epidermal elements are dragged into the skull, leading to the defect.

Imaging Findings

Characteristics on magnetic resonance imaging (MRI) are variable. Most images show fluid-like T1-weighted, T2-weighted, and fluid attenuated inversion recovery (FLAIR) signal, but some may appear slightly brighter. Restriction of diffusion usually indicates this diagnosis, but on occasion, highly cellular lesions may also cause restricted diffusion. They are nearly always bright on T2-weighted image, unless hemorrhagic. Constructive interference in steady state (CISS) and fast imaging employing steady-state acquisition (FIESTA) images differentiate epidermoids from arachnoid cysts by showing less intense signal. Epidermoids do not enhance. Recurrence rates are reported as high as 33%.

Other Calvarial Lesions

Of the benign skull neoplasms, osteomas are the most common, followed by hemangiomas. Fibrous dysplasia of the facial bones and skull is also more common than epidermoids of the calvaria.

Reference

Arana E, Latorre FF, Revert A, Menor F, Riesgo P, Liaño F, et al. Intradiploic epidermoid cysts. *Neuroradiology.* 1996;38(4):306-311.

Cross-Reference

Neuroradiology: The Requisites, 3rd ed, 69-71, 280-282, 282-283, 352, 371-373, 391-392, 445, 552.

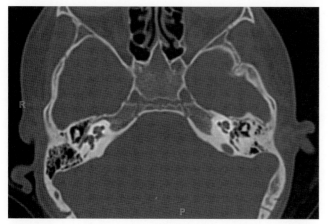

Figure 83-1

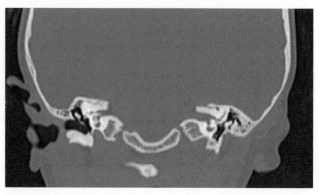

Figure 83-2

HISTORY: A child has a lifelong history of left-sided hearing loss.

1. Which of the following should be included in the differential diagnosis of these findings? (Choose all that apply).
   A. Internal auditory canal atresia
   B. External auditory canal (EAC) stenosis
   C. Macrotia
   D. EAC atresia and microtia
   E. EAC stenosis and microtia

2. Which of the following is/are *not* associated with external ear anomalies?
   A. Achondroplasia
   B. CHARGE syndrome
   C. Apert syndrome
   D. Cleidocranial monostosis
   E. A and C

3. Which of the following ear anomalies is associated with Down syndrome?
   A. Microtia with EAC stenosis
   B. Deformed middle ear ossicles
   C. Mastoid air cell underpneumatization
   D. Cochlear shortening and/or widened cochlear aqueduct
   E. All of the above

4. How often is congenital aural dysplasia bilateral?
   A. 0% to 25%
   B. 26% to 50%
   C. 51% to 75%
   D. >75%

See Supplemental Figures section for additional figures and legends for this case.

CASE 83

Microtia and External Auditory Canal Atresia

1. **D.** EAC atresia and microtia best characterize the findings depicted on these scans. No canal is visible, and so stenosis is not the condition.

2. **E.** Achondroplasia and Apert syndrome are not associated with external ear anomalies. CHARGE syndrome (coloboma of the eye, heart defects, atresia of the nasal choanae, retardation of growth and/or development, genital and/or urinary abnormalities, and ear abnormalities and deafness) has ear anomalies as the "E".

3. **E.** All of the ear anomalies listed are associated with Down syndrome. This disorder is also characterized by malformed vestibules and semicircular canals, as well as stenosis of the cochlear aperture.

4. **B.** Congenital aural dysplasia is bilateral in 26% to 50% of cases.

Comment

Incidence of Microtia

In descriptions of ear anomalies, the dysplasia of the pinna (auricle) of the ear should be distinguished from that of the EAC. Microtia is the condition in which the auricular structures are small and superficial (Figures S83-1 to S83-3). It is associated with EAC stenosis or atresia in approximately 75% of cases. Microtia is present in about 1 per 10,000 live births and is unilateral in more than 75% of cases. Mild microtia is more commonly associated with EAC stenosis, whereas severe microtia is usually associated with EAC atresia (79%) as opposed to stenosis (21%). For some reason, the right ear is affected more commonly than the left.

Syndromes Associated with Congenital Aural Dysplasia

The syndromes associated with congenital aural dysplasia include the following:

- Chromosome 18 deletion
- Cleidocranial dysostosis
- Crouzon syndrome
- Duane retraction
- Goldenhar syndrome
- Klippel-Feil syndrome
- Möbius syndrome
- Pierre Robin syndrome
- Thalidomide embryopathy
- Treacher Collins syndrome

Associations with Stenosis or Atresia of the External Auditory Canal

Inner ear anomalies occur in fewer than 15% of patients exhibiting EAC atresia. Anomalies that often coexist with EAC stenosis or atresia include (1) elongation of the scutum, (2) congenital epidermoid and acquired cholesteatomas, (3) facial nerve anterior malposition, (4) anomalous middle ear ossicles, (5) underpneumatization of the middle ear and mastoid antrum, and (6) anomalous development of the mandibular condyle.

Reference

Alasti F, Van Camp G. Genetics of microtia and associated syndromes. *J Med Genet.* 2009;46(6):361-369.

Cross-Reference

Neuroradiology: The Requisites, 3rd ed, 385-386.

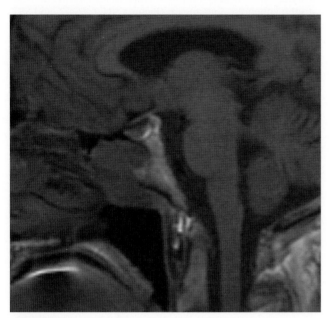

Figure 84-1

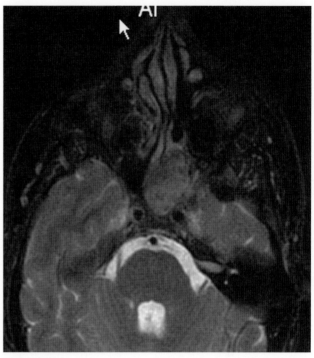

Figure 84-2

HISTORY: A teenaged boy presents with sudden onset of bleeding from the throat.

1. Which of the following should be included in the differential diagnosis? (Choose all that apply.)
   A. Nasopharyngeal carcinoma
   B. Juvenile nasopharyngeal angiofibroma
   C. Squamous cell carcinoma
   D. Lymphoma
   E. None of the above

2. What are the risk factors for nasopharyngeal carcinoma?
   A. Southeast American
   B. Infection with HSV-1
   C. Drinking alcohol
   D. Smoking
   E. Infection with human papillomavirus type 1

3. Which is the most precise description of the site of origin of this mass?
   A. Nasal cavity
   B. The nasopharynx
   C. The pterygopalatine fossa
   D. The nasopalatine canal
   E. The sphenopalatine foramen

4. Which foramen is inferomedial to the foramen rotundum?
   A. Vidian canal
   B. Foramen ovale
   C. Foramen spinosum
   D. Optic canal
   E. None of the above

See Supplemental Figures section for additional figures and legends for this case.

CASE 84

Juvenile Nasopharyngeal Angiofibroma

1. **B.** Juvenile nasopharyngeal angiofibroma should be included in the differential diagnosis. Lymphoma is possible but is not typical of the history provided. Nasopharyngeal carcinoma would be unusual in a teenager except those at risk, and lymphoma enhances on images less than this lesion. Squamous cell carcinoma is less common in the nasopharynx and unusual in a teenager.

2. **B.** Southeast Asian ancestry, Epstein-Barr virus exposure, and human immunodeficiency virus (HIV) infection are the risk factors for nasopharyngeal carcinoma. Alcohol and smoking are not risk factors for nasopharyngeal cancer.

3. **E.** The sphenopalatine foramen is considered the site of origin. From there, the pterygopalatine fossa and the nasopharynx are infiltrated.

4. **A.** The Vidian canal is inferomedial to the foramen rotundum. The foramen ovale and foramen spinosum are inferior and lateral. The optic canal is superior.

Comment

Characteristics of Juvenile Nasopharyngeal Angiofibroma

This case is not a typical growth pattern for juvenile nasopharyngeal angiofibroma (which is why it appears in the "Fair Game" section of this book). The typical juvenile nasopharyngeal angiofibroma has more nasopharyngeal and nasal cavity growth whereas this one seemed to turn north and head into the sphenoid sinus region (Figures S84-1, S84-2, and S84-3). These tumors originate from the sphenopalatine foramen, the medial egress from the pterygopalatine fossa, but they may extend through the various exits from the pterygopalatine fossa. Therefore, the Vidian canal, foramen rotundum, pterygomaxillary fissure, inferior orbital fissure, and palatine foramina must be scanned for tumor growth.

Main Findings

Juvenile nasopharyngeal angiofibroma typically afflicts teenaged boys, and the classical history is nasal bleeding. There is clearly a genetic predisposition involving the Y chromosome, inasmuch as the lesion is decidedly uncommon in girls. Treatment may be by excision, preceded by endovascular embolization to reduce blood loss. The classic teaching is that flow voids are seen in this lesion (as in paragangliomas), but that is not the experience of the author. However, this lesion enhances just as strongly as paraganglioma.

Reference

Lloyd G, Howard D, Lund VJ, Savy L. Imaging for juvenile angiofibroma. *J Laryngol Otol.* 2000;114(9):727-730.

Cross-Reference

Neuroradiology: The Requisites, 3rd ed, 383, 492.

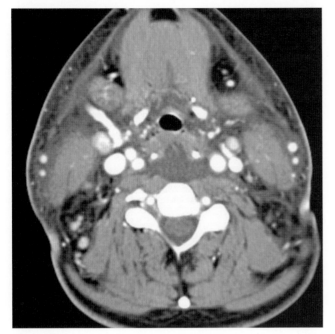

Figure 85-1

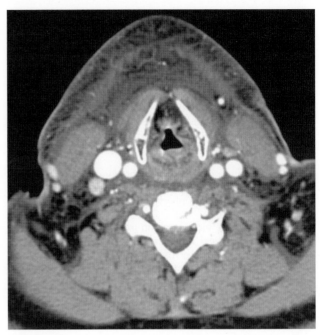

Figure 85-2

HISTORY: A young patient has pain while swallowing.

1. Which of the following should be included in the differential diagnosis? (Choose all that apply.)
   A. Pharyngeal abscess
   B. Peritonsillar abscess
   C. Retropharyngeal inflammatory process
   D. Osteomyelitis and diskitis complication

2. In what space would this lesion be localized?
   A. Parapharyngeal space
   B. Retropharyngeal space
   C. Prevertebral space
   D. Carotid space

3. What is the most common inflammatory condition in this space?
   A. Adenitis
   B. Retropharyngeal abscess
   C. Retropharyngeal phlegmon
   D. Calcific tendinitis

4. What is Lemierre syndrome?
   A. Sepsis after a tooth infection
   B. Increased coagulability that is caused by neoplasm
   C. Thrombophlebitis of the jugular vein that results from pharyngitis
   D. Torticollis that results from a retropharyngeal infection

See Supplemental Figures section for additional figures and legends for this case.

CASE 85

Retropharyngeal Inflammation

1. **C.** The condition depicted is a retropharyngeal inflammatory process, probably edema or phlegmon. Pharyngeal abscess occurs behind the pharynx, and peritonsillar abscess occurs behind the tonsils. It would not be osteomyelitis and diskitis complication because the longus muscles are not involved.

2. **B.** The lesion is centered between the mucosal compartment and the perivertebral compartment with the longus colli muscles: the retropharyngeal space.

3. **A.** Adenitis is the most common inflammatory condition of the retropharyngeal space. Inflammation of retropharyngeal lymph nodes may cause them to become necrotic, which in turn would lead to necrotizing retropharyngeal adenitis that simulates an abscess.

4. **C.** Lemierre syndrome is thrombophlebitis of the jugular vein that is a complication of pharyngitis.

Comment

Differentiation of Retropharyngeal Edema

Differentiating among retropharyngeal edema, cellulitis, phlegmon, abscess, and adenitis is difficult in many cases (Figures S85-1 and S85-2). Moreover, because more and more affected patients undergo a trial of intravenous antibiotics rather than transoral or transcervical surgical drainage (and even during surgery, the pathologic process may be confusing), the criteria for diagnosis are becoming blurred. A few tips are noted in the following table:

Entity	Imaging Hint
Necrotizing adenitis	Off midline, does not cross midline, often has irregular wall with edema extending into parapharyngeal space
Edema	Subtle, no mass effect, no rim enhancement, not infected, smooth
Cellulitis	Same as edema but more edema may extend into adjacent soft tissue and parapharyngeal space
Phlegmon	Mass effect, more of a collection, subtle or no enhancing of rim
Abscess	Mass effect, better defined rim, enhancement, convex margins, loss of definition with longus musculature
Lipoma	Fat density, mass effect, no enhancement

Causes of Retropharyngeal Edema

All the inflammatory entities above are usually detected as a result of a severe pharyngitis or tonsillitis or, less likely, a penetrating injury. The inflammatory process, if untreated, may evolve from edema to cellulitis to phlegmon to abscess with reactive and then suppurative adenopathy, which may also blur the margins and further obfuscate the diagnosis.

Reference

Al-Sabah B, Bin Salleen H, Hagr A, Choi-Rosen J, Manoukian JJ, Tewfik TL. Retropharyngeal abscess in children: 10-year study. *J Otolaryngol.* 2004;33(6):352-355.

Cross-Reference

Neuroradiology: The Requisites, 3rd ed, 499-500.

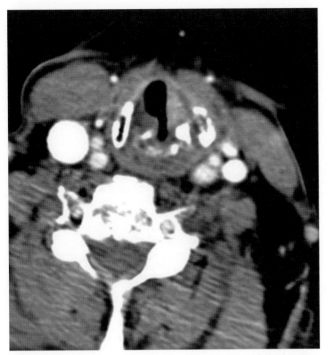

Figure 86-1

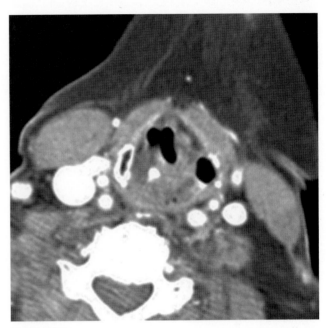

Figure 86-2

HISTORY: A middle-aged patient has had a 3-week history of change in voice that is unresponsive to decongestants.

1. Which of the following should be included in the differential diagnosis? (Choose all that apply.)
   A. Vocal cord paralysis
   B. Vocal cord cancer
   C. Vocal cord neurofibroma
   D. Laryngitis

2. Which of the following muscles may be atrophic in this patient?
   A. Thyroarytenoid muscle
   B. Thyrohyoid strap muscle
   C. Sternocleidomastoid muscle
   D. A and C
   E. All of the above

3. Which of the following is true?
   A. Most vocal cord paralyses result from vagus nerve lesions.
   B. Most vocal cord paralyses result from recurrent laryngeal nerve lesions.
   C. Most vocal cord paralyses result from superior laryngeal nerve lesions.
   D. Most vocal cord paralyses result from medullary lesions.

4. What is the most common etiologic factor in vocal cord paralyses?
   A. Idiopathic
   B. Infectious (e.g., viral)
   C. Iatrogenic/postsurgical
   D. None of the above

See Supplemental Figures section for additional figures and legends for this case.

CASE 86

Vocal Cord Paralysis

1. **A.** The cord is atrophic, which would be the case with vocal cord paralysis but not vocal cord cancer. Vocal cord neurofibroma is very rare. Laryngitis is not expected to cause these findings.

2. **A.** The thyroarytenoid muscle may be atrophic in this patient. None of the other muscles is innervated by the recurrent laryngeal nerve.

3. **B.** Most cases of vocal cord paralysis are due to lesions of the recurrent laryngeal nerve.

4. **C.** Iatrogenic/postsurgical entities most commonly cause vocal cord paralyses during thyroid or parathyroid surgery.

Comment

Signs of Vocal Cord Paralysis

The most common signs of vocal cord paralysis are dilation of the ipsilateral piriform sinus and vallecula, thickening and medialization of the ipsilateral aryepiglottic fold, and dilation of the ipsilateral laryngeal ventricle (Figures S86-1, S86-2, and S86-3), the latter of which reflects the atrophy of the underlying thyroarytenoid muscle. Anteromedial postion of the arytenoid cartilage is well demonstrated in these images as well. Cricothyroid muscle atrophy, one of the subtle and infrequently seen findings in vocal cord paralysis, may also be evident. Its presence is pathognomonic of vocal cord paralysis. While a single image of the vocal cord might raise concern about a vocal cord mass or polyp due to its asymmetry, the presence of the cricothyroid muscle atrophy clarifies the correct diagnosis.

Causes of Vocal Cord Paralysis

In this case, the cause of the vocal cord paralysis was a recurrent thyroid cancer that affected the right recurrent laryngeal nerve as it ascended from circling the right subclavian artery in the tracheoesophageal groove. The most common cause of vocal cord paralysis in most series is iatrogenic. Patients undergoing thyroidectomy and or parathyroidectomy, even when it is performed by the most skillful surgeons, have a 3% to 7% chance of awakening with recurrent laryngeal nerve palsy.

Reference

Paquette CM, Manos DC, Psooy BJ. Unilateral vocal cord paralysis: a review of CT findings, mediastinal causes, and the course of the recurrent laryngeal nerves. *Radiographics*. 2012;32:721-740.

Cross-Reference

Neuroradiology: The Requisites, 3rd ed, 453-455.

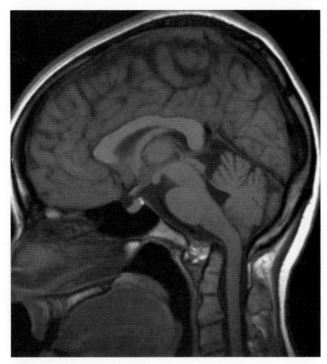

Figure 87-1

HISTORY: A patient is being evaluated with magnetic resonance imaging (MRI) of the brain for recurrent headaches.

1. What should be included in the differential diagnosis for this patient's abnormality? (Choose all that apply.)
   A. Basilar impression
   B. Basilar aneurysm
   C. Platybasia
   D. Basilar depression
   E. None of the above

2. The McGregor line is drawn between which two landmarks?
   A. Opisthion to basion
   B. Hard palate to anterior lip of foramen magnum
   C. Hard palate to posterior lip of foramen magnum
   D. Nasion to dorsum sella to plane of clivus
   E. None of the above

3. The Chamberlain line is drawn between which two landmarks?
   A. Opisthion to basion
   B. Hard palate to anterior lip of foramen magnum
   C. Hard palate to posterior lip of foramen magnum
   D. Nasion to dorsum sella to plane of clivus
   E. None of the above

4. The basal angle is drawn between which three landmarks?
   A. Opisthion to basion
   B. Hard palate to anterior lip of foramen magnum
   C. Hard palate to posterior lip of foramen magnum
   D. Nasion to dorsum sella to plane of clivus
   E. None of the above

See Supplemental Figures section for additional figures and legends for this case.

CASE 87

Basilar Impression

1. **A.** The abnormality in the image is most indicative of basilar impression. In the presence of an underlying bone disease, basilar invagination is indicated. Platybasia is flattening of the basal angle (Figure S87-1).

2. **E.** The McGregor line extends from the hard palate to the undersurface of the skull at the occipital bone. This line is used to measure the position of the odontoid process for basilar impression.

3. **C.** The Chamberlain line extends from the hard palate to the posterior margin of the foramen magnum. This line is also used to measure the position of the odontoid process for basilar impression.

4. **D.** The basal angle is formed from the nasion to the dorsum sella to the plane of the clivus. These lines are used to measure for platybasia.

Comment

Differences Between Basilar Invagination and Basilar Impression

The difference between the terms *basilar invagination* and *basilar impression* has been hotly debated, and they are rarely used appropriately. Cases in which the odontoid process is above either the McGregor line or the Chamberlain line by 5 mm are usually referred to as "basilar invagination." This is also considered upward migration of the vertebral elements. When the underlying bone is normal, however, the correct term is *basilar impression*; hence most congenital causes of odontoid elevation into the skull base produce basilar impression. These causes include such entities as Klippel-Feil and Down syndromes, achondroplasia, and occipitoatlantal fusions in which the bone density is normal. In contrast, in deformities "acquired" from such conditions as Paget disease, rheumatoid arthritis, hyperparathyroidism, rickets, and osteogenesis imperfecta, the bone is abnormal. In those cases, the more appropriate term is *basilar invagination*.

Determining the Basal Angle

The basal angle is measured from axes envisioned from the nasion to the dorsum sella and from the dorsum sella down the plane of clivus to the anterior margin of the foramen magnum (basion). If that angle is greater than 143 degrees (some authorities use 140 degrees), then the skull base is considered flattened (platybasia). The McRae line is the line defined by the anterior and posterior borders of the foramen magnum. The odontoid process is normally not above this line at all.

Determining Occipitoatlantal Dissociation

According to Cronin and colleagues (2007), the normal mean position of the odontoid process is 1.2 mm (median, 1.5 mm) below the Chamberlain line; 0.9 mm (median, 1.1 mm) below the McGregor line; and 4.6 mm (median, 4.8 mm) below the McRae line. At two standard deviations, the values are 4.8 for the Chamberlain line, 5.1 for the McGregor line, and 0.6 for the McRae line. To determine occipitoatlantal dissociation, the distance between the basion and spinal laminar line of C1 (BC) is divided by the distance between the anterior arch of C1 and the opisthion (AO). If BC/AO is greater than 1, occipitoatlantal dissociation is present.

Reference

Cronin CG, Lohan DG, Mhuircheartigh JN, Meehan CP, Murphy JM, Roche C. MRI evaluation and measurement of the normal odontoid peg position. *Clin Radiol.* 2007;62(9):897-903.

Cross-Reference

Neuroradiology: The Requisites, 3rd ed, 300.

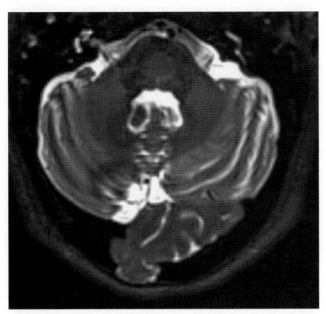

Figure 88-1

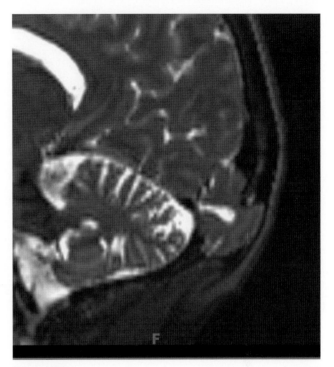

Figure 88-2

HISTORY: A child has a history of delayed development and seizures.

1. Which of the following should be included in the differential diagnosis? (Choose all that apply.)
   A. Meningocele
   B. Myelomeningocele
   C. Myelocele
   D. Meningoencephalocele

2. Which of the Arnold-Chiari malformations is associated with an occipital encephalocele?
   A. Type I
   B. Type II
   C. Type III
   D. Type IV

3. What is the difference between a basal encephalocele and a sincipital encephalocele?
   A. Basal encephalocele is not visible externally, whereas sincipital encephalocele is.
   B. Basal encephalocele is visible externally, whereas sincipital encephalocele is not.
   C. Basal and sincipital encephaloceles are defined by location.
   D. Basal encephalocele projects inferiorly, whereas sincipital encephalocele projects superiorly.

4. What is Miller-Dieker syndrome?
   A. Occipital encephalocele and Arnold-Chiari type I malformation
   B. Occipital encephalocele and lissencephaly
   C. Lissencephaly syndrome
   D. Lissencephaly and Arnold-Chiari type I malformation

See Supplemental Figures section for additional figures and legends for this case.

CASE 88

Occipital Encephalocele

1. **D.** Meningoencephalocele should be included in the differential diagnosis because the brain and meninges are herniating. No spinal cord herniation is present.

2. **C.** (Arnold)-Chiari type III malformation is associated with an occipital encephalocele. In this case, the image shows associated occipital lobe encephalocele. This is actually rare; usually cerebellar tissue is what herniates into the defect.

3. **A.** Basal encephaloceles are not visible externally, whereas sincipital encephaloceles are. This means that there is an external protuberance that can be observed without imaging.

4. **C.** Miller-Dieker syndrome is lissencephaly syndrome. Affected patients present with childhood seizures, developmental delay, spasticity, hypotonia, and feeding difficulties.

Comment

Associations with Occipital Encephaloceles

Occipital encephaloceles are classically associated with Arnold-Chiari type III malformation and thus are characterized by downward herniation of the medulla and cerebellum, in addition to the encephalocele (Figures S88-1 and S88-2). The neuroradiologist must be very wary of which tissue is herniated in an occipital encephalocele because it is possible for the torcula or other important venous structures to be included in the sac; this would pose a problem for the neurosurgeon. In occipital encephaloceles associated with Arnold-Chiari malformations, the herniated tissue is most commonly the cerebellum, whereas in those occurring without Arnold-Chiari malformations, the herniated tissue is most commonly cerebral cortex.

Manifestation of Encephaloceles

Most sincipital encephaloceles manifest along the nasal bridge or forehead. They also may contain vascular structures, including the superior sagittal sinus or even anterior cerebral arteries. Sincipital encephaloceles protrude, and so affected patients present earlier than do patients with basal encephaloceles. Encephaloceles may also be classified as primary, whereby the congenital lesion causes the skull defect, or as secondary, when the defect may be iatrogenic or a posttrauma occurrence (i.e., an event caused the encephalocele). Girls are more affected by occipital encephaloceles; boys are more affected by other encephaloceles than are girls. Basal and frontal encephaloceles are more common among people of Asian descent, but people of European descent have more occipital encephaloceles than any other type. Meckel-Gruber syndrome is an autosomal recessive syndrome that has a triad that consists of occipital encephalocele, large renal cystic dysplasia, and polydactyly. Affected patients may also have hepatic developmental defects, oral clefting, and pulmonary hypoplasia as a result of oligohydramnios.

Reference

David DJ, Proudman TW. Cephaloceles: classification, pathology, and management. *World J Surg.* 1989;13(4):349-357.

Cross-Reference

Neuroradiology: The Requisites, 3rd ed, 568-569.

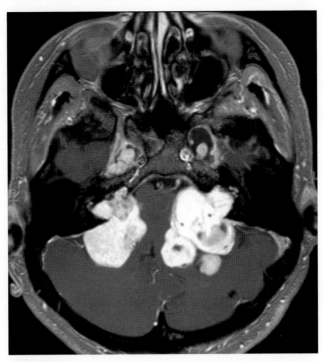

Figure 89-1

HISTORY: A 30-year-old man has bilateral hearing loss.

1. Which of the following should be included in the differential diagnosis? (Choose all that apply.)
   A. Bilateral vestibular schwannomas
   B. Subarachnoid seeding
   C. Bilateral meningiomas
   D. Neurofibromatosis type 1

2. Which is *not* a diagnostic criterion for confirming neurofibromatosis type 2 (NF-2) or including it in the differential diagnosis?
   A. Bilateral vestibular schwannomas
   B. Family history of NF-2 *and* either unilateral vestibular schwannomas or any two of the following tumor types: meningioma, glioma, schwannoma, juvenile posterior subcapsular lenticular opacity, juvenile cortical cataract
   C. Unilateral vestibular schwannoma plus at least two of any of the following: meningioma, glioma, schwannoma, juvenile posterior subcapsular lenticular opacity, juvenile cortical cataract
   D. All of the above

3. What single feature is the most reliable for distinguishing cerebellopontine angle schwannomas from meningiomas?
   A. Signal intensity
   B. Enhancement
   C. Location
   D. Dural tail

4. What percentage of vestibular schwannomas are entirely in the cerebellopontine angle cistern?
   A. 0% to 25%
   B. 26% to 50%
   C. 51% to 75%
   D. >75%

See Supplemental Figures section for additional figures and legends for this case.

CASE 89

Neurofibromatosis Type 2

1. **A.** Bilateral vestibular schwannomas should be included in the differential diagnosis. The appearance is not correct for subarachnoid seeding. Bilateral meningiomas are also unlikely to be present because no dural tails are visible.

2. **C.** The diagnostic criterion for NF-2 is (1) bilateral vestibular schwannomas or (2) family history of NF-2 *and* either unilateral vestibular schwannomas or any two of the following tumor types: meningioma, glioma, schwannoma, juvenile posterior subcapsular lenticular opacity, and juvenile cortical cataract.

3. **D.** Dural tails are specific for meningiomas; they are rare in schwannomas.

4. **A.** Vestibular schwannomas are entirely in the cerebellopontine angle cistern in 15% to 20% of cases.

Comment

Diagnostic Criterion for Neurofibromatosis Type 2

NF-2 is the definite diagnosis when a patient has bilateral vestibular schwannomas and is probably the diagnosis in a patient with a family history of NF-2 *and* either unilateral vestibular schwannomas *or* any two of the following tumor types: meningioma, glioma, schwannoma, juvenile posterior subcapsular lenticular opacity, and juvenile cortical cataract. NF-2 is caused by mutation in the gene encoding neurofibromin-2 (NF2; see OMIM reference), which is also called *merlin,* on chromosome 22q12.2 and is transmitted in an autosomal dominant manner. The mean age at onset of NF-2 is 20 to 25 years, and affected patients present with deafness. Café au lait spots occur in approximately 40% of cases, but very few patients have 6 or more such spots, as in neurofibromatosis type 1.

Incidence of Cranial Nerve Schwannomas with Neurofibromatosis Type 2

The acronym *MISME* (multiple inherited schwannomas, meningiomas, and ependymomas) is often applied to NF-2. That said, 95% of patients with NF-2 have a vestibular schwannoma (Figure S89-1). The fifth cranial nerve is the origin of only 1% to 8% of all intracranial schwannomas; the seventh and eighth cranial nerves are the origins in far more cases. Multiple schwannomas in concert with NF-2 account for about one third of cases of trigeminal schwannomas.

Features of Meningiomas

Meningiomas encase and narrow blood vessels and appear more dense on unenhanced computed tomography than schwannomas. On enhanced magnetic resonance imaging, intracranial meningiomas are characterized by a dural tail, a finding that is rare with schwannomas.

References

Rodriguez D, Young Poussaint T. Neuroimaging findings in neurofibromatosis type 1 and 2. *Neuroimaging Clin N Am.* 2004;14(2):149-170, vii.

607379: Neurofibromin 2; NF2. *OMIM.* Johns Hopkins University. Accessed January 10, 2014.

Cross-Reference

Neuroradiology: The Requisites, 3rd ed, 62-64, 380-382, 412, 567.

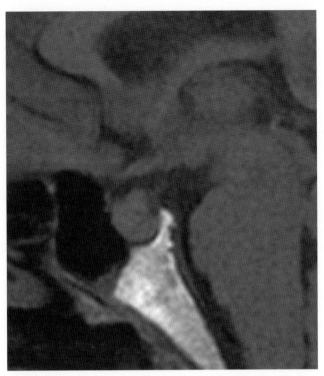

Figure 90-1

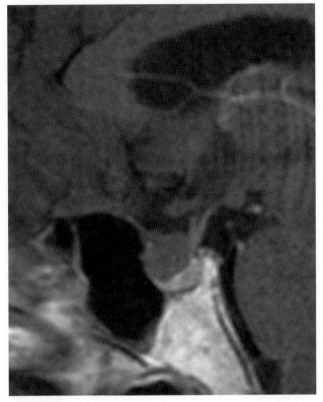

Figure 90-2

HISTORY: A patient is being evaluated for central hypothyroidism.

1. Which of the following should be included in the differential diagnosis? (Choose all that apply.)
   A. Hemorrhagic pituitary adenoma
   B. Craniopharyngioma
   C. Meningioma
   D. Rathke cleft cyst

2. What is the hormonal status most commonly associated with Rathke cleft cyst?
   A. No hormonal abnormalities
   B. Hypothyroidism
   C. Hyperprolactinemia
   D. Panhypopituitarism

3. What percentage of Rathke cleft cysts are confined to the sella?
   A. 0% to 20%
   B. 21% to 40%
   C. 41% to 60%
   D. >60%

4. What percentage of Rathke cleft cysts appear bright on T1-weighted images?
   A. 0% to 20%
   B. 21% to 40%
   C. 41% to 60%
   D. >60%

See Supplemental Figures section for additional figures and legends for this case.

CASE 90

Rathke Cleft Cyst

1. **D.** Rathke cleft cyst should be included in the differential diagnosis as it does not enhance and is slightly hyperintense before administration of gadolinium. This lesion seems separate from the gland. The lesion shows no enhancing foci, and so the diagnosis would not include craniopharyngioma or meningioma.

2. **A.** Only 35% to 40% of patients with Rathke cleft cysts have hormonal issues.

3. **A.** Approximately 5% of Rathke cleft cysts are confined to the sella. Most are suprasellar.

4. **C.** Approximately half of Rathke cleft cysts appear bright and half appear dark on T1-weighted images; some have mixed signal intensity.

Comment

Imaging Findings

Rathke cleft cysts are lesions that are typically found in the sella or the suprasellar region (usually both at once) and that can be distinguished from the adenohypophysis with high-resolution imaging. These lesions have variable signal intensity on T1-weighted images; nearly equal numbers are hypointense and hyperintense (Figures S90-1 and S90-2). On T2-weighted images, 75% of these cysts appear bright, but if the protein content of the cyst is high enough, even that may appear dark. The cysts do not enhance, and this confirms that the lesion is not a craniopharyngioma.

Symptoms of Rathke Cleft Cyst

Most affected patients present with headaches and no hormonal abnormalities, but in 35% to 40% of cases, these cysts manifest with mild pituitary hormonal abnormalities such as hypocortisolemia, panhypopituitarism, hypogonadism, hypothyroidism, and hyperprolactinemia, in order of frequency. In some patients, the cyst may rupture; such patients present with meningitic symptoms.

Cause of Rathke Cleft Cyst

The cause of Rathke cleft cyst is controversial: Some authorities ascribe the lesion to fluid contents derived from the neuroepithelium or endoderm or to metaplasia of adenohypophyseal cells. According to the classical description, however, Rathke cleft cysts arise from failure of obliteration of the lumen of the Rathke pouch, which should occur in the third to fourth week of gestation, having arisen from the primitive stomodeum. The anterior lobe of the pituitary gland and pars tuberalis are derived from the anterior wall of the Rathke pouch. Its posterior wall becomes the pars intermedia. The cleft between them, the Rathke cleft, should regress. When it does not regress, it persists and enlarges, usually in association with the pars intermedia of the pituitary gland, as the symptomatic Rathke cleft cyst.

Reference

Kim E. Symptomatic Rathke cleft cyst: clinical features and surgical outcomes. *World Neurosurg.* 2012;78(5):527-534.

Cross-Reference

Neuroradiology: The Requisites, 3rd ed, 282, 362, 371.

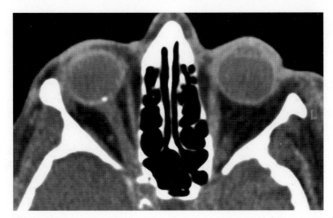

Figure 91-1

HISTORY: A middle-aged adult is being evaluated for sinusitis and papilledema.

1. Which of the following should be included in the differential diagnosis? (Choose all that apply.)
   A. Retinoblastoma
   B. Pseudotumor cerebri
   C. Optic neuritis
   D. Optic nerve head drusen

2. In what percentage of cases are optic nerve head drusen bilateral?
   A. 0% to 30%
   B. 31% to 60%
   C. 61% to 90%
   D. >90%

3. What is the potential significance of calcified drusen?
   A. They may cause no symptoms.
   B. Affected patients may have blind spots.
   C. Affected patients may have complete blindness.
   D. All of the above.

4. What do optic nerve head drusen most commonly mimic?
   A. Retinoblastoma
   B. Astrocytic hamartoma
   C. Papilledema
   D. Retinal hemangioblastoma

See Supplemental Figures section for additional figures and legends for this case.

CASE 91

Optic Nerve Drusen

1. **D.** Optic nerve head drusen often appear as a small calcification at the optic nerve insertion to the globe (Figure S91-1). The appearance in this image is unlikely to represent retinoblastoma in an adult. Pseudotumor cerebri and optic neuritis usually do not calcify.

2. **C.** Optic nerve head drusen are bilateral in 66% to 75% of cases.

3. **D.** Blind spots and blindness are possible, although rare, symptoms from calcified drusen. Drusen can also occur with no symptoms.

4. **C.** Optic nerve head drusen most commonly mimic papilledema, which usually prompts the neurologist to order scans. Calcified drusen do not mimic retinoblastoma in that there is no mass; moreover, retinoblastomas occur in young children, not at the age typical for drusen. Astrocytic hamartomas may calcify and may be visible as a mass, but they are less likely to occur at the optic nerve insertion. Retinal hemangioblastomas enhance on images and are hypervascular.

Comment

Incidence of Optic Nerve Drusen

The differential diagnosis of a calcified ocular *mass* includes retinoblastoma, astrocytic hamartomas (associated with tuberous sclerosis or neurofibromatosis), and choroidal osteoma. There is currently no treatment for optic nerve head drusen. They may occur sporadically or as a result of autosomal dominant inheritance. Whether their occurrence is sporadic or inherited, bilaterality is estimated to occur in 66% to 75% of cases. They occur most commonly in white persons. Optic disc drusen are more frequent in patients with retinitis pigmentosa, angioid streaks, Usher syndrome, Noonan syndrome, Alagille syndrome, and pseudoxanthoma elasticum.

Symptoms of Optic Nerve Drusen

With increasing age and size, these drusen may increasingly cause symptoms, but they may remain asymptomatic in some patients. Neovascularization may occur, leading to macular degeneration, as may compression and compromise of the nerve fibers and the vascular supply, leading to the following symptoms: visual field defects, vascular occlusion, and hemorrhage. Drusen may be a cause of acute ischemic optic neuropathy. On computed tomography, drusen may appear as a disorder seen in adults, but on ophthalmologic examination, drusen may be seen as mimicking papilledema, even in children. In such cases, they are known as "buried" drusen in younger children (preteen years) and can obscure the edges of the optic disc and cup. With increasing age, the drusen become more visible.

Reference

Sahin A, Cingü AK, Ari S, Cinar Y, Caça I. Bilateral optic disc drusen mimicking papilledema. *J Clin Neurol.* 2012;8(2):151-154.

Cross-Reference

Neuroradiology: The Requisites, 3rd ed, 322f, 327.

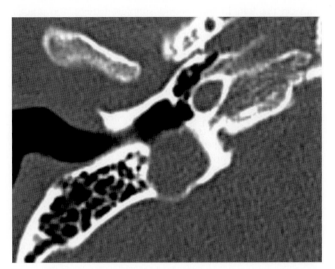

Figure 92-1

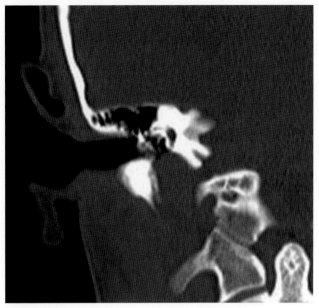

Figure 92-2

HISTORY: A young woman is being evaluated for pulsatile tinnitus in the right ear.

1. Which of the following should be included in the differential diagnosis? (Choose all that apply.)
   A. Glomus jugulare
   B. Aberrant internal carotid artery
   C. Cholesteatoma
   D. Dehiscent jugular bulb

2. How do dehiscent jugular bulbs manifest?
   A. Pulsatile tinnitus
   B. Neck mass
   C. Hemotympanum
   D. Fistula

3. During surgery for middle ear disease, in how many cases is a dehiscent jugular vein discovered?
   A. 0% to 10%
   B. 11% to 25%
   C. 26% to 50%
   D. >50%

4. How often is the right jugular bulb larger than the left?
   A. 0% to 20%
   B. 21% to 40%
   C. 41% to 60%
   D. >60%

See Supplemental Figures section for additional figures and legends for this case.

CASE 92

Jugular Vein Dehiscence

1. **D.** Incompleteness of the wall of the jugular bulb is characteristic of dehiscent jugular bulb. There is no mass here, and so glomus jugulare and cholesteatoma would not be included. Also, the structure is not the carotid artery, and so aberrant internal carotid artery could not be a diagnosis.

2. **A.** Dehiscent jugular bulbs manifest as pulsatile tinnitus with transmitted vascular sounds.

3. **A.** A dehiscent jugular vein is discovered only about 8% of the time as a normal variant.

4. **D.** The right jugular bulb is larger than the left in about 75% of individuals.

Comment

Types of Jugular Vein Anomalies

There are many different varieties of jugular vein anomalies in the temporal bone. The simplest is a high-riding jugular vein without dehiscence, which occurs when the jugular vein reaches the level of the internal auditory canal, above the inferior tympanic annulus, or above the basal turn of the cochlea (8.2%). These are more common on the right side than on the left. In the second simplest variety, the jugular bulb is dehiscent, and the sigmoid plate overlying the jugular vein's anterior wall is deficient (Figures S92-1 and S92-2). This anomaly may be observed at otoscopy as a retrotympanic, red, vascular mass. The more complex varieties include dehiscent jugular bulbs that communicate with structures other than the middle ear cavity, such as the endolymphatic sac, the facial nerve canal, or the semicircular canals. A diverticulum may protrude into the middle ear cavity and appear as a more focal mass. Of interest is that this is said to be more common on the left side. On otoscopy, this lesion may be mistaken for a paraganglioma or another vascular tumor. The jugular venous wave may not be evident at otoscopy to suggest a normal variant diagnosis.

Reference

Friedmann DR, Eubig J, Winata LS, Pramanik BK, Merchant SN, Lalwani AK. Prevalence of jugular bulb abnormalities and resultant inner ear dehiscence: a histopathologic and radiologic study. *Otolaryngol Head Neck Surg.* 2012;147(4):750-756.

Cross-Reference

Neuroradiology: The Requisites, 3rd ed, 385, 598.

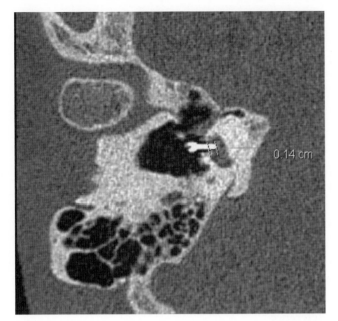

Figure 93-1

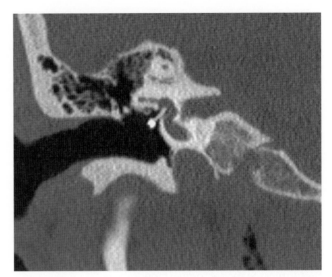

Figure 93-2

HISTORY: A patient has a history of bilateral mixed hearing loss, treated surgically.

1. Which of the following should be included in the differential diagnosis? (Choose all that apply.)
   A. Normal placement of the stapes prosthesis
   B. Malposition of the stapes prosthesis
   C. Dislocation of the stapes prosthesis
   D. Metallic foreign body

2. What is the most common reason for placement of a stapes implant or stapedectomy?
   A. Trauma
   B. Otosclerosis
   C. Cholesteatoma
   D. Tympanosclerosis

3. Through what structure is the stapes prosthesis inserted?
   A. Incus
   B. Round window niche
   C. Sinus tympani
   D. Oval window

4. What is the success rate for stapedectomy or stapedotomy?
   A. 0% to 25%
   B. 26% to 50%
   C. 51% to 75%
   D. >75%

See Supplemental Figures section for additional figures and legends for this case.

CASE 93

Stapes Implant

1. **A.** Normal placement of the stapes prosthesis should be included in the differential diagnosis. The implant protrudes less than 2.5 mm deep (measured at 1.4 mm) in the oval window, and it is in an appropriate position. It is still attached to the incus (Figures S93-1 and S93-2).

2. **B.** Otosclerosis is the most common indication for stapedectomy. The disease affects 10% of the population on autopsy specimens.

3. **D.** The stapes prosthesis is inserted into the oval window, through which the vestibule can be accessed.

4. **D.** Typical success rates for stapedectomy or stapedotomy are higher than 90%.

Comment

Performing Stapedectomy/Stapedotomy

Stapedectomy and stapedotomy are performed through the external auditory canal with the use of the operative microscope. After the stapes is dissociated from the malleus and incus, a laser is typically used to create a hole in the stapes footplate (stapedotomy) or to remove a portion of the footplate (stapedectomy). The stapes prosthesis is then attached to the incus, and the other portion is inserted through the oval window into the vestibule. Stapes implants vary in how they connect to the incus (hooks or anchors) and the material of which they are made. A graft is used to seal the connection of the prosthesis to the vestibule. Fat, fascia, veins, or blood sealants can be used. Possible complications after surgery include hearing loss, dizziness, cerebrospinal fluid leakage, and tinnitus.

Depth of Stapes Prosthesis Penetration

Yehudai and colleagues (2010) suggested that the depth of penetration of the stapes prosthesis into the vestibule had no impact on hearing results. In fact, they found that deeper penetration was *not* correlated with a worse hearing outcome. The mean depth was 2.4 mm into the vestibule. Compared with autopsy specimens, computed tomography (CT) tends to exaggerate the degree of penetration by slightly more than 0.5 mm. Some authorities have therefore stated that CT is not a useful means to assess depth of penetration. CT is useful only in detecting dislocation out of the vestibule.

Reference

Yehudai N, Masoud S, Most T, Luntz M. Depth of stapes prosthesis in the vestibule: baseline values and correlation with stapedectomy outcome. *Acta Otolaryngol.* 2010;130(8):904-908.

Cross-Reference

Neuroradiology: The Requisites, 3rd ed, 422, 424f.

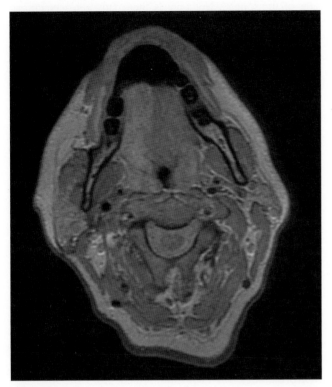

Figure 94-1

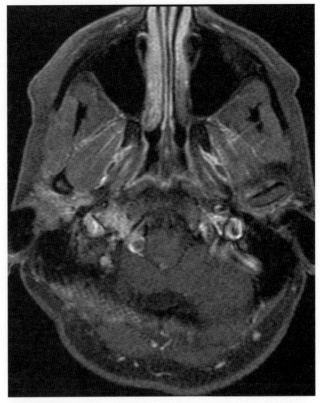

Figure 94-2

HISTORY: A patient presents with a headache.

1. Which of the following should be included in the differential diagnosis, in view of the combination of findings? (Choose all that apply.)
   A. Glomus jugulare
   B. Glomus vagale
   C. Hypoglossal schwannoma
   D. Nasopharyngeal carcinoma

2. On magnetic resonance imaging (MRI), what is the earliest finding of muscle denervation?
   A. Swelling: high signal on T2-weighted images
   B. Atrophy: decreased volume
   C. Fatty replacement: high signal on T1-weighted images
   D. Enhancement

3. What is the most common cause of tongue denervation?
   A. Trauma
   B. Neoplasms of the skull base
   C. Iatrogenic
   D. Brainstem stroke

4. Denervation atrophy with fatty replacement occurs in what time frame?
   A. Hours
   B. Days
   C. Weeks
   D. Months

See Supplemental Figures section for additional figures and legends for this case.

CASE 94

Hypoglossal Schwannoma and Tongue Atrophy

1. **C.** Hypoglossal schwannoma should be included in the differential diagnosis because the lesion is centered in the hypoglossal canal and the patient has tongue atrophy.

2. **A.** On MRI, the earliest finding of muscle denervation is swelling, which produces a high signal on T2-weighted images. The next finding is enhancement; the third finding is fatty replacement, which produces a high signal on T1-weighted images; and the last is atrophy, which appears as decreased tissue volume.

3. **B.** The most common cause of tongue denervation is neoplasms of the skull base, such as glomus tumors or intrinsic hypoglossal canal tumors. Of malignant lesions, most arise from the nasopharynx.

4. **C.** Denervation atrophy with fatty replacement occurs within weeks.

Comment

Imaging Findings

The images depict an example of a hypoglossal schwannoma arising in the canal and extending into the upper carotid space that has resulted in denervation atrophy of the right side of the tongue. Not only is there fatty replacement on the right side but also the bulk of the tongue is reduced ipsilaterally. The lesion has thus been there a long time (Figures S94-1, S94-2, and S94-3). Whereas hypoglossal canal schwannomas are uncommon, lesions at the skull base—whether paragangliomas, metastases, nasopharyngeal carcinomas, or meningiomas—generally are the most common cause of denervation atrophy of the tongue.

Pathophysiology

The sequence of events for muscular atrophy generally follows the pathophysiologic process. Initially, increased water content manifests as high signal on T2-weighted, fluid-attenuated inversion recovery (FLAIR), or short tau inversion recovery (STIR) sequences. Contrast then accumulates over time in the denervated muscle. Fatty infiltration and volume loss occur weeks later. In rare cases, pseudohypertrophy may occur in the late stages. The tongue may also prolapse into the oropharynx. When the tongue is paralyzed, the tongue deviates to the paralyzed side as a result of unbalanced muscle pull.

Reference

Kamath S, Venkatanarasimha N, Walsh MA, Hughes PM. MRI appearance of muscle denervation. *Skeletal Radiol.* 2008;37(5):397-404.

Cross-Reference

Neuroradiology: The Requisites, 3rd ed, 357-358, 598.

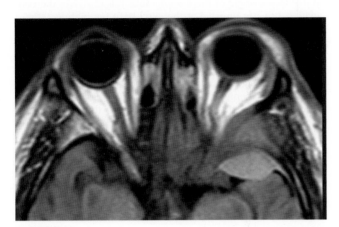

Figure 95-1

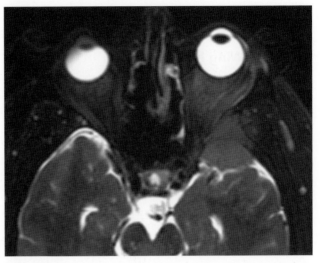

Figure 95-2

HISTORY: A 47-year-old woman presents with left orbital proptosis.

1. Which of the following should be included in the differential diagnosis? (Choose all that apply.)
   A. Fibrous dysplasia
   B. Metastasis
   C. Meningioma
   D. Epidermoid

2. What is the clinical significance of medial versus lateral sphenoid wing meningiomas?
   A. The medial ones are much harder to resect (because of proximity to the cavernous sinus), and the rate of cranial nerve involvement is higher.
   B. The lateral ones are much harder to resect (because of proximity to the middle cerebral artery branches), and the rate of cranial nerve involvement is higher.
   C. They are equally difficult to resect.
   D. They are not amenable to surgical resection.

3. Why is magnetic resonance imaging (MRI) superior to computed tomography (CT) for evaluating meningiomas?
   A. MRI better depicts malignant transformation.
   B. MRI better depicts calcified en plaque lesions.
   C. MRI is more likely to depict the small dural component of the intraosseous meningioma.
   D. MRI better depicts perineural spread.

4. Which of the following is true about meningiomas?
   A. Osteolysis is more common than hyperostosis.
   B. Osteolysis is less common than hyperostosis.
   C. Osteolysis and hyperostosis occur with equal frequency.
   D. None of the above.

See Supplemental Figures section for additional figures and legends for this case.

CASE 95

Sphenoid Wing Meningioma

1. **A, B, and C.** Fibrous dysplasia, metastases, and meningiomas can have this appearance on scans. Epidermoids do not enhance.

2. **A.** The medial ones are much harder to resect (because of proximity to the cavernous sinus and the optic nerve in the optic canal), and the rate of cranial nerve involvement is higher. Lateral ones are easier to resect.

3. **C.** MRI is more likely to depict the small dural component of the intraosseous meningioma, especially inasmuch as beam hardening off the sphenoid wing can occur with CT. Depiction of the dural components helps in the diagnosis.

4. **A.** Meningiomas may cause hyperostosis or osteolysis, but bone lysis is more common.

Comment

Variability of Hyperostosis

Hyperostosis of bone is visible in approximately one third of all meningiomas that are located along the anterior skull base, and it has been reported in a highly variable number of cases (4.5% to 45%). It seems that the variability of hyperostosis depends on the site of origin of the meningioma: It is rare over the convexities, but not unusual at the skull base (as high as 90% of cases of tumor along the sphenoid wing). Is it tumor in the bone or just reactive osteoblasts or hypervascularity that does it? The evidence favors a component of tumoral infiltration of the bone. Contrast enhancement of the bone on MRI is indicative of neoplastic infiltration. In fact, the whole idea of purely intraosseous meningiomas has been called into question because a piece of dural tissue adjacent to that bone almost always enhances (Figures S95-1, S95-2, and S95-3).

Associations with Osteoblastic Metastases

Osteoblastic metastases are most common with breast cancer and prostate cancer. Lung, bladder, and gastrointestinal primary lesions may cause osteosclerotic metastases, as can lymphoma. Chronic osteomyelitis, syphilis, and primary bone sarcomas can cause similar appearances.

Reference

Elder JB, Atkinson R, Zee CS, Chen TC. Primary intraosseous meningioma. *Neurosurg Focus.* 2007;23(4):E13.

Cross-Reference

Neuroradiology: The Requisites, 3rd ed, 59-62.

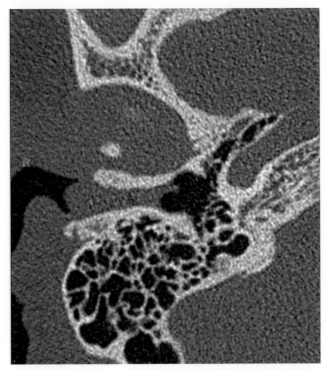

Figure 96-1

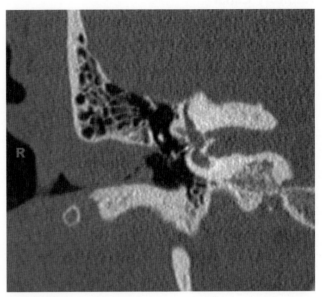

Figure 96-2

HISTORY: A patient complains of a sensation of fullness in the right ear.

1. Which of the following should be included in the differential diagnosis of a benign mass in the external auditory canal (EAC)? (Choose all that apply.)
   A. Cerumen impaction
   B. Cholesteatoma
   C. Ceruminoma
   D. Keratosis obturans

2. Which is *not* true of keratosis obturans?
   A. It is usually unilateral.
   B. It is painful.
   C. It is associated with bronchiectasis and sinusitis.
   D. It occurs in patients younger than 40 years.

3. Which is true of EAC cholesteatoma?
   A. It occurs in patients younger than 40 years.
   B. It may erode the EAC walls.
   C. It can be treated with irrigation and steroids.
   D. It is a pink lesion that blanches with insufflation.

4. What is true of ceruminomas?
   A. They start in the bony EAC.
   B. The World Health Organization reclassified them as ceruminous adenoma and pleomorphic adenoma.
   C. They manifest with otorrhea.
   D. They are uniformly benign.

See Supplemental Figures section for additional figures and legends for this case.

CASE 96

Cholesteatoma in the External Auditory Canal

1. **A, B, C, and D.** Cerumen impaction is the most common lesion of the EAC. Cholesteatoma may be acquired or congenital. Ceruminoma is a tumor of the cerumen producing glands in the EAC. Keratosis obturans can fill an EAC.

2. **A.** Keratosis obturans is typically a bilateral process (not unilateral). It is a painful condition associated with bronchiectasis and sinusitis. It occurs in patients younger than 40 years; it can simulate cystic fibrosis.

3. **B.** EAC cholesteatoma may erode the EAC walls, is seen in patients older than 40 years, must be treated surgically, and is pearly white.

4. **B.** The World Health Organization reclassified ceruminomas as ceruminous adenoma and pleomorphic adenoma. They are essentially a minor salivary gland tumor. They are found along the cartilaginous part of the external auditory meatus and manifest with obstruction and hearing loss.

Comment

Differential Diagnosis

The differential diagnosis of benign soft tissue masses in the EAC includes hemangiomas, venous vascular malformations, papillomas, hamartomas, and ceruminomas. Exostoses are also common, but they are bony. A congenital epidermoid lesion or an acquired cholesteatoma (particularly in individuals with EAC stenosis) may manifest as a pearly white mass in the EAC. Those lesions may develop from the classic middle ear cholesteatoma on an inflammatory basis, after trauma, after surgery, or they may occur also as a congenital skin rest. Spontaneous development has been reported as well. Otorrhea may occur. The EAC cholesteatoma usually erodes bone (not seen in this case), and intralesional bone spicules may be present.

Imaging Findings

EAC cholesteatomas (Figures S96-1 and S96-2) are a lot less common than cerumen impactions, exostoses, and keratosis obturans. They are hard to differentiate from those entities radiographically except by their enhancement characteristics: Only hemangiomas, adenomas, ceruminomas, and minor salivary gland tumors enhance. Diffusion-weighted imaging reveals a lesion that has restricted diffusion. Malignancies of the EAC are usually skin cancers, predominantly squamous cell carcinoma, basal cell carcinomas, and melanomas. Rhabdomyosarcomas may affect children. In rare cases, cholesterol granulomas may be confined to the EAC.

Diagnosing Malignant Otitis Externa

Because it is such a fulminant yet treatable disease, malignant otitis externa must be confirmed or ruled out whenever an EAC mass is detected. One should look for the cardinal signs of bone erosion, skull base invasion, and obliteration of parapharyngeal fat planes because the nature of the lesion in the ear may otherwise not be evident. A delay in diagnosis of malignant otitis externa can lead to death from diabetic ketoacidosis and sepsis.

Reference

White RD, Ananthakrishnan G, McKean SA, Brunton JN, Hussain SS, Sudarshan TA. Masses and disease entities of the external auditory canal: radiological and clinical correlation. *Clin Radiol.* 2012;67(2): 172-181.

Cross-Reference

Neuroradiology: The Requisites, pp 380, 382b, 382f, 387-388, 412, 567.

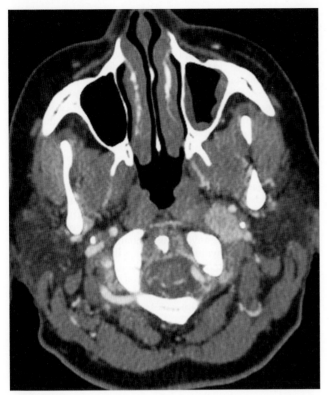

Figure 97-1

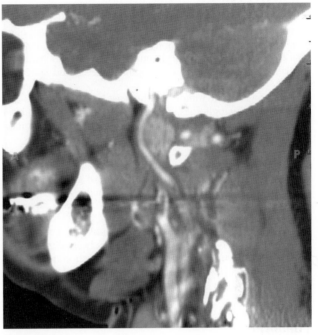

Figure 97-2

HISTORY: A 39-year-old man presents with hoarseness.

1. Which of the following should be included in the differential diagnosis? (Choose all that apply.)
   A. Schwannoma
   B. Glomus jugulare
   C. Lymphadenopathy
   D. Meningioma

2. What percentage of head and neck paragangliomas are glomus vagale tumors?
   A. 0% to 10%
   B. 11% to 25%
   C. 26% to 50%
   D. >50%

3. What is the rate of secretion of catecholamines for glomus vagale tumors?
   A. 0% to 10%
   B. 11% to 25%
   C. 26% to 50%
   D. >50%

4. Which of the following is not a component of Carney's triad?
   A. Gastric epithelioid leiomyosarcoma
   B. Pulmonary chondroma
   C. Pituitary adenoma
   D. Extra-adrenal paraganglioma

See Supplemental Figures section for additional figures and legends for this case.

CASE 97

Glomus Vagale

1. **A and C.** This lesion does not enter the jugular foramen and therefore is unlikely to represent a glomus jugulare tumor; because of the lesion's location in the carotid space, it is more likely to be a glomus vagale tumor. Schwannomas and lymph nodes also populate the carotid space.

2. **A.** Glomus vagale tumors are the least common (only 2.5%) of the paragangliomas. Carotid body tumors outnumber glomus jugulare tumors; these are the two most common paragangliomas.

3. **B.** Of the paragangliomas, 12.5% of glomus vagale varieties secrete catecholamines, whereas 16.7% of glomus jugulare tumors secrete catecholamines (the highest rate among paragangliomas).

4. **C.** Carney's triad comprises gastric epithelioid leiomyosarcoma (which is now known to actually be malignant gastrointestinal stromal tumor), pulmonary chondroma, and extra-adrenal paraganglioma, a form of multiple endocrine neoplasia.

Comment

Characteristics of Glomus Vagale Tumors

Glomus vagale tumors are head and neck paragangliomas. They are the third most frequent such neoplasms, after carotid body tumors and glomus jugulare tumors, but are more common than glomus tympanicum tumors. These tumors are found at the upper cervical regions below the jugular foramen but still in association with the carotid sheath (Figures S97-1 and S97-2). They may be distinguished from the other glomus tumors because (1) they push carotid sheath artery and jugular vein structures anteriorly rather than splaying them (as do carotid body tumors) and they less commonly invade the jugular foramen or jugular vein (as do glomus jugulare tumors). Glomus vagale tumors can arise anywhere along the course of the vagus nerve, but the majority, including the one in this case, arise near the ganglion nodosum, located at C1. Typical manifestations may include pulsatile tinnitus, hoarseness (because they affect the vagus nerve in ≈50% of cases), swallowing disorder, and, late in the disease process, a neck mass. More women than men are affected, and the incidence is highest among people aged 40 to 60 years. These tumors have a low rate of invasion into the jugular vein.

Secretion of Catecholamines

Glomus vagale tumors are hypervascular lesions, enhancing greatly on scans. In 12.5% of cases, they secrete catecholamine-like agents, and so hypertension may coexist. This characteristic may distinguish them from schwannomas of the vagus, which do not secrete any agents, enhance more variably, and have no flow voids within the tumor. Salt-and-pepper appearance on T2-weighted magnetic resonance imaging occurs when glomus vagale tumors are very large. The rate of surgical cure is 70% to 75%, but in 30% of cases, the disease recurs or residual disease, distant disease, and metachronous new lesions occur.

Carney's Triad

Carney's triad is gastric epithelioid leiomyosarcoma (which is now known to actually be malignant gastrointestinal stromal tumor), pulmonary chondroma, and extra-adrenal paraganglioma, a form of multiple endocrine neoplasia.

Reference

Erickson D, Kudva YC, Ebersold MJ, Thompson GB, Grant CS, van Heerden JA, et al. Benign paragangliomas: clinical presentation and treatment outcomes in 236 patients. *J Clin Endocrinol Metab.* 2001;86(11):5210-5216.

Cross-Reference

Neuroradiology: The Requisites, 3rd ed, 497-498.

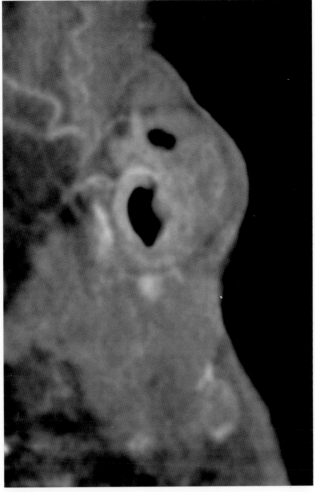

Figure 98-1

HISTORY: A patient presents with left ear ulceration, swelling and parotid palpable mass.

1. Which of the following should be included in the differential diagnosis? (Choose all that apply.)
   A. Malignant otitis externa
   B. Squamous cell carcinoma
   C. Pleomorphic adenoma
   D. Melanoma

2. What is the most common site of head and neck cancer?
   A. Oropharynx
   B. Oral cavity
   C. Larynx
   D. Skin

3. What percentage of skin cancers develop in or around the ear?
   A. 0% to 10%
   B. 11% to 20%
   C. 21% to 30%
   D. >30%

4. Which is considered a high-risk feature of skin cancer?
   A. Thickness of more than 5 mm
   B. Growth into the lower dermis
   C. Origin in the scalp
   D. Well-differentiated histologic feature

See Supplemental Figures section for additional figures and legends for this case.

CASE 98

Malignant Melanoma of the Ear

1. **B and D.** Squamous cell carcinoma (a common ear malignancy) and melanoma (which affects sun-exposed skin of the ear) should be included in the differential diagnosis.

2. **D.** The most common head and neck cancer is skin cancer. The oral cavity is the second most common site (because of the lips). The oropharynx is the third.

3. **A.** About 5% of skin cancers develop in or around the ear.

4. **B.** Both depth and size (more than 2 mm) of invasion into the lower dermis are high-risk features. In addition, cancers of the lip and ear are high-risk skin cancers. Poor differentiation is a high-risk feature.

Comment
Staging of Skin Cancers

The staging of skin cancers according to the American Joint Committee on Cancer is related to size and depth of the cancer:

TX	Primary tumor cannot be assessed
T0	No evidence of primary tumor
Tis	Carcinoma in situ
T1	Tumor 2 cm or less in greatest dimension
T2	Tumor more than 2 cm but not more than 5 cm in greatest dimension
T3	Tumor more than 5 cm in greatest dimension
T4	Tumor invasion of deep extradermal structures (i.e., cartilage, skeletal muscle, or bone)

Incidence of Melanoma of the Ear

Squamous cell carcinoma and basal cell carcinomas of the pinna of the ear are more common than melanomas, but this patient had a melanoma. The patient showed classic nodal drainage for ear cancers into the parotid lymph nodes (Figure S98-1). The median age at diagnosis of pinna cancer is in the 70s. Recurrences are more common with squamous cell carcinomas than with basal cell carcinomas. Of the cancers treated with radiation therapy, those in which tumor size exceeded 2 cm, those with higher T stage, those with cartilage necrosis, recurrent lesions, those with a field size exceeding 6 cm², and those for which treatment time was longer had an increased rate of local treatment failure.

Reference

Silva JJ, Tsang RW, Panzarella T, Levin W, Wells W. Results of radiotherapy for epithelial skin cancer of the pinna: the Princess Margaret Hospital experience, 1982-1993. *Int J Radiat Oncol Biol Phys.* 2000;47(2):451-459.

Cross-Reference

Neuroradiology: The Requisites, 3rd ed, 404.

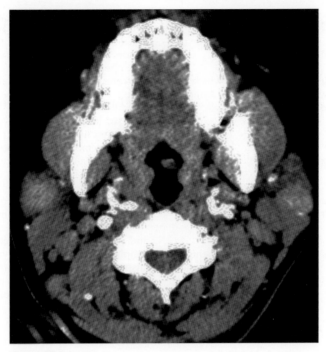

Figure 99-1

HISTORY: A 56-year-old man has a palpable neck mass below the left ear.

1. Which of the following should be included in the differential diagnosis? (Choose all that apply.)
   A. Lymph nodes
   B. Warthin tumors
   C. Pleomorphic adenomas
   D. First branchial cleft cysts

2. Which of the following is not one of the T stages designated by the American Joint Committee on Cancer (AJCC) for salivary gland tumors?
   A. T1: tumor 2 cm or less in greatest dimension
   B. T2: tumor greater than 2 cm but less than or equal to 4 cm in greatest dimensions
   C. T3: tumor greater than 6 cm
   D. T0: No primary tumor

3. What is the rate of malignant tumors of the parotid gland lesions in adults versus the rate of malignant tumors in children?
   A. 20% malignant in adults, 33% malignant in children
   B. 80% malignant in adults, 67% malignant in children
   C. 20% malignant in adults, 67% malignant in children
   D. 80% malignant in adults, 33% malignant in children

4. What is the second most common benign tumor of the parotid gland in adults?
   A. Pleomorphic adenoma
   B. Monomorphic adenoma
   C. Cylindroma
   D. Warthin tumor

See Supplemental Figures section for additional figures and legends for this case.

CASE 99

Warthin Tumors

1. **A and B.** In this patient, the lesions are bilateral, which is the case in 33% of patients with Warthin tumors. Lymph nodes may be inflammatory or neoplastic in origin and may also be bilateral.

2. **C.** T3 tumors are greater than 4 cm but it may be T3 also if there is extraparenchymal extension (outside the capsule of the gland).

3. **A.** Parotid gland lesions are malignant in 20% of adults and 33% in children. Mucoepidermoid carcinomas are most common.

4. **D.** Warthin tumor is the second most common benign tumor of the parotid gland, after pleomorphic adenoma. Monomorphic adenoma is less common, and cylindroma is rare.

Comment

Imaging Findings

In this case, the masses in the parotid glands appear bilateral on computed tomography (Figure S99-1). Although the findings on computed tomography are nonspecific, Warthin tumors—unlike other benign tumors of the parotid gland, which appear bright on T2-weighted scans—usually appear intermediate and inhomogeneous in signal intensity. The other names for this tumor—*papillary cystadenoma lymphomatosum, adenolymphoma, lymphomatous adenoma,* and *cystadenolymphoma*—refer to its varied histologic content, which have countervailing T2-weighted intensities. A predilection for the tail of the parotid gland is noted with Warthin tumors. Thus Warthin tumors' features include multiplicity, heterogeneity of the tumor on all pulse sequences, absence of strong enhancement, and a predilection for the parotid tail.

Risk Factors of Warthin Tumors

Data suggest that smoking is a risk factor for the development of Warthin tumors because patients with Warthin tumors are four times more likely to be smokers than are age-matched controls or patients with pleomorphic adenomas of the parotid glands. Number of packs per day and years of smoking appear to be correlated with the risk of developing Warthin tumors. Men are affected more often than women, at a rate of 5:1, which is in contrast to pleomorphic adenomas.

Warthin tumors have thin capsules, intratumoral septations, and, on occasion, hemorrhage. Hyperproteinaceous debris, lymphoid follicles, reactive lymphocytes, and cholesterol crystals may be present. Cystic areas are present in 30% of cases. Warthin tumors can occur in periparotid lymph nodes because they may arise within heterotopic salivary gland tissue in lymph nodes of the parotid or periparotid region.

Reference

Christe A, Waldherr C, Hallett R, Zbaeren P, Thoeny H. MR imaging of parotid tumors: typical lesion characteristics in MR imaging improve discrimination between benign and malignant disease. *AJNR Am J Neuroradiol.* 2011;32(7):1202-1207.

Cross-Reference

Neuroradiology: The Requisites, 3rd ed, 456-457, 482-484, 486-487, 494.

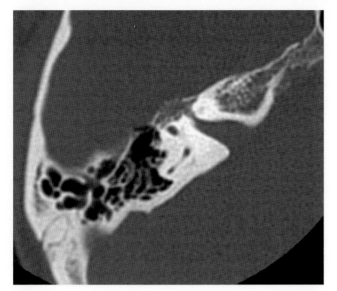

Figure 100-1

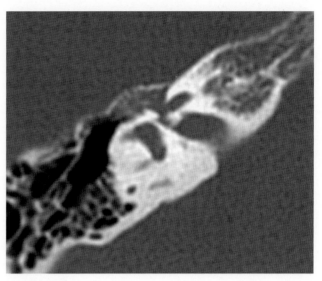

Figure 100-2

HISTORY: A 52-year-old woman presents with progressive facial paresis.

1. Which of the following should be included in the differential diagnosis? (Choose all that apply.)
   A. Schwannoma
   B. Paraganglioma
   C. Meningioma
   D. Hemangioma

2. Which part of the nerve is most commonly affected by facial nerve hemangioma?
   A. Intracanalicular
   B. Preganglionic, labyrinthine segment
   C. Geniculate ganglion
   D. Postganglionic

3. Which is true about resection of facial nerve hemangiomas?
   A. The bony lesion is separable from the nerve.
   B. The bony lesion is inseparable from the nerve.
   C. The bony lesion is sometimes easily and sometimes not easily separable from the nerve.
   D. These lesions are not amenable to surgical treatment.

4. What symptoms are most common with facial nerve hemangiomas?
   A. Usually no symptoms
   B. Facial nerve paresis/paralysis
   C. Tinnitus
   D. Facial twitching

See Supplemental Figures section for additional figures and legends for this case.

CASE 100

Facial Nerve Hemangioma

1. **D.** The appearance is a classic appearance and location for a facial nerve hemangioma. The bony reaction is atypical for a schwannoma or meningioma. The location and appearance are unusual for paraganglioma.

2. **C.** The geniculate ganglion is the segment most commonly affected by facial nerve hemangioma. The intracanalicular segment is the second most commonly affected. The postganglionic segment is the third most commonly affected. The preganglionic, labyrinthine segment is not commonly affected.

3. **C.** The bony lesion is sometimes easily and sometimes not easily separable from the nerve.

4. **B.** Facial nerve paresis/paralysis is a common early symptom. Facial twitching occurs in more than 50% of affected patients but not as frequently as facial nerve paresis. Tinnitus does occur but less frequently than facial nerve dysfunction.

Comment

Symptoms of Facial Hemangiomas

Despite their small size, facial nerve hemangiomas are often symptomatic in that they cause facial nerve motor dysfunction.

When a patient presents with facial nerve paralysis, one must consider such entities as Bell palsy, a common source of transient weakness caused by a viral neuritis, a parotid malignancy with or without perineural spread, trauma from temporal bone fractures, and facial nerve schwannomas. However, facial nerve hemangioma, found most commonly at the geniculate ganglion and next in the internal auditory canal, is yet another entity to consider.

Imaging Findings

These lesions are now considered to be largely bony lesions that are intimately associated with and sometimes not easily separable from the facial nerve (Figures S100-1 and S100-2). In such cases, grafting of the nerve is mandatory. At times these lesions have the full honeycomb appearance of a typical bony hemangioma. They enhance vividly and are particularly well demonstrated on both computed tomography and magnetic resonance imaging. When they arise in the internal auditory canal, they are typically accompanied by hearing loss. Histopathologically, they are not tumors; hence many authorities consider them benign venous vascular malformations.

Reference

Mijangos SV, Meltzer DE. Case 171: facial nerve hemangioma. *Radiology.* 2011;260(1):296-301.

Cross-Reference

Neuroradiology: The Requisites, 3rd ed, 403-405.

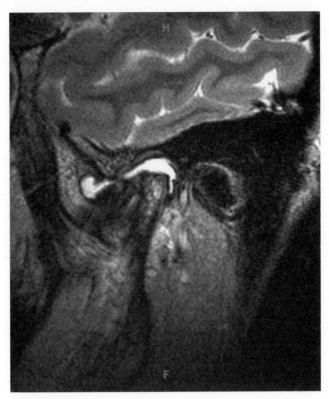

Figure 101-1

HISTORY: A 53-year-old woman presents with long-standing early morning jaw pain.

1. Which of the following should be included in the differential diagnosis? (Choose all that apply.)
   A. Rheumatoid arthritis
   B. Degenerative changes in the meniscus
   C. Synovial sarcoma
   D. Synovial chondromatosis

2. What is the significance of joint effusions in the presence of meniscal displacement?
   A. It hurts.
   B. It means there is medial or lateral meniscal displacement.
   C. It means that surgery is indicated.
   D. It means that splinting is likely to be ineffective.

3. With which of the following is the rate of associated effusions highest?
   A. Disk perforation
   B. Disk displacement anteriorly
   C. "Stuck" disks
   D. Beaking of the mandibular condyle

4. The temporomandibular joint (TMJ) consists of how many compartments?
   A. One
   B. Two
   C. Three
   D. Four

See Supplemental Figures section for additional figures and legends for this case.

CASE 101

Temporomandibular Joint Effusion

1. **A and B.** Degenerative changes in the meniscus are the most common cause of effusions. Rheumatoid arthritis may also cause a TMJ effusion. No mass or calcific foci are shown, and so synovial sarcoma and synovial chondromatosis should not be considered.

2. **A.** The size of the effusion is very closely correlated with pain, even more so than meniscal position. Of all meniscal displacements, anterior disk displacements have the highest rate of effusions. There is no correlation between effusion and meniscal displacement, whether medial or lateral. There is no implication that surgery or splinting is necessary.

3. **A.** Disk perforation produces the highest rate of effusions. There is no strong association with anterior disk displacement, "stuck" disks, or beaking of the mandibular condyle.

4. **D.** There are four parts: superior and inferior divisions of the joint space that are seen both anteriorly and posteriorly.

Comment

Pain Associations

The presence of a TMJ effusion (Figure S101-1) is very important in understanding the pain associated with meniscal abnormalities. Unfortunately, the correlation of meniscal displacement and pain is weak because of the high proportion of patients with asymptomatic anterior meniscal displacements. However, the volume of effusion and the degree of pain correspond much better. Distention of the joint capsule might stimulate nociceptive fibers, which results in increased pain. The risk for associated effusion is 2.8 times higher with anterior meniscal displacements with recapture than with normal joints. Anterior disk displacements without reduction have a 4.6 times greater rate of effusions.

Sites of Effusions in the Joint

Effusions may be present in all four separate compartments of the TMJ. The TMJ consists of superior and inferior components of the joint space both anterior to the meniscus and posterior to the meniscus. The irritation of the meniscus and synovial tissues by meniscal abnormalities is the most common source of effusions, but systemic diseases of joints, such as rheumatoid arthritis, gout, and pseudogout, may also predispose to joint effusions.

Reference

Roh HS, Kim W, Kim YK, Lee JY. Relationships between disk displacement, joint effusion, and degenerative changes of the TMJ in TMD patients based on MRI findings. *J Craniomaxillofac Surg.* 2012;40(3):283-286.

Cross-Reference

Neuroradiology: The Requisites, 3rd ed, 488-491.

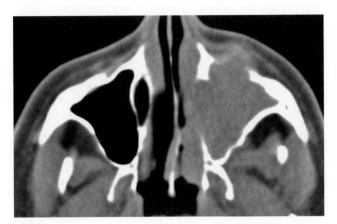

Figure 102-1

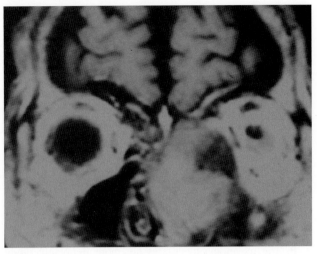

Figure 102-2

HISTORY: A 72-year-old man has nasal congestion and bleeding from the nose.

1. Which of the following should be included in the differential diagnosis? (Choose all that apply.)
   A. Metastatic renal cell carcinoma
   B. Metastatic choriocarcinoma
   C. Chondrosarcoma
   D. Primary sinonasal melanoma

2. What is the characteristic clinical feature of primary sinonasal melanoma?
   A. Nosebleeds
   B. Dural spread
   C. Rotatory nystagmus
   D. Black pigmentation

3. Do melanoma metastases in the brain more commonly appear bright on imaging as a result of hemorrhage or melanin?
   A. Melanin
   B. Hemorrhage
   C. Both melanin and hemorrhage equally
   D. Neither

4. Which of the following is a risk factor for melanoma of the skin?
   A. Sun exposure
   B. Smoking
   C. Human papillomavirus infection
   D. Alcohol abuse

See Supplemental Figures section for additional figures and legends for this case.

CASE 102

Sinonasal Melanoma

1. **A, B, and D.** The mass shown is probably a hemorrhagic or melanotic sinonasal lesion because it is bright on T1-weighted image—hemorrhage is characteristic of metastatic renal cell carcinoma and metastatic choriocarcinoma, but primary sinonasal melanoma may be bright as a result of either hemorrhage or melanin. Chondrosarcoma is not so uniformly bright on T1-weighted images.

2. **D.** Black pigmentation is the characteristic clinical feature of primary sinonasal melanoma, as seen endoscopically. Nosebleeds are a nonspecific sign. Dural spread is unlikely and not seen clinically, and rotatory nystagmus is not present.

3. **B.** The melanoma metastases are more frequently bright on T1-weighted images because of hemorrhage than because of melanin. There may be amelanotic melanomas that bleed.

4. **A.** Sun exposure is a risk factor for melanoma. Smoking, human papillomavirus infection, and alcohol abuse are not known risk factors.

Comment

Imaging Findings

Sinonasal melanoma is one of the tumors in this region of the body that radiologists inevitably encounter in a routine practice (Figure S102-1). The lesion may or may not contain melanin. It may or may not be hemorrhagic. It may have both hemorrhage and melanin. Thus this lesion may have a variety of appearances, often bright on T1-weighted images (Figure S102-2) and dark from blood and melanin on T2-weighted images. The lesion often destroys bone and has a predilection for the nasal septum and maxillary sinuses. Enhancement may be difficult to assess because the tumor often is bright on T1-weighted images without contrast, but both the nonbright and bright areas usually enhance and become "brighter" after gadolinium administration.

Prognosis

The prognosis for patients with sinonasal melanoma is not encouraging: The median disease-free interval is 18 months, the median length of survival is 23 months, and the mean rate of 5-year survival is 30%. Lesions in the maxillary and ethmoid sinuses progress to orbital and skull base invasion more often than do lesions in the nasal cavity. Hematogenous metastases can occur in up to 50% of cases. Skin melanomas far outnumber sinonasal melanomas in the head and neck. Surgical treatment is the mainstay of therapy.

Reference

Yousem DM, Li C, Montone KT, Montgomery L, Loevner LA, Rao V, et al. Primary malignant melanoma of the sinonasal cavity: MR imaging evaluation. *Radiographics*. 1996;16:1101-1110.

Cross-Reference

Neuroradiology: The Requisites, 3rd ed, 437-438.

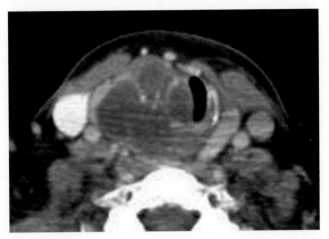

Figure 103-1

HISTORY: A 34-year-old patient presents with a 1-year history of voice changes.

1. Which of the following should be included in the differential diagnosis? (Choose all that apply.)
   A. Lymphoma
   B. Squamous cell carcinoma
   C. Chondrosarcoma
   D. Adenoid cystic carcinoma

2. What feature does *not* imply higher grade chondrosarcoma?
   A. Pain
   B. Size >3 cm
   C. Rapid growth
   D. Enhancement

3. What part of the larynx is involved most commonly with chondroid tumors?
   A. Epiglottis
   B. Thyroid cartilage
   C. Arytenoid cartilage
   D. Cricoid cartilage

4. What cartilage is most commonly affected by squamous cell carcinoma?
   A. Epiglottis
   B. Thyroid cartilage
   C. Arytenoid cartilage
   D. Cricoid cartilage

See Supplemental Figures section for additional figures and legends for this case.

CASE 103

Chondrosarcoma of the Larynx

1. **A and C.** Because the lesion is a submucosal mass, it could be lymphoma, as well as chondrosarcoma (although this lesion is without matrix). Because of the lack of mucosal mass, this is probably not squamous cell carcinoma or adenoid cystic carcinoma.

2. **D.** Enhancement does *not* imply higher grade. Pain and rapid growth are signs of aggressiveness, hence higher grade. Larger size (>3 cm) is also a feature of higher grade.

3. **D.** The cricoid cartilage is involved in 70% of all laryngeal chondrosarcomas. The thyroid cartilage is second most commonly involved; the arytenoid cartilage is third most commonly involved; and the epiglottis is not usually involved.

4. **B.** The thyroid cartilage is most commonly affected by squamous cell carcinoma usually from a laryngeal or hypopharyngeal primary tumor. The epiglottis is second most commonly affected, by either oropharyngeal or laryngeal primary tumors. The arytenoid cartilage is third and the cricoid cartilage is fourth most commonly affected.

Comment

Implications of Chondrosarcomas

Squamous cell carcinoma is the dominant tumor of the larynx, but the most common sarcoma of the larynx is the chondrosarcoma. It may or may not have a chondroid matrix, and it is more a submucosal primary tumor (Figure S103-1). Although sarcomas usually have poor prognoses, chondrosarcomas of the cricoid cartilage are usually low-grade tumors that are not life-threatening. They metastasize infrequently and late in the course. The problem, of course, is that the voice cannot be preserved when these cricoid cartilage tumors are surgically removed. For this reason, these tumors are treated late in their course when all other treatment fails, including incomplete resection to preserve the airway, breathing, and voice.

Features of Aggressive Pathologic Processes

Features that suggest that such tumors are more aggressive and of higher grade are pain, rapid growth, and larger size. The grading system from I to III, first described by Evans, is based on mitotic rate, cellularity, and nuclear size. The most common symptom is dysphonia (hoarseness). Men are affected more than women by a 3:1 ratio.

Incidence

Chondrosarcomas are the second most common sarcoma overall after osteosarcoma. They may arise within benign chondromas and occur more commonly in syndromic conditions such as Ollier disease. The rate of 5-year survival is 70%.

Reference

Policarpo M, Taranto F, Aina E, Aluffi PV, Pia F. Chondrosarcoma of the larynx: a case report. *Acta Otorhinolaryngol Ital.* 2008;28(1): 38-41.

Cross-Reference

Neuroradiology: The Requisites, 3rd ed, 380, 412, 567.

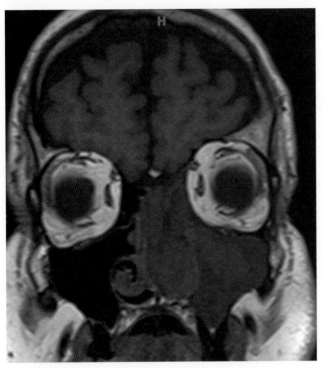

Figure 104-1

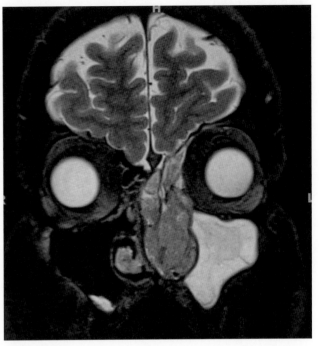

Figure 104-2

HISTORY: A patient has long-standing chronic sinusitis that had been treated medically by the family practitioner.

1. Which should be included in the differential diagnosis? (Choose all that apply.)
   A. Mucocele
   B. Obstructed secretions and mucocele
   C. Mucocele and polyps
   D. Inverted papilloma and mucocele
   E. Inverted papilloma and obstructed secretions

2. Which of the following is true?
   A. For an inverted papilloma, the term *cerebriform* refers to both its appearance on T2-weighted imaging and its enhancement characteristics.
   B. The most common site of origin of inverted papillomas is the nasal septum.
   C. Inverted papillomas are considered inflammatory lesions.
   D. Inverted papilloma is related to human papilloma type 1 (HPV-1) virus.
   E. All of the above.

3. With regard to inverted papillomas, what is the rate of coexistent squamous cell carcinoma?
   A. <15%
   B. 15% to 30%
   C. 31% to 45%
   D. 46% to 60%
   E. >60%

4. Which of the following are the two most common sites of origin of inverted papillomas?
   A. Sphenoid and maxillary sinuses
   B. Frontal and maxillary sinuses
   C. Nasal/septal and maxillary sinuses
   D. Nasal/septal and ethmoid sinuses
   E. Sphenoid and nasal sinuses

See Supplemental Figures section for additional figures and legends for this case.

CASE 104

Inverted Papilloma with Cancer

1. **E.** Inverted papilloma and obstructed secretions are the most likely diagnoses. The mass in the nasal cavity does not indicate mucocele or obstructed secretions alone. The lesion has no expansile nature, as would be expected of a mucocele. The enhancement pattern is not that of mucocele and polyps, which is more peripheral.

2. **A.** The term *cerebriform* refers to the appearance of an inverted papilloma on T2-weighted imaging, on which its signal intensities may look like gray matter and white matter in a crenated appearance. The term also refers to the gyriform enhancement pattern. Inverted papillomas are tumors that usually originate from the medial wall of the maxillary sinus.

3. **A.** The rate of coexistent squamous cell carcinoma is approximately 13%. Because of this, inverted papillomas are treated with aggressive extensive surgery for clean margins.

4. **C.** The two most common sites of origin of inverted papillomas are the medial wall of the maxillary sinus and the nasal septum.

Comment
Imaging Findings

Inverted papillomas can be readily distinguished from mucoceles or polyps by virtue of their distinctive bands of hypointensity and hyperintensity on T2-weighted images and their gyriform pattern of enhancement (Figures S104-1, S104-2, and S104-3). This *cerebriform* pattern is characteristic of inverted papillomas. Unfortunately, discerning which of the inverted papillomas coexists with squamous cell carcinoma (in approximately 13% of cases) is nearly impossible. Some authorities suggest that focal loss of the characteristic cerebriform appearance suggests malignant degeneration, but this observation is very subjective. The role of positron emission tomography is currently being examined for this purpose as well. To make matters worse, inverted papillomas often aggressively destroy the bony margins of the sinonasal cavity, including the cribriform plate. Therefore, they often are included in the differential diagnosis of squamous cell carcinomas and esthesioneuroblastomas. They do not usually have the same cystic features at the periphery as do esthesioneuroblastomas; however, only one third of esthesioneuroblastomas have such characteristic peripheral cysts. Obstructed secretions initially have typical low intensity on T1-weighted images and appear bright on T2-weighted images. With time, the signal increases on T1-weighted images. However, the peripheral rim enhancement pattern is reliable in ruling out neoplasms. Sinonasal polyposis, although it may have internal linear enhancement, does not enhance in a solid pattern in the way that inverted papillomas do.

Sites of Inverted Papillomas

The most common sites of origin of inverted papillomas are the lateral nasal wall/medial wall of the maxillary sinus and the nasal septum. They are occasionally multifocal. Imaging of inverted papillomas may depict apparent internal calcification; however, most authorities believe this to be destroyed bone rather than tumoral calcification. This opinion is supported on histologic study.

Reference

Jeon TY, Kim HJ, Chung SK, Dhong HJ, Kim HY, Yim YJ, et al. Sinonasal inverted papilloma: value of convoluted cerebriform pattern on MR imaging. *AJNR Am J Neuroradiol.* 2008;29(8):1556-1560.

Cross-Reference

Neuroradiology: The Requisites, 3rd ed, 687-688, 433-434, 456.

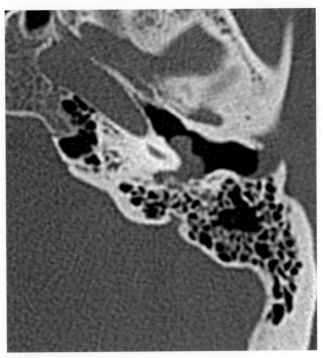

Figure 105-1

HISTORY: A young woman presents with a retrotympanic vascular mass and tinnitus.

1. Which of the following should be included in the differential diagnosis? (Choose all that apply.)
   A. Glomus jugulare
   B. Aberrant carotid artery
   C. Hemangioma
   D. Glomus tympanicum
   E. Facial nerve schwannoma

2. Which of the following is correct with regard to facial nerve hemangiomas?
   A. The most common sites are the geniculate ganglion region and tympanic segment.
   B. They usually manifest with facial muscle paralysis.
   C. Most are actually dural venous fistulas.
   D. They do not cause the bone to have a honeycomb appearance.
   E. None of the above.

3. Which of the following is *not* true of glomus tympanicum tumors?
   A. They are usually treated through a tympanotomy.
   B. Affected patients usually do not benefit from preoperative embolization.
   C. They and glomus jugulare are the most common tumors of the middle ear.
   D. They arise from the tympanic (Jacobson) nerve.
   E. None of the above.

4. Which of the following is true?
   A. Glomus tympanicum tumors have a salt-and-pepper appearance on T2-weighted images.
   B. Aberrant carotid arteries are often seen along the cochlear promontory.
   C. Jugular dehiscences are often seen along the cochlear promontory.
   D. Glomus jugulare tumors often are seen along the cochlear promontory.

See Supplemental Figures section for additional figures and legends for this case.

CASE 105

Glomus Tympanicum

1. **D.** Glomus tympanicum is the most likely diagnosis. The mass shown in the figure is too high to be glomus jugulare, and it is not the appropriate location for facial nerve schwannoma. In addition, the carotid canal is intact, so it would not be aberrant carotid artery.

2. **A.** The most common sites of facial nerve hemangiomas are the geniculate ganglion region and tympanic segment. They often cause the bone to have a honeycomb appearance. They usually do not present with facial muscle paralysis, and they are not dural venous fistulas.

3. **E.** Glomus tympanicum tumors arise from the tympanic nerve and are usually treated through a tympanotomy. Affected patients usually do not benefit from preoperative embolization, because the lesions are so small they rarely cause significant blood loss. They and glomus jugulare are the most common tumors of the middle ear.

4. **B.** Because of their small size, glomus tympanicum tumors usually do *not* have a salt-and-pepper appearance. The aberrant internal carotid artery is often seen in the same location as glomus tympanicum tumors, but the glomus jugulare and jugulare dehiscences are located around the jugular foramen and upper jugular wall, respectively.

Comment

Differential Diagnosis

For a retrotympanic vascular mass, the differential diagnosis may include glomus jugulare, glomus tympanicum, aberrant carotid artery, persistent stapedial artery, jugular bulb diverticulum, hemangioma, vascular metastasis, endolymphatic sac tumor, and many other lesions. Computed tomography helps narrow the scope of this differential diagnosis. Figure S105-1 is a characteristic image of a glomus tympanicum lesion. The lesion lies over the cochlear promontory, is often less than 1 cm in size, and is well-defined. On other images of the same study, one could see the intact carotid artery canal, jugular foramen, facial nerve canal, endolymphatic sac/vestibular aqueduct, and foramen spinosum; thus the other potential causes are virtually ruled out.

Incidence

Glomus tumors affect women more than men by a 3:1 ratio. This lesion is a tumor of adulthood, usually manifesting in early middle age. Patients with glomus tympanicum tumors usually have a history of pulsatile tinnitus, conductive hearing loss, or both. Multiple paragangliomas are reported in 5% to 25% of cases, and this is particularly true of patients with a family history of these tumors. The glomus tympanicum tumor may merge with the glomus jugulare tumor; in such cases, a lesion that spans from the jugular foramen into the middle ear cavity is called a *glomus jugulotympanicum tumor*. Over the cochlear promontory, the lesion usually arises from the tympanic nerve, an offshoot of the glossopharyngeal nerve and the inferior tympanic nerve. As opposed to glomus tympanicum tumors, which are treated via a transmembrane approach without preoperative embolization, treatment of glomus jugulare tumors begins with embolization, and they are treated as skull base tumors with more extensive surgery. If the glomus jugulare tumors grow into and around the carotid canal or cavernous sinus, treatment may involve attempts to partially resect the tumor and/or treat with focused radiation and embolization. Glomus tympanicum tumors that extend to the hypotympanum may be more challenging; surgery may need to be more aggressive than the transmembrane option.

Reference

Alaani A, Chavda SV, Irving RM. The crucial role of imaging in determining the approach to glomus tympanicum tumours. *Eur Arch Otorhinolaryngol.* 2009;266(6):827-831.

Cross-Reference

Neuroradiology: The Requisites, 3rd ed, 397.

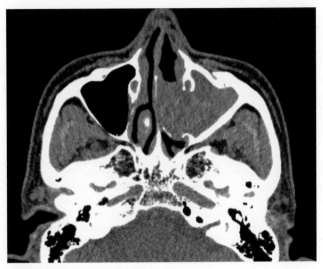

Figure 106-1

HISTORY: A young adult presents with sinonasal congestion.

1. Which of the following should be included in the differential diagnosis? (Choose all that apply.)
   A. Antrochoanal polyp
   B. Squamous cell carcinoma
   C. Inverted papilloma
   D. Allergic fungal sinusitis

2. Staging of antrochoanal polyps depends on which of the following?
   A. Occlusion of the maxillary sinus accessory ostium
   B. Occlusion of the maxillary sinus primary ostium
   C. Extension into the sphenoid sinus
   D. Extension into the ethmoid sinus

3. Which of the following is not associated with polyps?
   A. Cystic fibrosis
   B. Aspirin intolerance
   C. Nickel exposure
   D. Kartagener syndrome
   E. None of the above

4. What is the most common malignancy of the paranasal sinuses?
   A. Squamous cell carcinoma
   B. Inverted papilloma
   C. Adenoid cystic carcinoma
   D. Adenocarcinoma
   E. Melanoma

See Supplemental Figures section for additional figures and legends for this case.

CASE 106

Antrochoanal Polyp

1. **A and C.** Antrochoanal polyp is the most likely diagnosis. Because of the benign growth appearance and pattern, this mass is unlikely to be squamous cell carcinoma. However, inverted papilloma could be considered. The mass has no hyperdensity, and so the diagnosis would not include allergic fungal sinusitis.

2. **A.** Staging of antrochoanal polyps depends on occlusion of the maxillary sinus accessory ostium. Stage I: strictly an antronasal polyp; stage II: extension of polyp to the nasopharynx and full occlusion of the accessory ostium of the maxillary sinus by the polyp; stage III: extension of the polyp to the nasopharynx and only partial occlusion of the accessory ostium of the maxillary sinus by the neck of the polyp.

3. **E.** All of the entities listed are associated with polyps.

4. **A.** Squamous cell carcinoma is the most common malignancy of the paranasal sinuses. Adenocarcinoma is less common. Inverted papilloma is not a malignancy. Adenoid cystic carcinoma may arise in the sinonasal minor salivary glands.

Comment

Location and Appearance of Antrochoanal Polyps

Antrochoanal polyp is a sinonasal inflammatory polyp with a characteristic location and appearance in that it involves one of the maxillary sinuses and extends through the ostium of the maxillary sinus into the nasal cavity and posteriorly toward the nasopharynx (Figure S106-1). It usually occurs as a solitary polyp in the sinonasal fossa. The staging of antrochoanal polyps is based on whether the maxillary sinus accessory ostium is occluded by the stalk of the polyp (stage II is full occlusion, stage III is partial occlusion). Projection posteriorly into the nasopharynx is typical of this lesion.

Imaging Findings

The imaging characteristics of antrochoanal polyps includes enlargement of the maxillary sinus ostia. Usually the density is low on computed tomography. On magnetic resonance imaging, the lesion shows minimal peripheral enhancement, which distinguishes the antrochoanal polyp from both inverted papilloma and squamous cell carcinoma, which enhance in a solid manner. Inverted papillomas have a strong association with coexistent squamous cell carcinomas. This diagnosis is extremely difficult to make because some inverted papillomas have an appearance of aggressive bony erosion. However, the cerebriform appearance on T2-weighted images is suggestive of inverted papillomas, not of antrochoanal polyps.

Causes of Sinonasal Polyposis

The causes of sinonasal polyposis include cystic fibrosis, aspirin intolerance, nickel exposure, Kartagener syndrome, Peutz-Jeghers syndrome, and allergic fungal polyposis.

Reference

Cook PR, Davis WE, McDonald R, McKinsey JP. Antrochoanal polyposis: a review of 33 cases. *Ear Nose Throat J.* 1993;72(6):401-402, 404-410.

Cross-Reference

Neuroradiology: The Requisites, 3rd ed, 432.

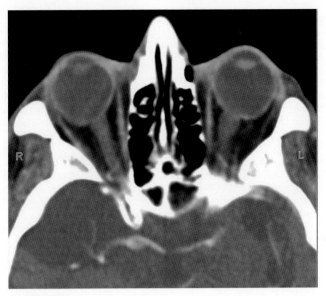

Figure 107-1

HISTORY: A 60-year-old nearsighted woman presents with recent worsening of visual blurring.

1. Which of the following should be included in the differential diagnosis? (Choose all that apply.)
   A. Retinoblastoma
   B. Choroidal melanoma
   C. Coloboma
   D. Staphyloma

2. What is the embryologic derivation of a coloboma?
   A. Failure of scleral fissure closure
   B. Failure of choroidal-retinal fissure closure
   C. Failure of ora serrata closure
   D. Failure of corneal closure

3. How is staphyloma different from coloboma?
   A. Staphylomas are weaknesses of the sclera.
   B. Staphylomas are weaknesses of the choroid.
   C. Staphylomas but not colobomas cause outpouchings.
   D. Staphylomas cause inpouchings.

4. Which of the following is *not* a cause of staphyloma?
   A. Axial myopia
   B. Glaucoma
   C. Scleritis
   D. Retinoblastoma

See Supplemental Figures section for additional figures and legends for this case.

CASE 107

Staphyloma

1. **C and D.** Staphyloma is the most likely diagnosis for adults. Coloboma is also possible, but it is usually more focal and pediatric. No masses are visible, and so the diagnosis would not include retinoblastoma or choroidal melanoma.

2. **B.** The embryologic derivation of a coloboma is failure of choroidal-retinal fissure closure. The most common manifestation of a coloboma is a keyhole defect in the iris.

3. **A.** Staphylomas are weaknesses of the sclera. Both staphyloma and coloboma cause outpouchings, and neither causes inpouchings.

4. **D.** Retinoblastoma is not a cause of staphyloma. The most common cause is axial myopia, and the second most common is glaucoma. Scleritis is a common cause of inflammatory staphylomas.

Comment

Appearance of Staphyloma

The appearances of coloboma and staphyloma overlap somewhat, but in their classic forms they are easily distinguishable. Classically, a coloboma is a cystic outpouching of choroid and retinal layers into the optic nerve head insertion in a child.

Many colobomas, however, are eccentric to the optic nerve insertion and protrude irregularly into the retrobulbar fat. The presence of other congenital lesions in association with colobomas, such as agenesis of the corpus callosum and the CHARGE syndrome (*c*oloboma, *h*eart defects, choanal *a*tresia, *r*etardation, *g*enitourinary abnormalities, *e*ar abnormalities), facilitates the diagnosis. Colobomas may be inherited in an autosomally dominant manner and are bilateral in 60% of cases. They may be associated with microphthalmos, optic nerve hypoplasia, or both.

Causes of Staphyloma

Most staphylomas are not congenital lesions. They result from stretching, or "ectasia," of the sclerouveal coats of the globe (Figure S107-1). The most common scenario of staphylomas is in a patient with severe axial myopia in which the sclera is thinned asymmetrically and the globe assumes an irregular shape. Any process—be it inflammatory, traumatic, or developmental (including glaucoma)—that can weaken the sclera may lead to a staphyloma. Staphylomas are usually off center to the optic disk, in a temporal position, and therefore are not similar to classic colobomas.

Reference

Osborne D, Foulks GN. Computed tomographic analysis of deformity and dimensional changes in the eyeball. *Radiographics*. 1985;153: 669-674.

Cross-Reference

Neuroradiology: The Requisites, 3rd ed, 324, 331.

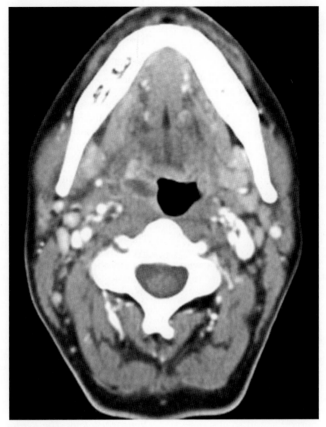

Figure 108-1

HISTORY: A young child has throat pain and fever.

1. Which of the following should be included in the differential diagnosis? (Choose all that apply.)
   A. Retropharyngeal abscess
   B. Squamous cell carcinoma
   C. Epiglottitis
   D. Peritonsillar abscess

2. Which is more common, a peritonsillar abscess or a tonsillar abscess?
   A. Peritonsillar abscess
   B. Tonsillar abscess
   C. Both equally common
   D. Peritonsillar abscess in children and tonsillar abscess in adults

3. What is the typical cause for low density on imaging of tonsillar crypts?
   A. Abscess
   B. Pus
   C. Peritonsillar abscess
   D. Mucous retention cysts

4. What is Lemierre syndrome?
   A. Infection of the submandibular region from dental abscess
   B. Infection of the oropharynx with thrombophlebitis and possible septic emboli
   C. Quincy: a peritonsillar abscess
   D. Peritonsillar abscess associated with carotid pseudoaneurysm

See Supplemental Figures section for additional figures and legends for this case.

CASE 108

Peritonsillar Abscess

1. **D.** Peritonsillar abscess should be included in the diagnosis. There is a lesion associated with the tissues adjacent to the tonsil. Squamous cell carcinoma is unlikely in a young child, and retropharyngeal abscess is located in the retropharyngeal space, not in the peritonsillar soft tissues. The lesion is not affecting the larynx; thus it is not epiglottitis.

2. **A.** Peritonsillar abscess is much more common than tonsillar abscess in adults and children.

3. **B.** Pus is the typical cause of low density in imaging of tonsillar crypts. Abscess, peritonsillar abscess, and mucous retention cysts are much less common.

4. **B.** Lemierre syndrome is infection of the oropharynx with thrombophlebitis and possible septic emboli. This may complicate pharyngitis.

Comment

Formation of Peritonsillar Abscesses

Peritonsillar abscesses form in the area between the palatine tonsil and its capsule. They are most common in young adults and account for more infections of the deep tissues than any other source (skin abscesses being more common). This is because pharyngitis and tonsillitis are so common. Fortunately, these infections respond well to antibiotics, and so abscesses are becoming less frequent, and percutaneous and intraoral drainage are becoming more of an emergency department–based procedure rather than urgent surgical resection.

Weber Glands

A strange little-known part of anatomy has been implicated in the causes of peritonsillar abscesses. Weber glands are a group of about 20 to 25 mucous minor salivary glands located between the tonsil (below) and the soft palate (above), where most peritonsillar abscesses develop. The ducts of these glands, which normally clear debris from the tonsils, may become obstructed, which leads to necrosis, inflammation, and peritonsillar abscesses. The bacteria involved include β-hemolytic *Streptococcus* organisms, *Staphylococcus aureus,* pneumococci, and *Haemophilus influenzae.*

Imaging Findings

The lesion depicted in Figure S108-1 is not a tonsillar abscess, even though the tonsil is clearly inflamed and enlarged. Usually the low-density appearance in the tonsils is only the exudate of purulent material in the tonsil and its crypts, not an abscess. Tonsillar abscesses are far less common than peritonsillar abscesses.

Reference

Capps EF, Kinsella JJ, Gupta M, Bhatki AM, Opatowsky MJ. Emergency imaging assessment of acute, nontraumatic conditions of the head and neck. *Radiographics.* 2010;30(5):1335-1352.

Cross-Reference

Neuroradiology: The Requisites, 3rd ed, 451.

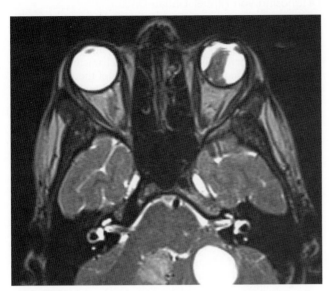

Figure 109-1

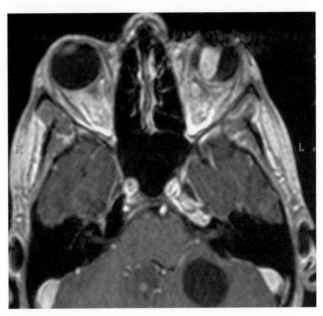

Figure 109-2

HISTORY: A 45-year-old patient has left visual blurring.

1. Which of the following should be included in the differential diagnosis? (Choose all that apply.)
   A. Retinoblastoma
   B. Melanoma
   C. Hemangioblastoma/retinal angioma
   D. Sarcoidosis

2. What percentage of patients with von Hippel–Lindau (VHL) disease have ocular hemangioblastomas or other vascular lesions?
   A. 0% to 20%
   B. 21% to 40%
   C. 41% to 60%
   D. >60%

3. In what percentage are the ocular lesions of VHL disease bilateral?
   A. 0% to 20%
   B. 21% to 40%
   C. 41% to 60%
   D. >60%

4. In what percentage of patients with VHL disease are the ocular manifestations the presenting symptoms?
   A. 0% to 20%
   B. 21% to 40%
   C. 41% to 60%
   D. >60%

See Supplemental Figures section for additional figures and legends for this case.

CASE 109

Ocular Hemangioblastoma in von Hippel–Lindau Disease

1. **B and C.** Melanoma with a posterior fossa metastasis and hemangioblastoma/retinal angioma (i.e., in a patient with a cerebellar hemangioblastoma in VHL disease) should be included in the diagnosis. Retinoblastoma is unlikely to develop in a 45-year-old person. Sarcoidosis has a predilection for the uveal tracts.

2. **C.** Ocular hemangioblastomas or other ocular vascular lesions are present in 45% to 60% of patients with VHL disease.

3. **C.** In 50% of patients with VHL disease, the lesions are bilateral.

4. **C.** The ocular manifestations are the presenting symptoms in 50% of patients with VHL disease.

Comment
Incidence

Ocular hemangioblastomas occur in 45% to 60% of patients who have VHL disease, are bilateral in 50%, and lead to the diagnosis by virtue of their manifestation in 50% of cases. In this case, the images show a unilateral ocular/retinal hemangioblastoma; at the edges of the images, cystic and solid masses in the posterior fossa represent cerebellar hemangioblastomas (Figures S109-1 and S109-2). The lesions typically appear in patients in their 20s and cause visual abnormalities. They may be multiple at initial presentation or may multiply in the follow-up period.

Diagnosing von Hippel–Lindau Disease

For formal diagnosis of VHL disease, the following must be manifest:
- In an individual with no known family history of VHL disease, there must be two or more characteristic lesions:
  - Two or more hemangioblastomas of the retina, spine, or brain or a single hemangioblastoma in association with a visceral manifestation (e.g., multiple kidney or pancreatic cysts)
  - Renal cell carcinoma
  - Adrenal or extra-adrenal pheochromocytomas
  - Endolymphatic sac tumors, papillary cystadenomas of the epididymis or broad ligament, or neuroendocrine tumors of the pancreas
- In an individual with a family history of VHL disease, there must be one or more of the following disease manifestations:
  - Retinal angioma
  - Spinal or cerebellar hemangioblastoma
  - Adrenal or extra-adrenal pheochromocytoma
  - Renal cell carcinoma
  - Multiple renal and pancreatic cysts

Reference

Dollfus H, Massin P, Taupin P, Nemeth C, Amara S, Giraud S, et al. Retinal hemangioblastoma in von Hippel–Lindau disease: a clinical and molecular study. *Invest Ophthalmol Vis Sci.* 2002;43(9): 3067-3074.

Cross-Reference

Neuroradiology: The Requisites, 3rd ed, 327-330.

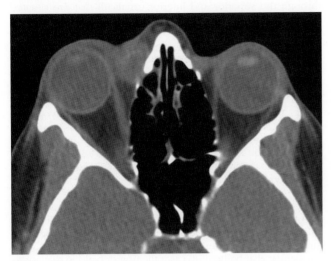

Figure 110-1

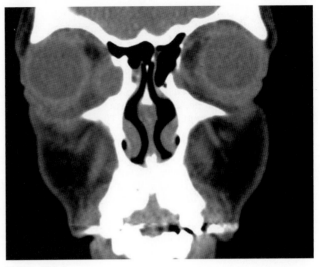

Figure 110-2

HISTORY: A patient presents with swelling along the right lacrimal sac.

1. Which of the following should be included in the differential diagnosis? (Choose all that apply.)
   A. Dacryon
   B. Dacryocystocele
   C. Dacryosialolithiasis
   D. Dacryocystitis

2. What group of pathogens accounts for most cases of dacryocystitis?
   A. Fungi
   B. Bacteria
   C. Viruses
   D. Parasites

3. Which of the following is *not* an autoimmune cause of dacryoadenitis?
   A. Sarcoidosis
   B. Wegener granulomatosis
   C. Sjögren syndrome
   D. Staphylococcus infection

4. Which valve is proximal and which is distal?
   A. Hasner valve is distal; Rosenmüller valve is proximal.
   B. Rosenmüller valve is distal; Hasner valve is proximal.
   C. Hasner valve is distal; Santorini valve is proximal.
   D. Bartholin valve is distal; Rosenmüller valve is proximal.

See Supplemental Figures section for additional figures and legends for this case.

CASE 110

Dacryocystitis

1. **D.** Dacryocystitis should be included in the differential diagnosis because the lacrimal sac is inflamed. There is no enlarged cyst or stone, and so dacryocystocele and dacryosialolithiasis should not be included. There is no such entity as a "dacryon."

2. **C.** Viruses are the most common pathogen and account for most cases of dacryocystitis. Bacteria are the second most common, staphylococci being the most common bacteria. Fungi and parasites are uncommon causes.

3. **D.** Staphylococcus infection is not an *autoimmune* cause of dacryoadenitis. Sarcoidosis, Wegener granulomatosis, and Sjögren syndrome all affect the lacrimal sac.

4. **A.** Hasner valve is distal, and Rosenmüller valve is proximal. Bartholin valves and Santorini valves do not exist.

Comment
Drainage of the Tears

Tears produced by the lacrimal system track medially and flow through the lacrimal punctum in each eyelid margin and through the superior and inferior canaliculi that are situated within the medial aspect of the upper and lower eyelids, and drain via the sinus of Maier into the lacrimal sac. The common canaliculus may have a functional one-way valve of Rosenmüller to prevent reflux into the canaliculi. From the sac, the tears drain via the valve of Krause into the nasolacrimal duct, through the valve of Hasner, and into the nasal cavity beneath the inferior turbinate. Obstruction of this drainage system results in epiphora and sometimes dacryocystitis (infection of the nasolacrimal sac). Dacryocystitis is usually caused by obstruction, which can occur after inflammation with subsequent scarring (Figures S110-1 and S110-2). Dacryoadenitis (inflammation of the lacrimal glandular tissue) can secondarily lead to orbital cellulitis or abscess.

Treatment of Dacryocystitis

Chronic dacryocystitis caused by obstruction of the ductal or valvular system may be treated with stents and nonsteroidal anti-inflammatory drugs. Compression, eye drops, and warm packs may also be helpful. Laser therapy or balloon dilatations via endoscopy are sometimes required as well.

Reference

Wald ER. Periorbital and orbital infections. *Infect Dis Clin North Am.* 2007;21(2):393-408, vi.

Cross-Reference

Neuroradiology: The Requisites, 3rd ed, 335-354.

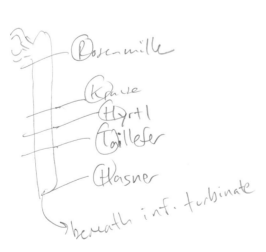

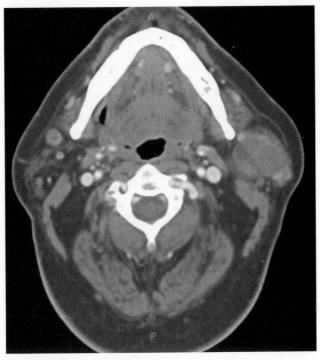

Figure 111-1

HISTORY: A patient seropositive for human immunodeficiency virus (HIV) presents with left periauricular swelling.

1. Which of the following should be included in the differential diagnosis? (Choose all that apply.)
   A. Benign lymphoepithelial lesions (cysts and nodules)
   B. First branchial cleft cyst
   C. Second branchial cleft cyst
   D. Sjögren disease

2. What do lymphoepithelial lesions in association with HIV suggest?
   A. The patient has acquired immunodeficiency syndrome (AIDS).
   B. The patient has lymphoma.
   C. The patient has a low white blood cell (WBC) count.
   D. They do not imply anything.

3. What other findings would suggest HIV-related cysts?
   A. Nasopharyngeal adenoidal enlargement
   B. Cervical adenopathy
   C. Tonsillar enlargement
   D. All of the above

4. What is the most common cause of lymphadenopathy of the parotid gland?
   A. Inflammation of the skin or ear
   B. Lymphoma
   C. Sinusitis
   D. Skin cancers

See Supplemental Figures section for additional figures and legends for this case.

CASE 111

Benign Lymphoepithelial Lesion

1. **A, B, and D.** Benign lymphoepithelial lesions (cysts and nodules) is the most likely diagnosis. First branchial cleft cyst is also a possible diagnosis. Sjögren disease can lead to parotid cysts and nodules. Second branchial cleft cysts do not occur in the parotid gland and therefore would not be included in the diagnosis.

2. **D.** The presence of lymphoepithelial lesions has no ramifications with regard to a patient's HIV status.

3. **D.** Nasopharyngeal adenoidal enlargement, cervical adenopathy, and tonsillar enlargement may all suggest HIV infection.

4. **A.** Inflammation of the skin or ear is the most common cause of lymphadenopathy of the parotid gland. Mastoiditis and otitis media may also be causative. Skin cancers are not as common as infections, and lymphoma is a rare diagnosis. Sinusitis does not cause drainage to the parotid nodes.

Comment

Benign Lymphoepithelial Lesion Associations

Because of the late encapsulation of the parotid gland embryologically, it is the only salivary gland that incorporates lymphoid tissue. Warthin tumors are of lymphatic origin. Cysts and nodules in the parotid glands may develop with HIV seropositivity, Sjögren syndrome, Warthin tumors, metastases (i.e., thyroid carcinoma), and sarcoidosis. There are three types of lymphoid infiltration of the parotid gland: (1) diffuse lymphocytic infiltration, (2) diffuse follicular lymphoid hyperplasia (as nodules), and (3) lymphoepithelial lesions (cysts and nodules) in HIV-positive patients (Figure S111-1). The lesions are caused by cystification within intraparotid nodes. Benign lymphoepithelial lesions (BLELs) can have cysts and nodules present as well. There is accompanying lymphocytic infiltration around the salivary ducts plus atrophy of the gland with BLELs of Sjögren syndrome. BLELs have thin, smooth walls, and when solitary, they are therefore indistinguishable from first branchial cleft cysts.

Patients with AIDS are prone to adenovirus, mycobacterial infection, and fungi in the parotid gland.

HIV-Related Cysts Treatment

Treatment options include fine-needle aspiration, sclerotherapy, surgery, radiotherapy, or medical therapy with highly active antiretroviral therapy (HAART). Many resolve with HAART alone.

Clinical Findings of Sjögren Syndrome

In Sjögren syndrome, parotid lesions have the potential to undergo malignant degeneration into lymphoma. The clinical findings in Sjögren syndrome are (1) the sicca syndrome (dry eyes, dry mouth, dry skin) and (2) a connective tissue disorder (rheumatoid arthritis). The entity occurs more commonly in women than in men (in a 9:1 ratio), usually in the fifth and sixth decades of life.

Clinical Findings of Kimura Disease

In Kimura disease, salivary gland and lymph node manifestations occur more often in men than in women (4:1) of Asian race. Nodes in the neck and parotid glands are enlarged and enhance dramatically on imaging. Eosinophilia may be present in the blood stream. Kikuchi-Fujimoto disease (subacute necrotizing histiocytic lymphadenitis) also manifests with cervical adenopathy and fever and usually resolves spontaneously; however, because affected patients are at risk for developing systemic lupus erythematosus, many authorities believe this to be an autoimmune disorder. Women are affected more than men.

Reference

Steehler MK, Steehler MW, Davison SP. Benign lymphoepithelial cysts of the parotid: long-term surgical results. *HIV AIDS (Auckl)*. 2012;4:81-86.

Cross-Reference

Neuroradiology: The Requisites, 3rd ed, 476-479.

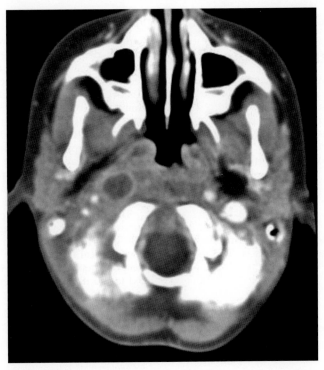

Figure 112-1

HISTORY: A child has throat pain and fever.

1. Which of the following should be included in the differential diagnosis? (Choose all that apply.)
   A. Retropharyngeal edema
   B. Retropharyngeal abscess
   C. Peritonsillar abscess
   D. Necrotizing adenitis

2. Which of these primary tumors has a predilection for retropharyngeal adenopathy?
   A. Cancer of the supraglottic larynx
   B. Cancer of the oral cavity
   C. Cancer of the esophagus
   D. Cancer of the thyroid

3. How are retropharyngeal abscesses and suppurative necrotizing adenitis treated?
   A. Both are treated with drainage.
   B. Both are treated with antibiotics without drainage.
   C. Retropharyngeal abscess is treated with drainage; necrotizing adenitis is not.
   D. Necrotizing adenitis is treated with drainage; retropharyngeal abscess is not.

4. Which demonstrates enhancement of the walls of the retropharyngeal space fascia on imaging?
   A. Retropharyngeal phlegmon
   B. Retropharyngeal edema
   C. Retropharyngeal adenitis
   D. Retropharyngeal abscess

See Supplemental Figures section for additional figures and legends for this case.

CASE 112

Necrotizing Adenitis of the Retropharynx

1. **D.** The location and appearance of the lesion is typical of necrotizing adenitis.

2. **D.** Thyroid cancer has a tendency to cause retropharyngeal adenopathy. However, the reasons are not well understood. Retropharyngeal adenopathy is rarely caused by cancers of the supraglottic larynx, oral cavity, and esophagus.

3. **C.** Retropharyngeal abscesses are usually treated with drainage (necrotizing adenitis is not). Both conditions are also treated with antibiotics.

4. **D.** Retropharyngeal abscess demonstrates enhancement of the walls of the retropharyngeal space fascia. This distinguishes the retropharyngeal abscess from the other entities when it is present.

Comment

Causes of Retropharyngeal Abscess

Retropharyngeal necrotizing adenitis may be a precursor to a retropharyngeal abscess as the nodes coalesce, extend outside the node capsule, and spill suppurative material into the retropharyngeal space. Streptococci are the usual pathogens, and the infection may start as a pharyngitis or adenitis of the retropharyngeal adenoidal lymphoid tissue. Affected patients complain of a sore throat and have fever and neck pain. Other lymph nodes in the upper neck may be enlarged as well.

Imaging Findings

Computed tomographic scans of retropharyngeal necrotizing adenitis demonstrate enlarged paramedian retropharyngeal lymph nodes with central low density that represents the necrosis (Figure S112-1). According to Fraser (2009), "Suppurative lymphadenitis is characterized by invasion of the lymph node by neutrophils, resulting in rapid swelling leading to capsular distention, edema, and ultimately tissue necrosis and liquefaction." If the nodes appear as rounded structures with intact capsules, as in this case, it is easier to distinguish retropharyngeal suppurative adenitis from abscess. Although these nodes might appear relatively easy to drain, intraoral aspiration or incision and drainage has variable success: Some drain, some do not.

The borders of the retropharyngeal space include (1) the buccopharyngeal fascia anteriorly, (2) the alar fascia posteriorly, and (3) the carotid sheaths and parapharyngeal space deep cervical fascia laterally. Pathogens in the alar fascia and the prevertebral fascia can travel to the lower mediastinum and to the diaphragm. Otherwise, the retropharyngeal space ends at the T3 level.

References

Al-Sabah B, Bin Salleen H, Hagr A, Choi-Rosen J, Manoukian JJ, Tewfik TL. Retropharyngeal abscess in children: 10-year study. *J Otolaryngol.* 2004;33(6):352-355.

Fraser IP. Suppurative lymphadenitis. *Curr Infect Dis Rep.* 2009;11(5): 383-388.

Cross-Reference

Neuroradiology: The Requisites, 3rd ed, 499-500.

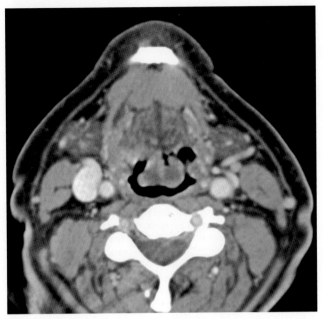

Figure 113-1

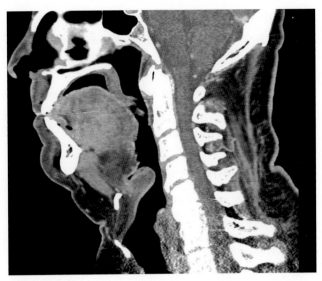

Figure 113-2

HISTORY: A young adult has fever, difficulty swallowing, and drooling.

1. Which of the following should be included in the differential diagnosis? (Choose all that apply.)
   A. Epiglottitis
   B. Supraglottitis
   C. Tonsillitis
   D. Peritonsillar abscess

2. What is the stereotypical organism associated with epiglottitis in children?
   A. Adenovirus
   B. Staphylococci
   C. Streptococci
   D. *Haemophilus influenzae*

3. Why do some authorities use the term *supraglottitis* rather than *epiglottitis?*
   A. *Supraglottitis* is general rather than specific.
   B. In addition to the epiglottis, the aryepiglottic folds and arytenoid cartilage may be primarily involved.
   C. *Supraglottitis* is a misnomer that should be avoided.
   D. The pharynx is also inflamed.

4. Why is computed tomography (CT) not used to diagnose acute epiglottitis in children?
   A. Airway compromise is possible during CT.
   B. Plain radiographs with the patient supine are just as efficacious as CT and deliver less radiation.
   C. The radiation dosage is too high with CT.
   D. Reactions to contrast are more severe in atopic patients.

See Supplemental Figures section for additional figures and legends for this case.

CASE 113

Supraglottitis

1. **A and B.** The epiglottis, which is part of the supraglottis, is swollen. The tonsil is not affected, and no abscess is present.

2. **D.** *H. influenzae* is the organism stereotypically associated with this diagnosis in children, although infection with this organism has become less frequent because of immunizations. Streptococci are the most common pathogens in adults.

3. **B.** The term *supraglottitis* may be preferred because, in addition to the epiglottis, the aryepiglottic folds and arytenoid cartilage may be primarily involved. In some cases, the epiglottis may not be affected as much as other components of the larynx.

4. **A.** CT should not be used to diagnose supraglottitis in children because of the risk of airway compromise. In pediatric patients, the inflamed airway can close when they are supine. In adults, the airway is wider with less lymphoid tissue, and so CT is safer in adults.

Comment

Symptoms of Epiglottitis

Most adult patients with epiglottitis have sore throat, odynophagia, and malaise. The diagnosis may be made by plain radiography (81.4% accurate) or flexible laryngoscopy (100%). Signs that suggest a need for immediate airway support include (1) drooling, (2) diabetes mellitus, (3) shorter onset of symptoms, (4) epiglottic abscess, (5) severe swelling of the epiglottis, and (6) arytenoid swelling. Vaccinations for H. Flu B have reduced the number of cases with that as a pathogen. Adults have more strep infections.

Imaging Findings

Supraglottitis is reemerging in adults, possibly because of the acquired immunodeficiency syndrome (AIDS) epidemic. It is a more indolent infection in adults than pediatric epiglottitis because adults can tolerate more supraglottic and prevertebral swelling than children can. The width of the epiglottis in an adult is normally less than one-third the anteroposterior width of the C4 vertebral body (Figures S113-1 and S113-2). Likewise, the width of the prevertebral tissue in an adult is normally less than half the anteroposterior width of the C4 vertebral body.

Epiglottitis occurs most commonly in the winter and has a bimodal age distribution of ages 0 to 8 years and 20 to 40 years. Fever, drooling, sore throat, dysphagia, stridor, and tachypnea are common. Two classical findings on lateral plain films are (1) the thumbprint appearance of the epiglottis, because of its thickness, and (2) hypopharyngeal distention, caused by airway obstruction. Anteroposterior plain radiographs are obtained only if croup is part of the differential diagnosis. Croup occurs in young children (<2 years old) and is usually caused by a viral illness. Pain is not a typical finding, and dysphagia is unusual with croup. The "steeple" sign of laryngeal narrowing can be seen on anteroposterior plain radiographic views of the airway of a patient with croup.

Reference

Verbruggen K, Halewyck S, Deron P, Foulon I, Gordts F. Epiglottitis and related complications in adults. Case reports and review of the literature. *B-ENT.* 2012;8(2):143-148.

Cross-Reference

Neuroradiology: The Requisites, 3rd ed, 449-452.

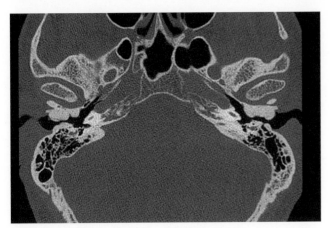

Figure 114-1

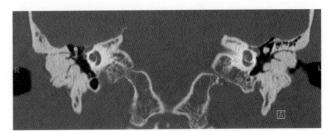

Figure 114-2

HISTORY: A patient presents with bilateral conductive hearing loss.

1. Which of the following should be included in the differential diagnosis? (Choose all that apply.)
   A. Malignant otitis externa
   B. Exostoses
   C. Osteomas
   D. Epidermoid

2. Of the following, who is a typical patient with external auditory canal (EAC) exostoses?
   A. Elderly person with diabetes
   B. Cold-water swimmer
   C. Patient with a history of colonic polyps
   D. Patient with a facial nevus

3. How are EAC cholesteatomas distinguished from keratosis obturans?
   A. Keratosis obturans is usually unilateral, develops in younger individuals, and is less painful than EAC cholesteatomas.
   B. Keratosis obturans is usually bilateral, develops in older individuals, and is more painful than EAC cholesteatomas.
   C. Keratosis obturans is usually unilateral, develops in older individuals, and is less painful than EAC cholesteatomas.
   D. Keratosis obturans is usually bilateral, develops in younger individuals, and is more painful than EAC cholesteatomas.

4. With which of the following is keratosis obturans not associated?
   A. Bronchiectasis
   B. Obstructive plugs in the EACs
   C. Sinusitis
   D. Sinonasal polyposis

See Supplemental Figures section for additional figures and legends for this case.

CASE 114

External Auditory Canal Exostoses

1. **B and C.** As the figures show, there is new bone growth, which indicates exostoses. The differential diagnosis also includes osteomas, although these bony tumors are rarely bilateral and not as smoothly narrowing the EAC. There are no erosions (bony overgrowth), and so malignant otitis externa would not be included. In addition, there is no soft tissue mass, and so epidermoid should not be included.

2. **B.** Cold-water swimmers develop bony overgrowths. Elderly diabetic patients are more likely to develop malignant otitis externa.

3. **D.** Keratosis obturans is usually bilateral, develops in younger individuals, and is more painful than EAC cholesteatomas. The pain may be severe. This lesion may erode bone.

4. **D.** Keratosis obturans is not associated with sinonasal polyposis. It is, however, associated with bronchiectasis and sinusitis, both of which occur frequently in patients with keratosis obturans.

Comments

Incidence and Cause of Exostoses

Because cold-water swimmers develop EAC exostoses (Figures S114-1 and S114-2), this condition is sometimes referred to as "surfer's ear," but it is not the external otitis ("swimmer's ear") that affects swimmers. The length of exposure is usually years of this type of swimming. The Scandinavian, New Zealand, and Australian literature is replete with studies of Arctic/Antarctic swimmers who develop exostoses. Surfer's ear can develop at any age, and its incidence is directly proportional to the amount of time spent in cold, wet, windy weather; thus it is also common in white water kayakers, snowboarders, divers, and jet skiers. The older a person is and the longer the person engages in the sport, the more likely the person is to develop exostoses. Even after surgical removal of the exostoses (and psychological counseling), patients who return to their cold-water habits develop new exostoses. Earplugs are usually protective. Patients may also develop external otitis that brings them in to their doctor, or they may have meatal blockage. The differential diagnosis includes keratosis obturans, epidermoids, acquired cholesteatomas, polyps, and osteomas.

Differences between Exostoses and Osteomas

Osteomas contain stroma and are usually pedunculated and more lateral than are exostoses. They are only rarely bilateral. Osteomas are found at the tympanosquamous or tympanomastoid suture line, characterized histologically by abundant discrete fibrovascular channels surrounded by irregularly oriented lamellated bone. True exostoses are sessile, flat, and medial and contain dense lamellar bone without fibrovascular channels. If a bone marrow space is visible on scans, the lesion is an osteoma. The other lesions (keratosis obturans, epidermoids, polyps, and cholesteatomas) do not usually calcify or ossify.

Reference

Moore RD, Schuman TA, Scott TA, Mann SE, Davidson MA, Labadie RF. Exostoses of the external auditory canal in white-water kayakers. *Laryngoscope.* 2010;120(3):582-590.

Cross-Reference

Neuroradiology: The Requisites, 3rd ed, 387-388.

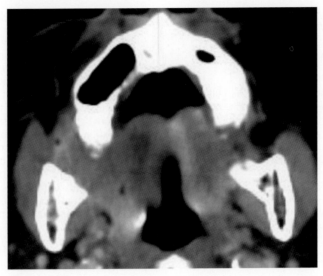

Figure 115-1

HISTORY: A 50-year-old patient complained of right-sided jaw pain and trismus.

1. Which of the following should be included in the differential diagnosis? (Choose all that apply.)
   A. Sialolithiasis
   B. Temporomandibular joint (TMJ) displacement
   C. Squamous cell carcinoma of the retromolar trigone
   D. Tetanus

2. What part of the aerodigestive system includes the retromolar trigone?
   A. The oral cavity
   B. The nasopharynx
   C. The oropharynx
   D. The hypopharynx

3. What structures of the palate are part of the oral cavity and of the oropharynx?
   A. The oral cavity includes the hard palate, and the oropharynx includes the soft palate.
   B. The oral cavity includes the hard palate, and the nasopharynx includes the soft palate
   C. The oropharynx includes both the hard and soft palates.
   D. The hypopharynx includes the hard palate, and oral cavity includes the soft palate.

4. What bony structure is often resected with a lesion of the retromolar trigone?
   A. The pterygoid plate
   B. The ascending ramus of the mandible
   C. The nasopalatine foramen
   D. The maxillary spine

See Supplemental Figures section for additional figures and legends for this case.

CASE 115

Squamous Cell Carcinoma of the Retromolar Trigone

1. **C.** The presence of a mass indicates squamous cell carcinoma of the retromolar trigone on the right. The presence of a stone (not here) would indicate sialolithiasis. TMJ displacement and tetanus are not present in this case.

2. **A.** The retromolar trigone is considered a part of the oral cavity.

3. **A.** The hard palate is part of the oral cavity, but the soft palate is part of the oropharynx. The oral tongue is also part of the oral cavity, but the base of the tongue is part of the oropharynx. This is based in part on embryologic derivation.

4. **B.** The ascending ramus of the mandible is often resected with a lesion of the retromolar trigone because it is at the posterior margin of the retromolar trigone. It is rare for the pterygoid plate to be resected with a lesion of the retromolar trigone.

Comment

Relevant Anatomy

The retromolar trigone is a critical site for squamous cell carcinoma. The retromolar trigone is located behind the maxillary tuberosity and the ascending ramus of the mandible. It usually contains fat and nerves. Because it sits at the junction of the maxilla and the mandible, cancer there often invades one or both of these bony structures (Figure S115-1). The nearby pterygoid muscles are also vulnerable to cancers in this region, and invasion is common. A retromolar trigonal cancer may also ascend or spread along the pterygomandibular raphe, which passes by the pterygopalatine fossa. From this location, the tumor may infiltrate the branches of the second division of the fifth cranial nerve. Perineural growth of tumor may direct the tumor into the orbit, the infratemporal fossa, the cavernous sinus, or the middle cranial fossa. One minor salivary gland malignancy, adenoid cystic carcinoma, is notorious for just such spread. Thus a tumor of the retromolar trigone may necessitate resection of the maxilla, mandible, orbit, temporal bone, and masticator space. Furthermore, the site is not readily approachable surgically, even for a limited resection, and the mandible often must be rotated laterally for access to the tumor. The operation often performed for retromolar trigonal cancers consists of hemimandibulectomy with resection of the pterygoid and masseter muscles and an ipsilateral neck dissection. Nodal spread is usually to levels 1 (submandibular-submental nodes) and 2 (higher jugular nodes above the hyoid bone).

Treatment of Retromolar Trigonal Cancer

Modern options for treatment are controversial. When imaging reveals no bone invasion, surgery and radiotherapy individually are satisfactory options, but outcomes may be better with combined therapy. Instead of the segmental mandibulectomy in these cases, other authorities advocate marginal mandibulectomy. The treatment of grade N0 neck nodes follows the primary treatment.

Odontogenic infection can simulate a tumor in the bone marrow on magnetic resonance imaging. It can lead to marrow signal abnormalities, low on T1-weighted images and bright on T2-weighted images.

Reference

Ayad T, Guertin L, Soulières D, Belair M, Temam S, Nguyen-Tân PF. Controversies in the management of retromolar trigone carcinoma. *Head Neck.* 2009;31(3):398-405.

Cross-Reference

Neuroradiology: The Requisites, 3rd ed, 461-462.

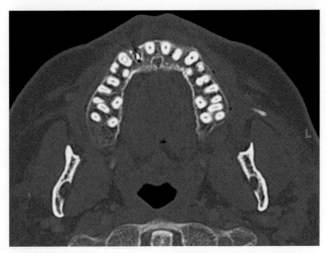

Figure 116-1

HISTORY: A patient presents with left facial swelling and pain.

1. Which of the following should be included in the differential diagnosis? (Choose all that apply.)
   A. Facial fracture
   B. Dental caries
   C. Facial cellulitis
   D. Parotid duct stone

2. Which of these disease processes do *not* predispose a patient to parotid sialolithiasis?
   A. Sarcoidosis
   B. Sjögren syndrome
   C. Hyperparathyroidism
   D. Alcoholism

3. What is the incidence of multiple salivary stones?
   A. 0% to 20%
   B. 21% to 40%
   C. 41% to 60%
   D. >60%

4. Nonpainful enlargement of the parotid glands (sialosis) can occur with what state?
   A. Sarcoidosis
   B. Sjögren syndrome
   C. Hyperparathyroidism
   D. Alcoholism

See Supplemental Figures section for additional figures and legends for this case.

CASE 116

Parotid Duct Stone

1. **D.** The diagnosis should include parotid duct stone in the distal left Stensen duct. Facial fractures, dental caries, and facial cellulitis are not visible on the image.

2. **D.** Alcoholism does not predispose a patient to parotid sialolithiasis unless dehydration coexists. Sarcoidosis, Sjögren syndrome, and hyperparathyroidism all do. Hyperparathyroidism also leads to renal stones.

3. **B.** The incidence of multiple salivary stones is 25%. This is more of an issue, however, in the submandibular glands and ducts.

4. **D.** Nonpainful enlargements of the parotid glands (sialosis) can occur with alcoholism. Sarcoidosis, Sjögren syndrome, and hyperparathyroidism do not cause the parotid glands to enlarge, although they may cause various other problems (see Comment section).

Comment

Treatment of Parotid Duct Stones

A stone is identified in the left Stensen duct (Figure S116-1), just posterior to the zygomaticus muscle before it enters the buccal mucosa. Sublingual and minor salivary gland calculi are distinctly uncommon. Calcifications in lymph nodes, tonsils, and vessels should be ruled out before calculi in these glands are diagnosed. The need for sialography to diagnose calculi is currently rare: Unenhanced computed tomography can reveal most calculi reliably even if their density is minimally different from surrounding tissue. Most submandibular calculi appear within the duct, rather than in the glandular parenchyma. Focal masslike firmness of the submandibular gland caused by chronic sialadenitis from calculus disease (Küttner tumor) may simulate a neoplasm. When the gland is affected with calculus and pain and swelling are limited to the duct orifices, treatment is easier; it may consist of manual manipulation or surgical excision. Stones within the glandular parenchyma may necessitate glandular removal if the patient cannot tolerate the symptoms. Bilateral glandular sialolithiasis is problematic in that bilateral glandular removal may lead to permanent dryness of the mouth, which is uncomfortable and may lead to dental caries.

Using Ultrasonography to Evaluate Salivary Gland Stones

Ultrasonography is an excellent means for evaluating salivary gland stones. The sensitivity, specificity, accuracy, and positive and negative predictive values of ultrasonography in the detection of calculi are 77%, 95%, 85%, 94%, and 78%, respectively. The numbers are even better for stones larger than 3 mm. Multiple small distal calculi, however, are hard to identify. Because of the low sensitivity and negative predictive values, ultrasonography is not reliable for ruling out calculi. Hence computed tomography continues to be the best test. No contrast is required; in fact, contrast in vessels may simulate calculi, and so unenhanced scans are best.

Reference

Terraz S, Poletti PA, Dulguerov P, Dfouni N, Becker CD, Marchal F, et al. How reliable is sonography in the assessment of sialolithiasis? *AJR Am J Roentgenol.* 2013;201(1):W104-W109.

Cross-Reference

Neuroradiology: The Requisites, 3rd ed, 479-480.

CASE 117

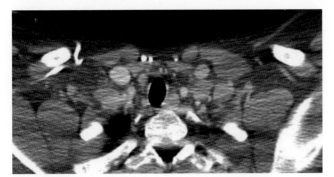

Figure 117-1

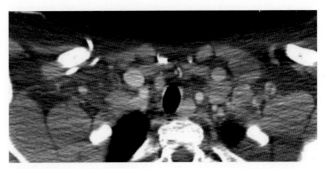

Figure 117-2

HISTORY: A young woman presents with palpable neck masses.

1. Which of the following should be included in the differential diagnosis? (Choose all that apply.)
   A. Lymphoma
   B. Thyroid cancer
   C. Breast cancer
   D. Lung cancer

2. What is the typical appearance of lymphomatous cervical adenopathy?
   A. Large round lymph nodes without necrosis
   B. Large necrotic nodes
   C. Small necrotic nodes
   D. Most commonly as a Waldeyer ring mass

3. Can lymphomatous lymph nodes enhance dramatically on imaging?
   A. Yes
   B. No
   C. Only after radiation therapy
   D. Only after bevacizumab (Avastin) therapy

4. What is the typical histologic variety of lymphoma in the neck?
   A. Hodgkin disease is more common than non-Hodgkin lymphoma.
   B. Burkitt lymphoma is more common than Hodgkin disease.
   C. Non-Hodgkin lymphoma is more common than Hodgkin disease.
   D. Non-Hodgkin lymphoma and Hodgkin disease occur equally frequently.

See Supplemental Figures section for additional figures and legends for this case.

CASE 117

Neck Lymphoma

1. **A, B, C, and D.** Lymphoma is a source of bilateral lower neck nodes. Thyroid cancer may manifest as nodal disease, and breast cancer and lung cancer may manifest with supraclavicular adenopathy.

2. **A.** Lymphomatous cervical adenopathy typically appears as large round lymph nodes without necrosis. This characteristic distinguishes them from squamous cell nodes, which may be the same size but are more frequently necrotic.

3. **A.** Lymphomatous lymph nodes can enhance dramatically, particularly those of the angiofollicular variety of lymphoma. They can enhance before treatment or after therapy.

4. **C.** Non-Hodgkin lymphoma is more common than Hodgkin disease. Burkitt lymphoma is rare except in Africa.

Comment

Causes of Neck Masses

The most common cause of neck mass in young adults is cervical adenopathy, and the malignancy to be considered is lymphoma. Nodal necrosis is distinctly uncommon in patients with Hodgkin disease and is only a little more frequent in those with non-Hodgkin lymphoma. The submental, retropharyngeal, submandibular, internal jugular, supraclavicular (Figures S117-1 and S117-2), and spinal accessory chains are frequently involved with lymphoma.

Incidence of Neck Lymphoma

Nearly 75% of patients with Hodgkin disease present with a neck node, but concurrent disease in the chest is common. Non-Hodgkin lymphoma affects extranodal neck tissue (Waldeyer ring) more frequently than does Hodgkin disease, and approximately 50% of patients with nodal disease have systemic dissemination. Isolated nodal disease is more characteristic of Hodgkin disease than of non-Hodgkin lymphoma, whereas isolated extranodal manifestation is the hallmark of non-Hodgkin lymphoma. Lymphoma accounts for 10% to 15% of malignancies of the orbit, 8% in the paranasal sinuses, 5% in the tonsils, less than 1% in the salivary glands, 2% in the thyroid gland, and less than 5% in the soft tissues. Diffuse large-cell lymphoma is the most common variety of non-Hodgkin lymphoma in the neck. There are several differences between Hodgkin disease and non-Hodgkin lymphoma besides the higher prevalence of extranodal disease with non-Hodgkin lymphoma (4% vs. 23%). The median age at diagnosis of Hodgkin disease is in the third decade of life, whereas for non-Hodgkin lymphoma, it is in the seventh decade. The rate of solitary node involvement for both is less than 35%, although it is less common in Hodgkin disease. Mediastinal involvement is two to three times more common with Hodgkin disease than with non-Hodgkin lymphoma, but the opposite is true for abdominal adenopathy. The overall rate of survival is much better with Hodgkin disease.

Imaging Findings

In a patient with a squamous cell carcinoma neck node and in whom a primary tumor is not apparent on clinical and endoscopic evaluation, imaging elucidates the primary tumor in many cases. For cases in which the primary tumor is not present somewhere in the upper aerodigestive system such as the nasopharynx, tonsils, piriform sinus, or base of the tongue, one should consider the thyroid gland, the breast, the lungs, and the esophagus as potential primary sites. Positron emission tomography (PET) may be of some benefit in searching for an occult primary tumor; it has been said that PET reveals the aerodigestive system primary tumor in 25% of cases that went undetected by conventional imaging.

Reference

Urquhart A, Berg R. Hodgkin's and non-Hodgkin's lymphoma of the head and neck. *Laryngoscope.* 2001;111(9):1565-1569.

Cross-Reference

Neuroradiology: The Requisites, 3rd ed, 472.

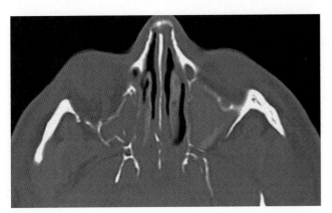

Figure 118-1

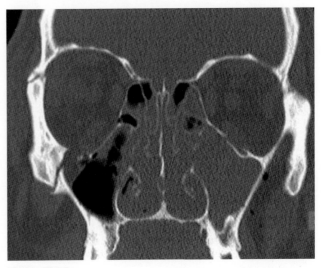

Figure 118-2

HISTORY: The statement "man versus baseball bat" is written on an emergency department requisition, suggesting facial trauma.

1. Which of the following should be included in the differential diagnosis? (Choose all that apply.)
   A. Trimalar fracture
   B. Nasoethmoidal strut fracture
   C. Le Fort–type fractures
   D. Normal

2. What structure or structures are invariably fractured with Le Fort fractures?
   A. Maxilla
   B. Pterygoid plates
   C. Orbital floor
   D. Nasal bones

3. In which types of Le Fort fractures is the medial orbital wall fractured?
   A. Types I and II
   B. Types II and III
   C. Types I and III
   D. None of the above

4. Which Le Fort fracture is associated with nasal bone fractures?
   A. Type I
   B. Type II
   C. Type III
   D. None of the above

See Supplemental Figures section for additional figures and legends for this case.

CASE 118

Le Fort Fracture Types

1. **C.** The diagnosis is Le Fort–type fractures. Le Fort type III fracture on the right side is demonstrated with fractures across lateral and medial orbital walls. Zygomatic attachment fractures are not being demonstrated, so the diagnosis would not include trimalar fractures. In addition, nasoethmoidal strut fractures are not shown.

2. **B.** Pterygoid plates are fractured with Le Fort fractures; they are the sine qua non of Le Fort fractures.

3. **B.** The medial orbital wall is fractured in Le Fort types II and III fractures. Fractures of the maxilla to the medial aspect of the orbit characterize type II, and fractures of the lateral and medial aspects of the orbit characterize type III.

4. **D.** The Le Fort classification does not specifically include nasal bone fractures.

Comment

Associations with Le Fort Fractures

Rhea and Novelline (2005) emphasized that each of the Le Fort fractures is associated with one unique fracture:
- Type I: the anterolateral margin of the nasal fossa
- Type II: the inferior orbital rim
- Type III: zygomatic arch

Le Fort type I fractures predominantly involve the lower maxilla and do not usually involve the orbits, whereas Le Fort type II fractures affect inferior and medial aspects of the orbit (Figures S118-1 and S118-2). Le Fort type I fracture is referred to as the *floating palate fracture* because the fracture crosses from medially at the nasal septum to the maxilla above the teeth and below the zygomaticomaxillary junction and includes the pterygoid plates. This fracture is often bilateral. Le Fort type II fracture is often termed the *pyramidal fracture* because it crosses the body of the maxilla down the midline of the hard palate; through the rim, floor, and medial wall of the orbit; and into the nasal cavity. Le Fort type III fractures, which cross from the lateral to medial aspects of the orbit, are the fracture constellations in which "craniofacial dissociation" may occur; that is, the facial bones inferiorly are relatively disconnected from the skull above.

Relevant Anatomy

Common to all of these fractures is extension across the pterygoid plates. Trimalar fractures affect the attachments of the zygoma to the maxilla, the frontal bone, and the sphenoid bone. They create a lateral divot out of the side of the face, dissociating the lateral orbit, zygoma, and lateral edge of the maxilla from the rest of the face. It is possible for a patient to have one type of Le Fort fracture on one side and another type of Le Fort fracture on the other side, as well as multiple Le Fort fractures ipsilaterally.

Reference

Rhea JT, Novelline RA. How to simplify the CT diagnosis of Le Fort fractures. *AJR Am J Roentgenol.* 2005;184(5):1700-1705.

Cross-Reference

Neuroradiology: The Requisites, 3rd ed, 189-190.

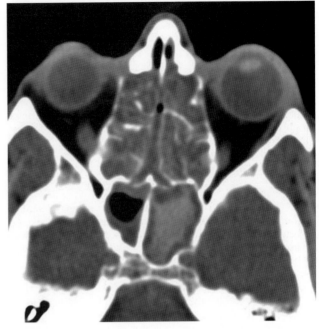

Figure 119-2

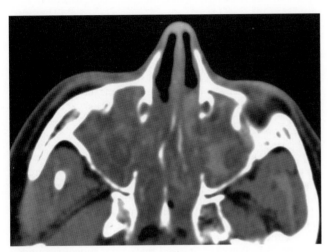

Figure 119-1

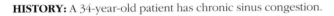

HISTORY: A 34-year-old patient has chronic sinus congestion.

1. Which of the following should be included in the differential diagnosis? (Choose all that apply.)
   A. Cystic fibrosis
   B. Aspirin triad syndrome
   C. Sinonasal polyposis
   D. Allergic fungal sinusitis

2. What is the success rate of functional endoscopic sinus surgery in patients with sinonasal polyposis treated with total ethmoidectomy?
   A. 0% to 25%
   B. 26% to 50%
   C. 51% to 75%
   D. >75%

3. What is the incidence of abnormalities in the paranasal sinuses (i.e., mucosal thickening, air-fluid levels, polypoid excrescences) on computed tomographic scans of children with no clinical signs and symptoms of sinusitis?
   A. 0% to 25%
   B. 26% to 50%
   C. 51% to 75%
   D. >75%

4. Which of the following is *not* correct?
   A. A solitary discrete area of increased density is probably caused by an inflammatory lesion.
   B. Multifocal calcifications or densities are just as likely to be found in a tumor as in an inflammatory lesion.
   C. Diffuse increased density is usually seen in fibroosseous benign bony lesions.
   D. Erosive lesions are most common in neoplasms.

See Supplemental Figures section for additional figures and legends for this case.

CASE 119

Sinonasal Polyposis

1. **A, B, C, and D.** Cystic fibrosis causes sinus opacification with polyps. Aspirin triad syndrome is associated with nasal polyps, asthma, and hypersensitivity to aspirin. Sinonasal polyposis is common in atopic patients. Allergic fungal sinusitis is often associated with polyps.

2. **D.** Of patients with sinonasal polyposis treated with total ethmoidectomy, 80% experience symptomatic improvement as a result of functional endoscopic sinus surgery.

3. **B.** The incidence of abnormalities in the paranasal sinuses (i.e., mucosal thickening, air-fluid levels, polypoid excrescences) on computed tomographic scans of children with no clinical signs and symptoms of sinusitis is reported to be 40%.

4. **D.** Polyps and other inflammatory conditions erode sinus walls more frequently than do tumors because they are so much more common. Because of this, the presence of bony erosion is not a reliable indicator of a malignant process. The type of erosion and the enhancement characteristics on magnetic resonance imaging are most helpful.

Comment

Samter Triad and Kounis-Zavras Syndrome

The Samter triad is the constellation of asthma, nasal polyposis (Figures S119-1 and S119-2), and aspirin sensitivity. Its prevalence rates are 0.3% of the general population and between 5% and 10% of asthmatic patients. Histologic features are benign eosinophilic polyps with edematous stroma and markedly thickened basement membranes. Kounis-Zavras syndrome, also known as *Kounis syndrome*, is a cause of angina pectoris or acute coronary syndrome secondary to coronary vasospasm in response to an allergen. The Samter triad and Kounis-Zavras syndrome may occur together.

Associations with Chronic Sinusitis

Chronic sinusitis may be associated with asthma, polyps, eosinophilia, cystic fibrosis, Kartagener syndrome, and allergies. Aspirin sensitivity may also be a component of the illness. Alternatively, chronic sinusitis may result from anatomic variations in sinonasal and osteomeatal anatomy that predispose the ostia to occlusions. Mucoperiosteal thickening, mucous retention cysts, osteitis, and polypoid mucosa may be evident on computed tomography.

Associations with Polyps

Polyps are common in patients with Churg-Strauss syndrome, allergic fungal sinusitis, cilia dyskinetic (Kartagener) syndrome, and Young syndrome. Nasal polyps are more common in patients with nonallergic asthma than in those with allergic asthma. The diagnosis of polyps should be considered when mass effect or ostial widening is associated with sinonasal opacification. Polypoid mucosal thickening suggests rounded excrescences off the mucosal surface.

Reference

Chen BS, Virant FS, Parikh SR, Manning SC. Aspirin sensitivity syndrome (Samter's triad): an unrecognized disorder in children with nasal polyposis. *Int J Pediatr Otorhinolaryngol.* 2013;77(2): 281-283.

Cross-Reference

Neuroradiology: The Requisites, 3rd ed, 432-433.

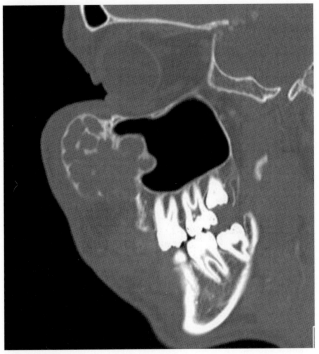

Figure 120-1

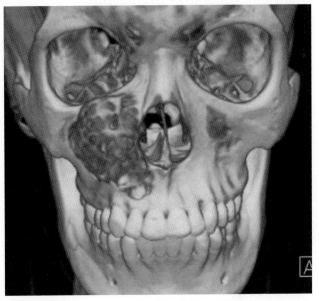

Figure 120-2

HISTORY: A patient presents with facial swelling anterior to the maxilla.

1. Which of the following should be included in the differential diagnosis? (Choose all that apply.)
   A. Giant cell tumor
   B. Aneurysmal bone cyst
   C. Giant cell reparative granuloma (GCRG)
   D. Osteoma

2. With which of the following are GCRGs of the mandible associated?
   A. Teflon-Proplast meniscus prostheses
   B. Carious teeth
   C. Dental trauma/tooth extraction
   D. All of the above

3. What is the ratio of peripheral GCRGs (of the gingiva or alveolar soft tissues) to central GCRGs (of the maxilla and mandible)?
   A. 1:4
   B. 1:2
   C. 2:1
   D. 4:1

4. Features that distinguish GCRGs from giant cell tumors include which of the following?
   A. GCRGs are more common in older patients, have a predilection for the mandible and maxilla, and affect the molar regions.
   B. GCRGs are more common in male patients, have a predilection for the mandible and maxilla, and are unilocular lesions.
   C. GCRGs are more common in younger patients, have a predilection for the mandible and maxilla, and affect the molar regions.
   D. GCRGs are more common in younger patients, have a predilection for the mandible and maxilla, and affect the premolar regions.

See Supplemental Figures section for additional figures and legends for this case.

CASE 120

Giant Cell Reparative Granuloma

1. **A, B, and C.** Giant cell tumors and aneurysmal bone cysts appear as bubbly bone lesions on computed tomography. GCRGs should also be included in the differential diagnosis. The appearance is too bubbly for pure osteoma, and the maxilla is an uncommon site for osteomas.

2. **D.** GCRGs of the mandible are associated with Teflon-Proplast meniscus prostheses, carious teeth, and dental trauma/tooth extraction. They are more common than many other giant cell–containing bone lesions, including aneurysmal bone cysts and giant cell tumors.

3. **D.** Peripheral GCRGs (of the gingiva or alveolar soft tissues) are four times more common than central GCRGs (of the maxilla and mandible).

4. **D.** GCRGs are more common in younger patients, have a predilection for the mandible and maxilla, and affect the premolar regions. Women are more commonly affected by GCRGs, presumably as a result of hormonal effects.

Comment

Imaging Findings

GCRGs of the head and neck most commonly occur in the mandible and maxilla (Figures S120-1 and S120-2). The temporal bone and paranasal sinuses are the second most common sites in the head and neck. The small bones of the hands and feet may also be affected. GCRG is a disease of adolescence, usually occurring in girls, and may be hormonally responsive inasmuch as they expand with pregnancy. Mixed signal intensity and density (owing to blood products and hemosiderin), inhomogeneous enhancement, and lysis of the bone are typical. GCRGs are more commonly multilocular lesions that leave the peripheral cortical bone intact. Most authorities believe the lesion to result from traumatic or iatrogenic causes that incite intraosseous hemorrhage. The differential diagnosis often includes pigmented villonodular synovitis, giant cell tumors, ameloblastoma, aneurysmal bone cysts, fasciitis, and synovial chondromatosis.

Histologic Features of Giant Cell Reparative Granulomas

Histologic study reveals giant cells, osteoid matrix, and foci of hemorrhage. The prognosis is excellent (as opposed to some of the other entities in the differential diagnosis). Treatment is surgical (curettage), but the rate of recurrence is 25% to 33%.

Reference

Murphey MD, Nomikos GC, Flemming DJ, Gannon FH, Temple HT, Kransdorf MJ. From the archives of AFIP. Imaging of giant cell tumor and giant cell reparative granuloma of bone: radiologic-pathologic correlation. *Radiographics*. 2001;21(5):1283-1309.

Cross-Reference

Neuroradiology: The Requisites, 3rd ed, 568-569.

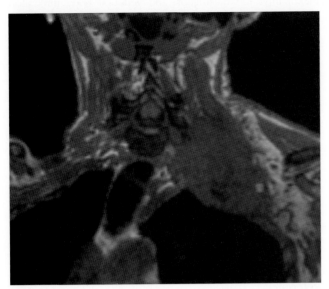

Figure 121-1

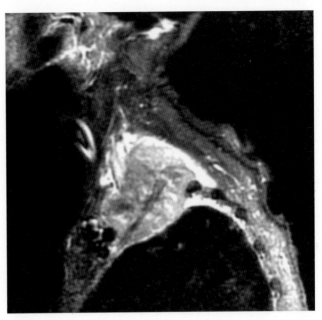

Figure 121-2

HISTORY: A patient presents with left-sided Horner syndrome.

1. Which of the following should be included in the differential diagnosis? (Choose all that apply.)
   A. Schwannoma
   B. Meningioma
   C. Pancoast tumor
   D. Metastatic adenopathy

2. What is the most common organ of origin and histologic type of a Pancoast tumor?
   A. The lung; small cell carcinoma
   B. The lung; non–small cell carcinoma
   C. Lymphoma; diffuse histiocytic
   D. Breast; adenocarcinoma

3. What infections may mimic a Pancoast tumor?
   A. Actinomycosis
   B. *Nocardia* infection
   C. Tuberculosis
   D. Fungal infection
   E. All of the above

4. Which non–lung parenchyma neoplasms most often progress to a Pancoast tumor?
   A. Breast cancer
   B. Lymphoma
   C. Mesothelioma
   D. Sarcoma

See Supplemental Figures section for additional figures and legends for this case.

CASE 121

Pancoast Tumor

1. **C.** Pancoast tumor emanates from the superior lung, as seen in the figures. Schwannomas and meningiomas are not as infiltrative or aggressive appearing. Metastatic adenopathy is unlikely to develop in this location.

2. **B.** The lung is the most common organ of origin and non–small cell carcinoma is the most common histologic type of a Pancoast tumor. The tumor passes upward to invade the brachial plexus, the sympathetic nervous system, or both.

3. **E.** Actinomycosis, *Nocardia* infection, tuberculosis, and fungal infection all may mimic a Pancoast tumor. All are capable of producing a virulent mass in the lung apex and chest wall.

4. **B.** After lung cancer, lymphoma most often progresses to a Pancoast tumor (although it is rare). Mesothelioma, breast cancer, and sarcoma are also rare origins of Pancoast tumors. In children, a neuroblastoma may manifest with a Pancoast-like configuration.

Comments

Manifestations of Pancoast Tumors

The superior sulcus (Pancoast) syndrome may include ipsilateral arm pain in the C8-T2 distribution and atrophy of the hand muscles, in addition to Horner syndrome and brachial plexopathy. Rib destruction and vertebral body infiltration also may occur. The lung cancers are usually non–small cell carcinomas.

Treatment of Pancoast Tumors

Often patients receive preoperative and postoperative irradiation (the latter for patients with incomplete resections). Among patients with incomplete resection, large adenopathy, or malignant invasion of ribs, rates of long-term survival are poor. Two of the most common sites of postoperative residual tumor with a Pancoast carcinoma are the brachial plexus and the supra-aortic vessels. Therefore, tumor spread to and around these sites must be assessed radiologically. In this case (Figures S121-1 and S121-2), disease clearly encases vascular structures and, because the extent of the tumor posteriorly is analogous to what is seen here anteriorly, the brachial plexus is also in jeopardy (seen best on the sagittal scan). Rib erosion in Pancoast tumors occurs in 50% of cases, with equal involvement of the first or second rib, and the third rib is eroded in 20% of cases.

Reference

Archie VC, Thomas CR Jr. Superior sulcus tumors: a mini-review. *Oncologist.* 2004;9(5):550-555.

Cross-Reference

Neuroradiology: The Requisites, 3rd ed, 504-505.

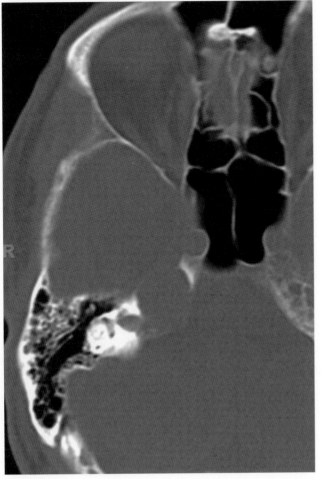

Figure 122-1

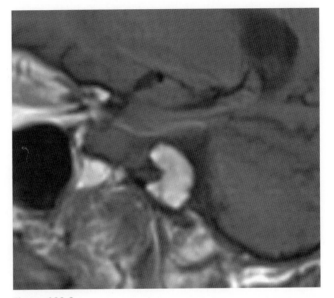

Figure 122-2

HISTORY: A young adult patient presents with right-sided tinnitus and hearing loss.

1. Which of the following should be included in the differential diagnosis? (Choose all that apply.)
   A. Aneurysm
   B. Mucocele
   C. Cholesterol granuloma
   D. Schwannoma

2. What lesion of the petrous apex has the most restricted diffusion?
   A. Petrous apicitis
   B. Epidermoid
   C. Schwannoma
   D. Aneurysm

3. What is the danger in not treating a cholesterol granuloma of the petrous apex?
   A. Pseudoaneurysms of the petrous carotid artery
   B. Chemical meningitis
   C. Septic thrombophlebitis
   D. All of the above

4. In what percentage of patients is the petrous apex aerated?
   A. 0% to 20%
   B. 21% to 40%
   C. 41% to 60%
   D. >60%

See Supplemental Figures section for additional figures and legends for this case.

CASE 122

Cholesterol Granuloma

1. **B and C.** The lesion is in a classic location and has the signal intensity for cholesterol granuloma, appearing bright on T1-weighted images. Mucocele is also a possibility, although it is fairly rare in the petrous apex. Aneurysms are not embedded in the petrous apex, and the schwannomas do not often appear bright on unenhanced T1-weighted images.

2. **B.** Epidermoid produces a bright signal on diffusion-weighted images and demonstrates restricted diffusion on apparent diffusion coefficient maps. In rare cases, it also produces a bright signal on T1-weighted images.

3. **D.** Pseudoaneurysms of the petrous carotid artery, chemical meningitis, and septic thrombophlebitis may all be caused by cholesterol granuloma of the petrous apex through destruction, invasion, and dehiscence. Pseudoaneurysms can cause erosion of the carotid canal. Septic thrombophlebitis may involve the petrosal sinuses, jugular veins, or both.

4. **B.** The petrous apex is aerated in 30% of affected patients. Fatty infiltration of the apex is probably just as common.

Comment

Treatment of Cholesterol Granulomas

Cholesterol granulomas (also known as *blue dome cysts, chocolate cysts, cholesterol cysts,* and *giant cholesterol cysts*) appear characteristically bright on T1-weighted scans and are more dense than epidermoids on computed tomography (Figures S122-1, S122-2, and S122-3). Cholesterol granulomas are the most common primary expansile lesion of the petrous apex. At the author's institution, cholesterol granulomas may be drained endoscopically by placement of drainage catheters from the sphenoid sinus into the petrous apex. The option for this treatment depends on the proximity of those two structures to each other and the degree of aeration of the two. This procedure is not definitive surgery, but because of the nearness of cholesterol granulomas to the carotid arteries, the fifth cranial nerve, the sixth cranial nerve, and the petrosal sinuses, most patients opt for the least invasive surgery that relieves symptoms. The alternative is skull base surgery. Drainage with or without removal of the cyst lining can be achieved through the transcanal infracochlear, transmastoid infralabyrinthine, middle fossa, translabyrinthine, and transotic approaches. Paluzzi and colleagues (2012) categorized cholesterol granuloma treatment as three options:

- Type A (for larger cholesterol granulomas that extend medially): transclival approach, with the possibility of lateralizing the paraclival internal carotid artery
- Type B (for cholesterol granulomas with lateral and inferior extension below the petrous internal carotid artery): infrapetrous approach
- Type C (for very lateral cholesterol granulomas): open approach

Epidermoids

Congenital cholesteatomas are actually epidermoids of the temporal bone, as opposed to acquired cholesteatomas, which develop in the middle ear. In the temporal bone, epidermoids may develop in the middle ear, near the geniculate ganglion, and at the petrous apex; cholesterol granulomas are usually confined to the petrous apex or postoperative cavities. Epidermoids are caused by congenital epithelial rests, and the temporal bone is the most common site of occurrence in the calvaria. Calvarial epidermoids are of low density with well-defined borders on computed tomography. Low intensity is usually seen on T1-weighted scans; rarely do they appear bright on T1-weighted scans. They appear bright on diffusion-weighted images with restricted diffusion. Treatment for these two entities is different. Epidermoids necessitate complete removal.

Reference

Paluzzi A, Gardner P, Fernandez-Miranda JC, Pinheiro-Neto CD, Scopel TF, Koutourousiou M, et al. Endoscopic endonasal approach to cholesterol granulomas of the petrous apex: a series of 17 patients: clinical article. *J Neurosurg.* 2012;116(4):792-798.

Cross-Reference

Neuroradiology: The Requisites, 3rd ed, 411-413.

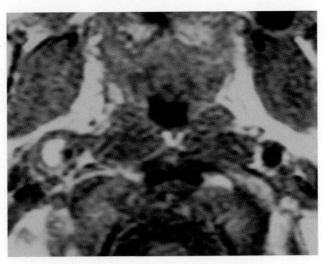

Figure 123-1

HISTORY: The patient presents with right-sided neck pain after a motor vehicle collision.

1. Which of the following should be included in the differential diagnosis? (Choose all that apply.)
   A. Paraganglioma
   B. Schwannoma
   C. Internal jugular vein thrombosis
   D. Carotid dissection

2. What are the likely symptoms in a patient with this entity?
   A. Neck pain, neurologic deficit (stroke), Horner syndrome, and/or transient ischemic attacks
   B. Neck pain, neurologic deficit (stroke), Gradenigo syndrome, and/or transient ischemic attacks
   C. Trigeminal neuralgia, neurologic deficit (stroke), Horner syndrome, and/or transient ischemic attacks
   D. Neck pain, neurologic deficit (stroke), Horner syndrome, and/or Lemierre syndrome.

3. What disease entity does not predispose the patient to carotid artery dissection?
   A. Fibromuscular dysplasia
   B. Marfan syndrome
   C. Ehlers-Danlos syndrome
   D. Hunter syndrome

4. Dissection affects which portion of the carotid artery most frequently?
   A. Common
   B. Cervical internal
   C. External
   D. Intracranial internal

See Supplemental Figures section for additional figures and legends for this case.

CASE 123

Carotid Dissection

1. **D.** A clot in the wall indicates carotid dissection. There is no mass, and so paraganglioma and schwannoma should not be included in the diagnosis.

2. **A.** The most likely symptoms of carotid dissection include neck pain, neurologic deficit (stroke), Horner syndrome, and/or transient ischemic attacks.

3. **D.** There is no association between carotid artery dissection and Hunter syndrome. Fibromuscular dysplasia, Marfan syndrome, and Ehlers-Danlos syndrome all predispose the patient to carotid artery dissection.

4. **B.** The cervical portion of the internal carotid artery is most frequently subject to dissection, in 68% of cases; the petrous portion is affected least commonly.

Comment

Manifestation of Carotid Dissection

Dissection causes approximately 10% of vascular strokes in patients younger than 20 years; as a cause of stroke in this age group, it is second to sickle cell disease. Patients may present with strokes, transient ischemic attacks, headache, neck pain, or Horner syndrome, or they may have no symptoms and the dissection is incidentally discovered, for example, after motor vehicle collisions. In rare cases, the manifestation is an enlarging neck mass, presumed to be a pseudoaneurysm. Dissection of the intracranial arteries is uncommon; it usually affects the middle cerebral artery and accounts for fewer than 10% of all dissections. Bilateral vascular dissections of either the carotid artery or the vertebral arteries have been reported in up to 28% of cases. The V_2 and V_3 portions of the vertebral artery are most commonly affected.

Imaging Findings

Magnetic resonance angiography (MRA) is probably the best study for detecting internal carotid artery dissection (Figure S123-1). Fat-suppression is particularly helpful in visualizing the wall hematoma opposite a dark (suppressed) background on unenhanced T1-weighted scans. There are areas in which magnetic resonance imaging (MRI) is fraught with problems: at any place where the vessel begins to turn in plane (seen with the vertebral arteries at the C1-C2 level and the petrous portion of the carotid artery), as a result of flow-related enhancement, or in the presence of huge atherosclerotic plaque with intra-plaque hemorrhage. In most cases, however, MRI is an efficacious study. On MRA, the radiologist should look at the raw data source images and include phase-contrast MRA (in which the high-intensity wall hematoma is nulled, unlike the time-of-flight MRA) if confusion exists. Monitoring affected patients with MRI and MRA for the development of pseudoaneurysms is warranted because rupture of the carotid artery or thrombo-embolism from the aneurysm can be catastrophic.

Treatment for Carotid Dissection

To treat dissections, most clinicians initiate anticoagulation with aspirin or other antiplatelet drugs. For symptomatic cervical carotid artery dissection with pseudoaneurysms or strokes, endovascular treatment has become popular. Stents to keep the carotid artery open or to prevent pseudoaneurysm can be used but are usually reserved for patients in whom emboli enter into the intracranial circulation even after medical treatment or in those who have an enlarging pseudoaneurysm.

Reference

Rodallec MH, Marteau V, Gerber S, Desmottes L, Zins M. Craniocervical arterial dissection: spectrum of imaging findings and differential diagnosis. *Radiographics*. 2008;28:1711-1728.

Cross-Reference

Neuroradiology: The Requisites, 3rd ed, 495-497.

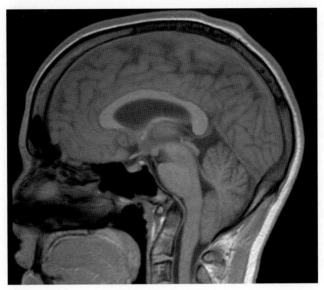

Figure 124-1

HISTORY: A patient presented with frequent headaches.

1. Which of the following should be included in the differential diagnosis? (Choose all that apply.)
   A. Platybasia
   B. Basilar invagination
   C. Chiari type I malformation
   D. Klippel-Feil syndrome

2. Which of the following is the correct definition of the basal (Weneke) angle?
   A. The angle formed by a line from the nasion to the basion and a line from the basion to the opisthion of the foramen magnum
   B. The angle formed by a line from the hard palate to the tuberculum sellae and a line from the tuberculum sellae down the plane of the clivus to the anterior margin of the foramen magnum
   C. The angle formed by a line from the nasion to the tuberculum sellae and a line from the tuberculum sellae down the plane of the clivus to the anterior margin of the foramen magnum
   D. The angle formed by a line from the hard palate to the tuberculum sellae and a line from the tuberculum sellae down the plane of the clivus to the posterior margin of the foramen magnum

3. What is the normal value for the basal angle?
   A. ≤110 degrees
   B. ≤125 degrees
   C. ≤135 degrees
   D. ≤143 degrees

4. What are not common causes of platybasia?
   A. Paget disease
   B. Down syndrome
   C. Achondroplasia
   D. Fibrous dysplasia

See Supplemental Figures section for additional figures and legends for this case.

CASE 124

Basilar Invagination, Platybasia, Chiari Type I Malformation

1. **A, B, and C.** The basal angle is greater than normal, which indicates platybasia. The odontoid rides far above the McGregor line, which indicates basilar invagination. The tonsils are low, which indicates Arnold-Chiari type I malformation. No fusion anomaly is present, and so Klippel-Feil syndrome should not be included in the diagnosis.

2. **C.** The basal (Weneke) angle is the angle formed by a line from the nasion to the tuberculum sellae and a line from the tuberculum sellae down the plane of the clivus to the anterior margin of the foramen magnum.

3. **D.** The normal value for the basal angle is less than 143 degrees.

4. **D.** Fibrous dysplasia is not a common cause of platybasia. Paget disease is a common cause in adults; Down syndrome is a common cause in children; and achondroplasia is a common cause in people with dwarfism.

Comment

Relevant Anatomy

Platybasia refers to flattening of the basal angle, whereas *basal invagination* reflects superior extensions of the odontoid process through the plane of the hard palate and foramen magnum. The basal (Weneke) angle is used to define platybasia and is the angle formed by the lines from the nasion to the tuberculum sellae and from the tuberculum sellae down the plane of the clivus to the anterior margin of the foramen magnum.

The Chamberlain line (from the hard palate to the posterior margin of the foramen magnum) and the McGregor line (from the hard palate to the undersurface of the occiput) are used to define basilar invagination. In basilar invagination, the dens lies more than 5 mm above these two lines. Basilar invagination is more common than platybasia, and Chiari type I malformations may occur with either entity. Depending on the severity of the disorder (usually based on the degree of spinal cord compression), operative decompression may be required. This is particularly true if atlantoaxial dislocation coexists, as in patients who have Down syndrome, Morquio syndrome, and other congenital disorders.

Manifestation of Basilar Invagination, Platybasia, and Chiari Type I Malformation

The concurrence of basilar invagination, platybasia, and Chiari type I malformation, as in this patient (Figure S124-1), suggests that skull base development is linked with the rhombencephalon. Compression of the brainstem or cervical portion of the spinal cord may lead to cranial nerve symptoms, gait abnormalities, myelopathy, or pain syndromes. In rare cases, ischemia of the vertebrobasilar system may be the presenting finding, usually in the more severe cases. Surgical decompression is reserved for the more severe degrees of basilar invagination and platybasia. Causes of platybasia include Paget disease, osteomalacia, renal osteodystrophy, Down syndrome, achondroplasia, and osteogenesis imperfecta.

Reference

Ghosh PS, Taute CT, Ghosh D. Teaching neuroImages: platybasia and basilar invagination in osteogenesis imperfecta. *Neurology.* 2011; 77(18):e108.

Cross-Reference

Neuroradiology: The Requisites, 3rd ed, 300-301.

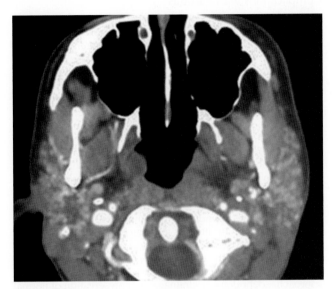

Figure 125-1

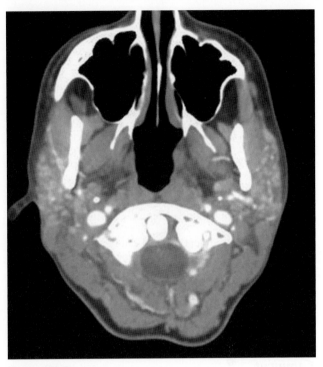

Figure 125-2

HISTORY: A patient presents with bilateral jaw fullness and discomfort, pain, and inflammation.

1. Which of the following should be included in the differential diagnosis? (Choose all that apply.)
   A. Sialadenitis
   B. Sialosis
   C. Parotitis
   D. Sialocele

2. What is the most common cause of parotitis?
   A. Sarcoidosis
   B. *Pseudomonas* infection
   C. Human immunodeficiency virus (HIV) infection
   D. Mumps

3. What is the clinical hallmark of parotitis?
   A. Purulent material that can be expressed from the Stensen duct
   B. Purulent material that can be expressed from the Wharton duct
   C. Elevated white blood cell count and superficial cellulitis over the ear
   D. All of the above

4. Of the bacterial causes of parotitis, which two are most common?
   A. *Mycobacterium tuberculosis* and staphylococci
   B. *Haemophilus influenzae* and streptococci
   C. Streptococci and staphylococci
   D. *Pseudomonas* organisms and staphylococci

See Supplemental Figures section for additional figures and legends for this case.

CASE 125

Parotitis

1. **A and C.** *Sialadenitis* is the generic term for salivary glandular inflammation, and parotitis is parotid inflammation. Sialosis is glandular enlargement but is usually not painful or accompanied by inflammation. Sialocele is usually manifested as a cyst that is connected to the ductal system.

2. **D.** Mumps is the most common cause of parotitis (paramyxovirus). Sarcoidosis is a cause but is not common. *Pseudomonas* infection is not associated with parotitis. HIV infection is not a usual cause of painful inflammation, but cysts and lymphoepithelial nodules can occur here.

3. **A.** In parotitis, purulent material can be expressed from the Stensen duct. This is usually bacterial. The Stensen duct is the duct of the parotid gland.

4. **C.** Streptococci and staphylococci are the most common bacterial causes of parotitis. *M. tuberculosis* is next most common.

Comment

Causes of Parotitis

The parotid gland may appear inflamed with many causes of cervical adenitis because of drainage to intraparotid lymph nodes and hence sialadenitis (Figures S125-1 and S125-2). Paramyxovirus, which causes mumps, is the most common viral cause, and staphylococci and streptococci are the most common bacterial causes. Worldwide, *M. tuberculosis* and other mycobacteria may also cause parotitis. Nontuberculous mycobacterial parotitis probably affects the gland via nodal spread. HIV infection usually does not cause acute parotitis, but it does cause a gnawing ache from the benign lymphoepithelial cysts and lymphoid aggregates. Nonetheless, the most common noninfectious cause of salivary gland inflammation of any type is sialolithiasis: stone disease.

Complications with Parotitis

Parotitis often presents a quandary for clinicians. Parotid inflammation is often misinterpreted as neoplastic on parotid cytologic study, and parotid neoplasms often induce an inflammatory reaction. Furthermore, any surgery on the parotid gland is complicated by the presence of the facial nerve coursing through the gland: In an inflamed gland, it is very hard to dissect the nerve cleanly without a greater risk of injury and subsequent paralysis. Surgery is performed only when a well-defined abscess is identified and the cytologic or bacteriologic studies absolutely confirm infection.

Parotid abscesses may arise from marked ductal ectasis and retrograde infection, primary parenchymal involvement, or suppuration and consolidation of intraparotid or periparotid lymph nodes. Diabetic patients and older debilitated adults are predisposed to abscesses. In many cases, a trial of intravenous antibiotics is undertaken in the hopes that the abscess will resolve or in an attempt to reduce the infection around the abscess so that the wall of the collection "matures." A soggy parotid gland filled with purulent material is not conducive to dissecting vital cranial nerves. The surgical approach—débridement, drainage, and preservation of normal parotid tissue—is vastly different from neoplasm removal, in which a cuff of normal tissue is removed without violation of the lesion's capsule.

Reference

Yousem DM, Kraut MA, Chalian AA. Major salivary gland imaging. *Radiology.* 2000;216:19-29.

Cross-Reference

Neuroradiology: The Requisites, 3rd ed, 479-480.

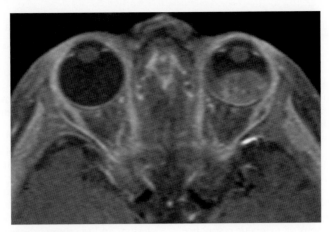

Figure 126-1

HISTORY: A 19-month-old child is referred with left-sided leukocoria.

1. Which of the following should be included in the differential diagnosis? (Choose all that apply.)
   A. Melanoma
   B. Retinoblastoma
   C. Metastasis
   D. Hemangioma

2. What percentage of retinoblastomas are bilateral?
   A. 0% to 20%
   B. 21% to 40%
   C. 41% to 60%
   D. >60%

3. What percentage of retinoblastomas show calcification?
   A. 0% to 20%
   B. 21% to 40%
   C. 41% to 60%
   D. >60%

4. What percentage of retinoblastomas are associated with a pineal region mass?
   A. 0% to 20%
   B. 21% to 40%
   C. 41% to 60%
   D. >60%

See Supplemental Figures section for additional figures and legends for this case.

CASE 126

Retinoblastoma

1. **B.** In a 19-month-old with leukocoria, the diagnosis is retinoblastoma until proven otherwise. For ocular masses, melanoma would be included in the diagnosis for an adult. Metastasis is the correct diagnosis in lung and breast cancer, and hemangioma is the diagnosis for a red lesion.

2. **B.** Of all retinoblastomas, 21% to 40% are bilateral. Most of these are familial lesions and occur in children.

3. **D.** More than 60% of retinoblastomas show calcification. Approximately 90% of lesions calcify, but the calcification may (as in this case) not be obvious on magnetic resonance imaging.

4. **A.** A small percentage of retinoblastomas (0% to 20%) are associated with a pineal region mass. That pineal mass is the source of the term *trilateral retinoblastoma* when the ocular lesions are bilateral.

Comment

Retinoblastomas in Infancy

Retinoblastomas are the most common ocular tumors of infancy (Figure S126-1). They also rank as one of the most common infantile malignancies, along with teratomas, neuroblastomas, and nephroblastomas. Retinoblastomas may be congenital in approximately 35% of cases; in 90% of this subset, they are bilateral. Calcification is very common.

Hereditary Retinoblastoma

Trilateral retinoblastomas are pineal region tumors that occur in patients with hereditary retinoblastoma. These typically manifest at the ages of 4 to 7 years, approximately 2 years after the initial presentation with retinoblastoma. Patients with hereditary retinoblastomas are also at risk for sarcomas (often in the irradiated field) and melanomas.

Treatment of Retinoblastomas

Treatment options for retinoblastomas include (1) enucleation (for large tumors); (2) radiation therapy, including intensity-modulated radiation therapy, stereotactic radiotherapy, proton beam radiation therapy, and plaque radiotherapy, in which brachytherapy radioactive seeds are applied to the tumor from the scleral surface of the globe; (3) cryotherapy to freeze the lesion; and (4) thermotherapy delivered by a laser beam and chemotherapy delivered via the cerebrospinal fluid or sub-tenon space through the extraocular muscles and nerves into the globe. Chemoreduction therapy can be combined with other therapies for effective treatment of larger lesions. In some academic programs, researchers are experimenting with direct instillation of chemotherapeutic agents into the ophthalmic artery by intra-arterial catheter injection.

Reference

Rao AA, Naheedy JH, Chen JY, Robbins SL, Ramkumar HL. A clinical update and radiologic review of pediatric orbital and ocular tumors. *J Oncol.* 2013;2013:975908.

Cross-Reference

Neuroradiology: The Requisites, 3rd ed, 321-323, 327-328.

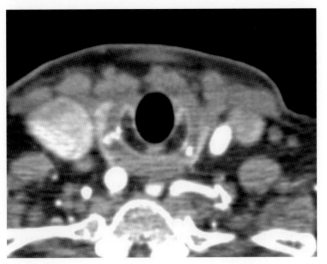

Figure 127-1

Figure 127-2

HISTORY: This is the arterial phase of a four-dimensional computed tomography (CT) for a diagnosis of hyperparathyroidism.

1. Which of the following should be included in the differential diagnosis? (Choose all that apply.)
   A. Parathyroid adenoma
   B. Thyroid adenoma
   C. Parathyroid hyperplasia
   D. Parathyroid carcinoma

2. Which of the following is the correct description of four-dimensional CT for parathyroid adenomas?
   A. Computed tomographic angiography with maximum-intensity projections of the thyroid gland
   B. Thin-section CT with three-dimensional reformatting and computed tomographic angiography
   C. Early-, late-, and delayed-phase CT of the thyroid bed
   D. Unenhanced early arterial phase, late phase, and delayed enhanced CT in a three-dimensional package

3. Which of the following is the drawback of sestamibi imaging for parathyroid adenomas?
   A. Lack of sensitivity
   B. Lack of specificity
   C. Frequent missing of neck lesions
   D. Radiation dosage

4. What is the benefit of preoperative localization of parathyroid adenomas?
   A. Decreased operating room times
   B. Need for only unilateral exploration of the neck
   C. Decreased rates of morbidity
   D. All of the above

See Supplemental Figures section for additional figures and legends for this case.

CASE 127

Parathyroid Adenoma

1. **A.** The lesion on the images is on the left, below the thyroid gland, and posterior. Therefore, the diagnosis should be parathyroid adenoma (not thyroid adenoma). Because it is a single lesion, the diagnosis would not include parathyroid hyperplasia. Parathyroid carcinoma is very rare, seen in 1% of patients with hyperparathyroidism.

2. **D.** Four-dimensional CT for parathyroid adenomas comprises unenhanced CT, early arterial phase enhanced CT, late phase enhanced venous CT, and delayed enhanced CT in a three-dimensional package. The idea is to distinguish the parathyroid adenomas from thyroid nodules and lymph nodes by reviewing these phases.

3. **A.** The drawback of sestamibi imaging for parathyroid adenomas is lack of sensitivity. Sestamibi imaging for parathyroid adenomas is excellent in the neck (not in the chest). Unfortunately, the anatomic localization also is lacking with sestamibi.

4. **D.** The benefits of preoperative localization of parathyroid adenomas include decreased operating room times, the need for only unilateral exploration of the neck, and decreased rates of morbidity. Nonetheless, some surgeons explore without any imaging at all and still have reasonable success.

Comment

Causes of Hyperparathyroidism

Hyperparathyroidism is most commonly caused by a solitary parathyroid adenoma (Figures S127-1, S127-2, and S127-3). If that were the only cause, imaging would be highly accurate with ultrasonography, technetium sestamibi imaging, CT, and magnetic resonance imaging. Unfortunately, hyperparathyroidism may also be caused by multiple adenomas, as well as by parathyroid hyperplasia with multiple nontumorous enlarged glands. All of the modalities have an issue with parathyroid hyperplasia. In addition, hormonally active parathyroid carcinomas, which are rare, can cause hyperparathyroidism.

Benefits of Four-Dimensional Computed Tomography

Four-dimensional CT has been advocated to help with the diagnosis of parathyroid disease of all types. Four-dimensional multiphase CT includes a scan of the neck without contrast, followed by contrast administration with arterial, venous, and delayed-phase scanning, whose aim is to capture the temporal changes in the enhancement of the adenomas. Parathyroid adenomas have high vascularity; thus arterial enhancement and washout occur, which allows differentiation from lymph nodes (which do not enhance early) and other potential mimickers.

Benefits of Technetium Sestamibi Scans

Technetium sestamibi nuclear medicine studies are performed with an early and delayed scanning technique. The adenomas show radiotracer uptake that, on delayed scanning, remains present even as the thyroid gland washes out. Initially, the thyroid gland itself may obscure visualization of the adenoma, but as the thyroid washes out, the parathyroid adenoma uptake becomes more apparent. Sestamibi scanning can be combined with subtraction techniques or single-photon emission computed tomography (SPECT) to enhance visualization of adenomas.

Reference

Chazen JL, Gupta A, Dunning A, Phillips CD. Diagnostic accuracy of 4D-CT for parathyroid adenomas and hyperplasia. *AJNR Am J Neuroradiol.* 2012;33(3):429-433.

Cross-Reference

Neuroradiology: The Requisites, 3rd ed, 507.

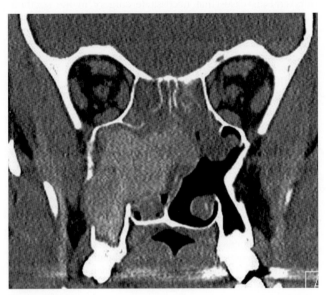

Figure 128-1

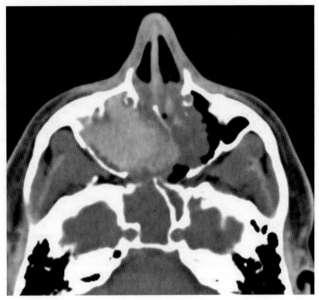

Figure 128-2

HISTORY: A patient suffers from chronic nasal congestion.

1. Which of the following should be included in the differential diagnosis? (Choose all that apply.)
   A. Hematoma
   B. Chronic rhinosinusitis
   C. Allergic fungal rhinosinusitis (AFRS)
   D. Fungus ball
   E. Juvenile angiofibroma

2. AFRS is not associated with which of the following?
   A. Increased levels of immunoglobulin E (IgE)
   B. Eosinophilia
   C. Allergic bronchopulmonary aspergillosis
   D. Cold climate
   E. Nasal polyps

3. The characteristic hyperdense sinus content in AFRS represents which one of the following?
   A. Inspissated secretions
   B. Milk of calcium
   C. Hemorrhagic inflammatory infiltrate
   D. Eosinophilic mucin
   E. Byproducts of fungal metabolism

4. Which of the following is a criterion for the diagnosis of AFRS?
   A. Appearance of sinusitis on computed tomography (CT) in addition to eosinophilia
   B. Appearance of sinusitis on CT in addition to eosinophilia and increased IgE levels
   C. Appearance of sinusitis on CT in addition to positive fungal cultures
   D. Histologic demonstration of eosinophilic mucin
   E. Histologic demonstration of fungal hyphae in eosinophilic mucin

See Supplemental Figures section for additional figures and legends for this case.

Allergic Fungal Sinusitis

1. **C.** The most likely diagnosis is AFRS. Chronic rhinosinusitis is a possibility, but hyperattenuating material is characteristic of AFRS. The diagnosis does not include hematoma. In addition, this is an unenhanced computed tomographic scan showing hyperdense secretions, not an enhancing mass, and so juvenile angiofibroma is unlikely as well. Fungus ball usually involves a single sinus.

2. **D.** AFRS is associated with increased IgE levels, eosinophilia, allergic bronchopulmonary aspergillosis, and nasal polyps. Cold climate does not affect the incidence of AFRS; it can occur in all climates.

3. **D.** The characteristic hyperdense sinus content in AFRS represents eosinophilic mucin. Inspissated secretions can look similar. Although trace metal elements (fungal metabolism byproducts) can be present, they are not large enough in quantity to generate hyperdensity on CT.

4. **E.** The diagnosis of AFRS requires histologic demonstration of fungal hyphae in eosinophilic mucin. The appearance of sinusitis on CT in addition to eosinophilia is a common finding in patients with atopy. The appearance of sinusitis on CT and positive fungal cultures are also common because people have fungi in their nose. The appearance of sinusitis on CT, eosinophilia, and increased IgE levels are not specific enough to diagnose AFRS. Histologic demonstration of eosinophilic mucin is not a strong enough indicator of AFRS.

Comment

Manifestation of Allergic Fungal Rhinosinusitis

AFRS is a noninvasive form of fungal infection involving the nose and sinuses. It is common, accounting for 6% to 9% of rhinosinusitis cases that necessitate surgery in the southern states. It is much less common in the northern part of the United States. Patients present with symptoms of chronic rhinosinusitis and exhibit features of hypersensitivity, including eosinophilia, increased serum IgE levels, and atopy.

Imaging Findings

On imaging, opacification of the paranasal sinuses with hyperattenuating material is characteristic (Figures S128-1 and S128-2). The involved sinuses often exhibit expansion with thinning and remodeling of the bony walls, sometimes with focal dehiscences. In some patients, involvement is unilateral, but more commonly, all paranasal sinuses are involved bilaterally. Sinus contents show markedly decreased signal on T2-weighted magnetic resonance images with variable, but often bright, T1 signal and generally no enhancement other than a thin rim of mucosal enhancement along the periphery of the air cells. The sinus contents have the consistency of peanut butter in surgical specimens. The definitive diagnosis of AFRS can be made only when the histologic examination demonstrates fungal hyphae in the allergic mucin, which corresponds to hyperattenuating or T2-hypointense material, and lack of mucosal invasion.

Reference

Manning SC, Merkel M, Kriesel K, Vuitch F, Marple B. Computed tomography and magnetic resonance diagnosis of allergic fungal sinusitis. *Laryngoscope*. 1997;107(2):170-176.

Cross-Reference

Neuroradiology: The Requisites, 3rd ed, 430-431.

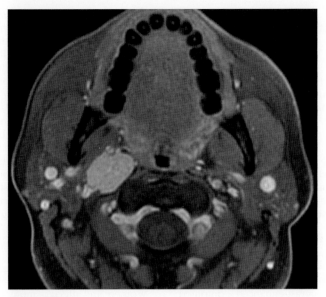

Figure 129-1

HISTORY: This patient has moderate difficulty swallowing solid foods.

1. Which of the following should be included in the differential diagnosis? (Choose all that apply.)
   A. Schwannoma
   B. Neurofibroma
   C. Paraganglioma
   D. Lymphadenopathy

2. Which one of the following locations is atypical for a paraganglioma?
   A. The jugular foramen
   B. The carotid bifurcation
   C. The middle ear
   D. The sinonasal cavity

3. What percentage of head and neck paragangliomas are vasoactive (i.e., secrete vasoactive substances)?
   A. 0% to 5%
   B. 6% to 10%
   C. 11% to 15%
   D. >15%

4. What is the most common head and neck paraganglioma?
   A. Glomus tympanicum
   B. Glomus jugulare
   C. Carotid body tumor
   D. Glomus vagale

See Supplemental Figures section for additional figures and legends for this case.

CASE 129

Carotid Body Tumor

1. **A, B, C, and D.** Carotid sheath tumors include schwannoma, neurofibroma, and paraganglioma. The lesion could also represent lymphadenopathy, although this is less likely because of the absence of a primary aerodigestive tumor.

2. **D.** The sinonasal cavity is not a common site for paragangliomas. The jugular foramen is a common site for a glomus jugulare; the carotid bifurcation, for a carotid body tumor; and the middle ear, for a glomus tympanicum. That said, paragangliomas can occur in unusual locations, including the spinal column.

3. **A.** Of all head and neck paragangliomas, 3% to 4% are vasoactive (i.e., secrete vasoactive substances). For this reason, they are screened before angiographic procedures, but not necessarily before contrast-enhanced computed tomography.

4. **C.** Carotid body tumor is the most common head and neck paraganglioma. Glomus jugulare is the second most common, just behind carotid body tumor. Glomus vagale and glomus tympanicum are not very common.

Comment

Paragangliomas in the Head and Neck

Carotid body tumors are the most common of the four frequent varieties of paragangliomas in the head and neck (Figure S129-1). Like pheochromocytomas, these tumors are derived from neural crest chromaffin cells that have the capacity to secrete (at a rate of 3% to 4%) vasoactive agents, although they are less prevalent than pheochromocytomas. The substance secreted by carotid body tumors is norepinephrine, which may dramatically influence the patient's blood pressure during administration of iodine-based contrast agents for computed tomography or angiography.

Incidence of Carotid Body Tumors

Among paragangliomas that occur sporadically, the incidence of multiplicity is about 15%, but of hereditary paragangliomas, the incidence of multiplicity may exceed 50%. The hereditary form may affect as many as one third of all patients with head and neck paragangliomas. Malignant paragangliomas, defined as those that metastasize, occur in 3% of all cases. Although magnetic resonance imaging is an excellent means for evaluating multiple paragangliomas, conventional angiography may be the best test, and indium-111–octreotide scintigraphy has a sensitivity of 88% to 97% and a specificity of 75% to 82%.

Features of Carotid Body Tumors

Women are affected more commonly than men by carotid body tumors; the mean age at presentation is between 40 and 50 years. A neck mass, difficulty swallowing, or hoarseness may be the presenting symptom. Surgical therapy is usually curative; the rate of recurrence after incomplete resection is 5%.

Reference

Colen TY, Mihm FG, Mason TP, Roberson JB. Catecholamine-secreting paragangliomas: recent progress in diagnosis and perioperative management. *Skull Base.* 2009;19(6):377-385.

Cross-Reference

Neuroradiology: The Requisites, 3rd ed, 494-499.

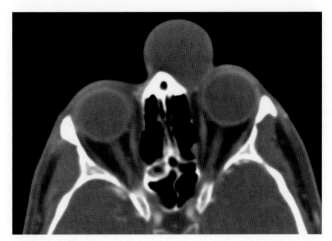

Figure 130-1

HISTORY: A computed tomographic scan was ordered for an 8-year-old patient with a mass protruding from the nasal tip.

1. Which of the following should be included in the differential diagnosis? (Choose all that apply.)
   A. Encephalocele
   B. Nasal glioma
   C. Dermoid
   D. Epidermoid
   E. Sebaceous cyst

2. Which of the following statements is correct in regard to nasal gliomas?
   A. They are usually grade I according to the World Health Organization (WHO).
   B. They are more commonly intranasal than extranasal.
   C. They have a cerebrospinal fluid connection intracranially.
   D. They have a fibrous connection intracranially.
   E. They have a white matter connection intracranially.

3. Which of the following statements is correct in regard to nasal epidermoids?
   A. They are not tumors.
   B. They may have connections to the intracranial compartment.
   C. They are also called *epidermal inclusion cysts.*
   D. All of the above.

4. What is the most common site of head and neck dermoids?
   A. Nose
   B. Periorbital area
   C. Oral cavity
   D. None of the above

See Supplemental Figures section for additional figures and legends for this case.

CASE 130

Nasal Epidermoid

1. **A, C, D, and E.** The diagnosis includes encephalocele, dermoid, epidermoid, and sebaceous cyst. Since it is a cystic lesion, nasal glioma should not be included. Otherwise, for solid lesions, vascular tumors (hemangiomas) and vascular malformations would be included too.

2. **D.** Nasal gliomas have a fibrous connection intracranially. Sixty percent are extranasal and 40% intranasal; both may have a fibrous connection to the intracranial compartment but not to the meninges.

3. **D.** All of the statements are true. Epidermoids are congenital rests or remnants.

4. **B.** Head and neck dermoids are most commonly periorbital. The oral cavity is the second most common site, and the nose is third.

Comment

Relevant Anatomy

After the primitive diverticulum in the prenasal space touches the skin of the tip of the nose, it regresses intracranially, and it may drag ectodermal elements back with it (Figure S130-1). Incomplete regression of the ectodermal elements of the embryonic frontonasal diverticulum may trap nonglial tissue. In doing so, it may create a tract between the nasal bone and the septum. Cells trapped in this tract may proliferate, producing a dermoid or an epidermoid. More than 50% of head and neck dermoids are found in the periorbital region; 25%, in the oral cavity; and 13%, in the nasal cavities. Of isolated cysts, only 10% communicate with the intracranial compartment via a sinus. Potential complications include meningitis, brain abscess, thrombosis of the cavernous sinus, periorbital cellulitis, nasal abscesses, fistulas, and epidural abscesses.

Terminology

Other terms used for epidermoid cysts include (1) *follicular infundibular cysts,* (2) *epidermal cysts,* (3) epidermal inclusion cysts (implanted epidermal elements in the dermis), (4) *sebaceous cyst* (which implies that the cyst is of sebaceous origin), and (5) milia (very small, superficial epidermoid cysts). If the cysts include dermal elements, they are called *dermoids.* This was an epidermoid.

Reference

Valencia MP, Castillo M. Congenital and acquired lesions of the nasal septum: a practical guide for differential diagnosis. *Radiographics.* 2008;28:205-223.

Cross-Reference

Neuroradiology: The Requisites, 3rd ed, 280-282, 282-283, 352, 371-373, 445.

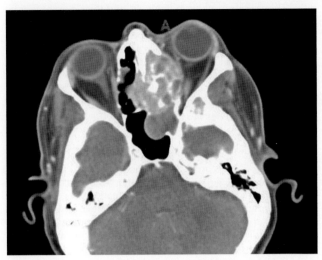

Figure 131-1

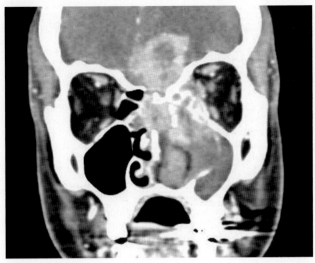

Figure 131-2

HISTORY: An elderly woman presents with headaches and nasal congestion.

1. Which of the following should be included in the differential diagnosis? (Choose all that apply.)
   A. Squamous cell carcinoma
   B. Sinonasal undifferentiated carcinoma (SNUC)
   C. Olfactory neuroblastoma
   D. Rhabdomyosarcoma
   E. Melanoma

2. What imaging finding is *not* demonstrated?
   A. Intracranial spread
   B. Intraorbital spread
   C. Obstructed secretions
   D. Bone destruction
   E. Cavernous sinus invasion

3. What is the unusual feature of SNUC that distinguishes it from other sinonasal cancers?
   A. Early metastases
   B. Retropharyngeal lymphadenopathy
   C. Dural/leptomeningeal spread
   D. Perineural spread
   E. Subarachnoid seeding

4. What is the rate of 5-year survival with SNUC?
   A. 0% to 20%
   B. 21% to 40%
   C. 41% to 60%
   D. 61% to 80%
   E. >80%

See Supplemental Figures section for additional figures and legends for this case.

CASE 131

Sinonasal Undifferentiated Carcinoma

1. **A, B, C, and E.** The most likely diagnosis is squamous cell carcinoma. Olfactory neuroblastoma, SNUC, and melanoma are less common than squamous cell carcinoma but may appear similar on imaging (although this lesion is relatively large for melanoma, which manifests earlier in life). Rhabdomyosarcoma is rare except in children and would not occur in an elderly woman.

2. **E.** The images do not depict the cavernous sinus, and the location of the lesion is more anterior than that. The imaging findings demonstrated include intracranial spread, intraorbital spread, obstructed secretions, proptosis, extraocular muscle invasion, and bone destruction.

3. **C.** Dural/leptomeningeal spread is an unusual feature that is characteristic of SNUC, as opposed to other sinonasal cancers. This makes surgical treatment much more complicated and chemoradiation therapy a frequent occurrence.

4. **A.** The rate of 5-year survival with SNUC is 0% to 20%. This is one of the worst cancers of the sinonasal cavity, partly because of its aggressiveness and intracranial growth pattern.

Comment

Incidence of Sinonasal Undifferentiated Carcinomas

SNUCs are highly aggressive lesions of the sinonasal cavity that are more common in men than in women by a 2.5:1 ratio. They occur in older individuals, and their manifestations include nasal congestion, epistaxis, diplopia, pain, and headache. The symptoms are rapidly progressive. They are relatively rare cancers of the sinonasal cavity as 60% to 70% of sinonasal malignancies are squamous cell carcinomas, 10% to 20% are adenocarcinomas, and the rest are esthesioneuroblastomas, adenoid cystic carcinomas, other salivary gland origin tumors, melanoma, lymphoma, and rhabdomyosarcomas. Smoking and exposure to wood dust, formaldehyde, nickel, chromium, and asbestos are risk factors for sinonasal cancers.

Imaging Findings

On imaging, SNUCs are large tumors that often span one or more sinonasal regions (Figures S131-1 and S131-2). Intraorbital and intracranial spread at presentation is common. A recent review reported dural invasion in 50% of cases, cavernous sinus spread in 30%, periorbital invasion in 43%, and orbital invasion in 30%. Nodal disease, however, was present in only 10% to 30% of patients.

Treatment and Survival Rates

Treatment is usually the intensive combination of surgery, chemotherapy, and radiation therapy. SNUC is, however, relatively radioresistant. Two-year survival rates are usually quoted as 40% to 50%, and 5-year disease-free survival is very rare.

Reference

Enepekides DJ. Sinonasal undifferentiated carcinoma: an update. *Curr Opin Otolaryngol Head Neck Surg.* 2005;13(4):222-225.

Cross-Reference

Neuroradiology: The Requisites, 3rd ed, 436.

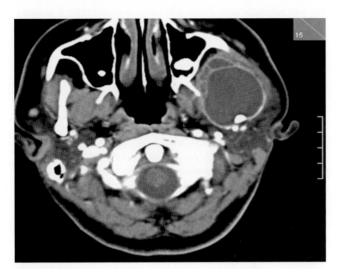

Figure 132-1

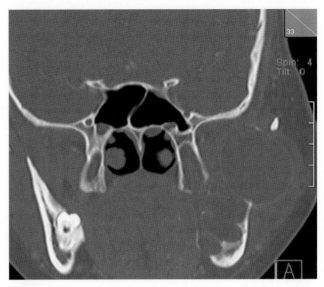

Figure 132-2

HISTORY: A patient has a palpable mass and left-sided jaw pain.

1. Which of the following should be included in the differential diagnosis? (Choose all that apply.)
   A. Dentigerous cyst
   B. Radicular cyst
   C. Odontogenic keratocyst
   D. Complex odontoma
   E. Ameloblastoma

2. What condition is associated with odontogenic keratocysts (keratocystic odontogenic tumor [KOT])?
   A. Gorham syndrome
   B. Gotham syndrome
   C. Blue rubber bleb nevus syndrome
   D. Gorlin syndrome
   E. Gardner syndrome

3. How can apparent diffusion coefficient maps differentiate KOTs from ameloblastomas?
   A. ADCs are higher in nonenhancing portions of ameloblastomas than of KOTs.
   B. ADCs are lower in nonenhancing portions of ameloblastomas than of KOTs.
   C. ADCs are higher in enhancing portions of ameloblastomas than of KOTs.
   D. All of the above.
   E. None of the above.

4. Which of the following is true?
   A. Ameloblastomas have more solid and more enhancing components than KOTs.
   B. Approximately 5% of ameloblastomas metastasize.
   C. Multicystic ameloblastoma is more common than unicystic ameloblastoma in the maxilla.
   D. The prognosis in metastatic ameloblastoma is excellent despite the metastases.

See Supplemental Figures section for additional figures and legends for this case.

CASE 132

Ameloblastoma

1. **E.** The image is most compatible with ameloblastoma because of the multiloculated cystic and solid components. The other lesions are more often associated with unerupted teeth (dentigerous), carious teeth (radicular), and solid components (odontomas).

2. **D.** Gorlin syndrome is associated with odontogenic keratocysts (KOTs). Gorham syndrome is associated with idiopathic vanishing bone; blue rubber bleb nevus syndrome, with cutaneous and gastrointestinal hemangiomas; and Gardner syndrome, with osteomas and colonic polyps.

3. **A.** ADC values are higher in the nonenhancing portions of ameloblastomas than of KOTs. This may be attributable to fluid components.

4. **A.** Ameloblastomas are more commonly solid. Metastasis, which portends a worse prognosis, occurs in only 2% of ameloblastomas. Although one thinks of ameloblastoma when lesions are multicystic, ameloblastomas are more commonly unicystic than multicystic when in the maxilla. Thus unilocularity cannot rule out maxillary ameloblastomas.

Comment

Implications of Ameloblastomas

Ameloblastomas usually affect the mandible in the molar region. They have both solid and cystic components, and magnetic resonance imaging in particular may also reveal solid enhancing areas (Figures S132-1, S132-2, S132-3, and S132-4). The non-enhancing components have higher apparent diffusion coefficient values than those of KOTs because KOTS have higher levels of desquamated keratin, which raises the cyst viscosity and lowers the ADC value. If the jaw lesion is multicystic with solid components, it is probably ameloblastoma. If the lesion is unilocular and along the long axis of the mandible, it is probably KOT, although ameloblastomas are also often unilocular.

Associations with Ameloblastomas

A number of dental lesions are associated with syndromes. KOT is associated with Gorlin basal cell nevus syndrome. Osteomas, supernumerary teeth, and sebaceous cysts are associated with Gardner syndrome. Cherubism is associated with Noonan syndrome. Patients with the syndrome of synovitis, acne, pustulosis, hyperostosis, and osteitis (SAPHO syndrome) may have periosteal reactions along the mandible. Down syndrome is characterized by dental caries. Fibrous dysplasia occurs with McCune-Albright syndrome.

Odontogenic Tumors

Odontomas are the most common dense lesions of the jawbones, accounting for more than two thirds of such lesions reported. Compound odontomas affect the maxilla and produce cystic areas with small, toothlike radiodensities on imaging, whereas complex odontomas affect the mandible and are more solidly dense and calcified. Ameloblastoma is the second most common odontogenic tumor (with the exclusion of KOTs, whose status as tumors is still being debated). Of all ameloblastomas, 80% affect the mandible, and 80% of those in the mandible are multilocular (40% in the maxilla). Of the multilocular tumors, 80% recur.

Reference

Sumi M, Ichikawa Y, Katayama I, Tashiro S, Nakamura T. Diffusion-weighted MR imaging of ameloblastomas and keratocystic odontogenic tumors: differentiation by apparent diffusion coefficients of cystic lesions. *AJNR Am J Neuroradiol.* 2008;29(10):1897-1901.

Cross-Reference

Neuroradiology: The Requisites, 3rd ed, 456, 492.

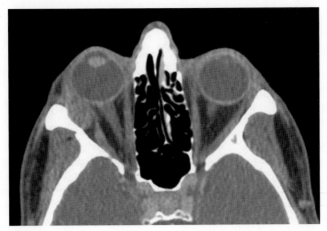

Figure 133-1

HISTORY: A 43-year-old woman has mild proptosis.

1. Which of the following should be included in the differential diagnosis? (Choose all that apply.)
   A. Adenoid cystic carcinoma
   B. Pleomorphic adenoma
   C. Dacryocystocele
   D. Sarcoidosis

2. Name the three groupings of lacrimal fossa masses.
   A. Salivary gland tumors, squamous cell carcinomas, and ductal epithelial lesions
   B. Salivary gland tumors, granulomatous lesions, and ductal epithelial lesions
   C. Ductal lesions, germ cell lesions, and lymphoid lesions
   D. Salivary gland epithelial tumors, germ cell tumors, and lymphoid lesions

3. In what percentage of cases of orbital pseudotumor is the lacrimal gland involved?
   A. 0% to 25%
   B. 25% to 50%
   C. 51% to 75%
   D. >75%

4. Is remodeling of the bone suggestive of benignity in lacrimal gland tumors?
   A. Yes, as in pleomorphic adenoma
   B. Yes, as in dermoid
   C. No, as in lymphoma
   D. No, as in squamous cell carcinoma

See Supplemental Figures section for additional figures and legends for this case.

CASE 133

Lacrimal Gland Mass: Pleomorphic Adenoma

1. **A, B, and D.** Adenoid cystic carcinoma is the most common malignancy of the lacrimal gland. Pleomorphic adenoma is the most common benign tumor of the lacrimal gland. Sarcoidosis is one of many granulomatous processes that can affect the lacrimal gland. No cyst is present, and so the differential diagnosis should not include dacryocystocele.

2. **D.** The three major types of lacrimal fossa masses are salivary gland epithelial tumors, germ cell tumors, and lymphoid lesions. These three generic groups account for 90% of lacrimal gland tumors. Epithelial lesions are most common.

3. **A.** The lacrimal gland is involved in about 15% of orbital pseudotumor cases. Most cases affect the ocular and retrobulbar structures, but the eyelids can also be involved.

4. **C.** Lymphoma in the orbit is frequently associated with bony remodeling. It seems to be less aggressive in this location. In malignant lesions such as lymphoma and adenoid cystic carcinoma, the bones of the lacrimal fossa are often remodeled.

Comment
Categories of Lacrimal Gland Lesions

Lacrimal gland lesions are usually grouped into three classic categories: (1) salivary gland epithelial tumors (pleomorphic adenoma (Figure S133-1), adenoid cystic carcinoma, malignant mixed tumors, mucoepidermoid carcinomas, adenocarcinoma), (2) germ cell tumors (dermoids), and (3) lymphoid/granulomatous lesions (lymphoma, sarcoid, pseudotumor, Wegener granulomatosis). The lacrimal gland is similar to the parotid gland in that it can have tumors of salivary gland origin and lymphoproliferative disease. The two glands may share the same disease, including sarcoidosis, Sjögren syndrome, Wegener granulomatosis, Mikulicz disease, lymphoma, pleomorphic adenoma (the most common benign tumor), and adenoid cystic carcinoma (the most common malignant tumor). In addition, the lacrimal fossa may be the site of the epidermoid-dermoid line of lesions. In contrast, lacrimal sac tumors (on the other side of the orbit) are often of epithelial origin, such as squamous cell carcinomas or transitional cell carcinomas. Mucoepidermoid carcinoma is the most common minor salivary gland tumor to affect the lacrimal sac.

Manifestations of Lacrimal Gland Lesions

In more than half of patients with lymphoma in their lacrimal glands, it is a manifestation of systemic disease, usually non-Hodgkin lymphoma. In contrast, lymphoma of the conjunctiva is usually localized to that site. The lacrimal fossa is the most common site of lymphoma in the orbit but represents only 15% of all orbital lymphomas because so many orbital sites may be involved. It often has a benign appearance with remodeled bone.

Inflammation Associated with Lacrimal Gland Lesions

The nonepithelial mass lesions of the lacrimal gland are either inflammatory or lymphoproliferative. Chronic infection (dacryoadenitis) may manifest as a lacrimal gland mass lesion. On imaging, idiopathic orbital inflammation (orbital pseudotumor) that involves the lacrimal gland is usually indistinguishable from other mass lesions or inflammatory processes. Painful eye and steroid responsiveness are informative clinical clues to the diagnosis. Granulomatous inflammatory lesions, such as sarcoidosis and Wegener granulomatosis, are also relatively frequent in the lacrimal gland and can cause unilateral or bilateral uniform enlargement of the glands. Sjögren disease usually manifests with bilateral involvement of the gland. Lymphoproliferative disorders can manifest as unilateral or bilateral gland involvement that can be limited to the orbit and may be the first manifestation of the systemic disease or metastasis of known systemic lymphoma.

Reference
Jung WS, Ahn KJ, Park MR, Kim JY, Choi JJ, Kim BS, et al. The radiological spectrum of orbital pathologies that involve the lacrimal gland and the lacrimal fossa. *Korean J Radiol.* 2007;8(4): 336-342.

Cross-Reference
Neuroradiology: The Requisites, 3rd ed, 353-355.

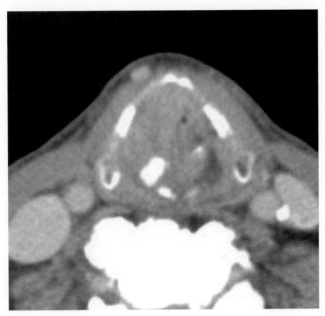

Figure 134-1

HISTORY: A 64-year-old patient presents with a change in voice quality.

1. Which of the following should be included in the differential diagnosis? (Choose all that apply.)
   A. Squamous cell carcinoma with arytenoid cartilage invasion
   B. Squamous cell carcinoma without arytenoid cartilage invasion
   C. Laryngitis
   D. Paget disease

2. What percentage of normal patients have asymmetric arytenoid sclerosis?
   A. 0% to 10%
   B. 11% to 20%
   C. 21% to 30%
   D. >30%

3. With which cartilage is the presence of sclerosis least informative in suggesting tumoral invasion?
   A. The thyroid cartilage
   B. The epiglottis
   C. The cricoid cartilage
   D. The arytenoid cartilage

4. Which finding on computed tomography (CT) is not useful for diagnosing cartilaginous invasion?
   A. Irregular ossification
   B. Soft tissue entering into the strap muscles
   C. Erosion of cartilage
   D. Obliteration of medullary space of cartilage

See Supplemental Figures section for additional figures and legends for this case.

CASE 134

Arytenoid Sclerosis with Laryngeal Carcinoma

1. **A and B.** Squamous cell carcinoma with and without arytenoid cartilage invasion should be included in the diagnosis. Sclerosis does not necessarily imply invasion. Laryngitis does not cause arytenoid sclerosis, and Paget disease does not involve laryngeal cartilages.

2. **B.** About 13% of normal patients have asymmetric arytenoid sclerosis. This may be a normal variant and can be seen on trauma cervical spines in the emergency department nearly every day. It should not be investigated in that setting when a mass is not present.

3. **A.** The presence of sclerosis in the thyroid cartilage is least informative in suggesting tumoral invasion. The presence of sclerosis in the cricoid cartilage and arytenoid cartilage is more reliable; however, 13% of normal patients may have sclerosis in these locations.

4. **A.** Because irregular ossification of the thyroid cartilage on CT is very common, it is not useful for diagnosing cartilaginous invasion. Soft tissue entering into the strap muscles, erosion of cartilage, and obliteration of medullary space imply a tumor (an aggressive tumor if soft tissue has been invaded).

Comment

Incidence of Arytenoid Sclerosis

Arytenoid sclerosis, calcification, and/or ossification may be seen in 13% of symptom-free patients who do *not* have cancer (Figure S134-1). This finding is more common in women than in men, and there is a left-sided predominance. In patients with cancer and arytenoid sclerosis, the positive predictive value for tumor infiltration is only about 55%, the sensitivity is 68%, and specificity is approximately 80%.

Magnetic resonance imaging (MRI) has been found to be more sensitive (89% vs. 66%) but less specific (94% vs. 84%) than CT for cartilage invasion. MRI tends to be more accurate in evaluation of cricoid and arytenoid cartilages, whereas CT is more accurate in evaluation of thyroid cartilage. However, in no study has MRI or CT achieved more than 80% accuracy for predicting thyroid cartilage invasion with cancer because of its propensity for reactive change from neighboring tumor and because of the variable ossification. In general, however, the greater the degree of cartilaginous invasion (from perichondrial to intracartilaginous to extracartilaginous), the higher the rate of detectability.

Imaging Findings

With MRI, the diagnosis of cartilage invasion is confirmed by abnormal marrow signal on T1-weighted images, fat-suppressed T2-weighted images, and enhancement on fat-suppressed, T1-weighted images in cartilage that simulates the primary tumor's signal intensity. Nonetheless these MR imaging findings can also occur purely as a result of reactive changes, particularly in the thyroid cartilage. Similarly, sclerosis and erosion of the cartilage without invasion may be visible on CT. This is important because the presence of cartilage invasion usually precludes radiation therapy as the primary therapeutic modality, or it may be predictive of radiation treatment failure. The potential for perichondritis in patients treated for cancer in the cartilage and concomitant airway collapse is devastating. For similar reasons, voice conservation therapy is contraindicated with cartilaginous invasion (particularly of the cricoid and arytenoid cartilages). The patient requires total laryngectomy.

Reference

Zan E, Yousem DM, Aygun N. Asymmetric mineralization of the arytenoid cartilages in patients without laryngeal cancer. *AJNR Am J Neuroradiol.* 2011;32(6):1113-1118.

Cross-Reference

Neuroradiology: The Requisites, 3rd ed, 672-677.

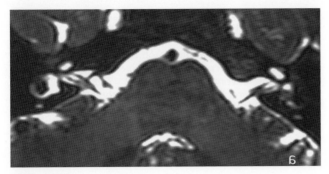

Figure 135-1

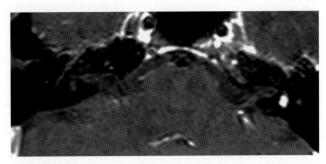

Figure 135-2

HISTORY: This patient complains of left-sided hearing loss and vertigo.

1. Which of the following should be included in the differential diagnosis? (Choose all that apply.)
   A. Schwannoma
   B. Inflammation/labyrinthitis
   C. Mondini malformation
   D. Endolymphatic sac tumor

2. What is not included in the differential diagnosis of a contrast-enhancing mass in the cerebellopontine angle cistern?
   A. Schwannomas of the seventh and eighth nerves
   B. Meningioma
   C. Subarachnoid seeding
   D. Bell palsy

3. What percentage of acoustic (or vestibular) schwannomas are purely intracanalicular?
   A. 1% to 25%
   B. 26% to 50%
   C. 51% to 75%
   D. >76%

4. Which of the following is *not* true?
   A. Criteria for the diagnosis of neurofibromatosis type 2 (NF-2) are as follows: (1) bilateral vestibular schwannomas or (2) having a first-degree relative with NF-2 and either an acoustic schwannoma or two of the following: nonacoustic schwannomas, neurofibromas, meningiomas, or gliomas.
   B. The most common cause of labyrinthitis in children is meningitis.
   C. Diffuse enhancement of the membranous labyrinth on contrast-enhanced T1-weighted images is always abnormal and associated with marked hearing loss.
   D. Autoimmune labyrinthitis is bilateral in 90% of cases.

See Supplemental Figures section for additional figures and legends for this case.

CASE 135

Intralabyrinthine Schwannoma

1. **A and B.** The diagnosis should include left-sided schwannoma and inflammation/labyrinthitis. Schwannoma usually occurs in the internal auditory canal or cerebellopontine angle cistern, but in rare cases it occurs in the vestibule. Inflammation/labyrinthitis has infectious and noninfectious causes. The location is wrong for endolymphatic sac tumor, which is usually in the mastoid or petrous bone, not in the vestibule, and Mondini malformation is not present, inasmuch as the cochlear partitioning is unaffected.

2. **D.** Bell palsy would not be included in the diagnosis because in that condition, the facial nerve does not usually enhance in the cerebellopontine angle cistern. Instead, the internal auditory canal or labyrinthine portion of the cranial nerve VII enhances. Schwannomas of the seventh and eighth nerves are the most common enhancing tumors in the cerebellopontine angle cistern, and meningioma is the second most common.

3. **A.** Of acoustic (or vestibular) schwannomas, 20% are purely intracanalicular. About 75% are both intracanalicular and extracanalicular.

4. **D.** Autoimmune labyrinthitis is bilateral in only approximately 50% of cases. On imaging, this condition is usually manifested as bilateral cochlear enhancement, but it can affect all parts of the inner ear.

Comment

Symptoms of Schwannomas

Intralabyrinthine schwannomas (ILSs) are rare tumors that arise from the distal branches of the cochlear, superior vestibular, or inferior vestibular nerves within the cochlea, vestibule, or semicircular canals or a combination of these (Figures S135-1 and S135-2). Patients with cochlear schwannomas typically present with unilateral hearing loss that progresses slowly to complete deafness. Vertigo is present in fewer than 50% of affected patients, whereas vestibular ILSs manifest primarily with vertigo and imbalance, with or without accompanying hearing loss.

Imaging Findings

ILSs are usually small tumors, and high-resolution T2-weighted and contrast-enhanced T1-weighted images are critical in making the diagnosis. The signal characteristics of these tumors are similar to schwannomas in the internal auditory canal, but because they are surrounded by the labyrinthine fluid, they appear hyperintense on unenhanced T1-weighted images and hypointense on T2-weighted images, in comparison with the labyrinthine fluid. On T2-weighted images, ILSs appear as either a focal filling defect in the labyrinthine fluid or complete focal replacement of the fluid signal; T1-weighted images with contrast show intense enhancement (see Figure S135-2). ILSs show slow growth on imaging follow-up. Surgical resection is considered only when there is no residual hearing.

Associations with Neurofibromatosis Type 2

NF-2 is one of a number of diseases that have been linked to mutations on chromosome 22, including DiGeorge syndrome, Schindler disease, chronic myelogenous leukemia, Ewing sarcoma, peripheral primitive neuroectodermal tumors, meningiomas, metachromatic leukodystrophy, and sporadic vestibular schwannomas. NF-2 is transmitted in an autosomal dominant manner with more than 90% penetrance. More than 50% of patients with NF-2 also develop a meningioma in their lifetime. Cystic components of vestibular schwannomas are reported in 4% of cases, and they appear to have a faster growth rate than do purely solid schwannomas. Causes of replacement of labyrinthine fluid signal and/or enhancement include the following:

- ILS
- Labyrinthitis
- Wegener granulomatosis
- Leukemia
- Cogan syndrome
- Systemic lupus erythematosus
- Behçet disease

Reference

Tieleman A, Casselman JW, Somers T, Delanote J, Kuhweide R, Ghekiere J, et al. Imaging of intralabyrinthine schwannomas: a retrospective study of 52 cases with emphasis on lesion growth. *AJNR Am J Neuroradiol.* 2008;29(5):898-905.

Cross-Reference

Neuroradiology: The Requisites, 3rd ed, 565-569.

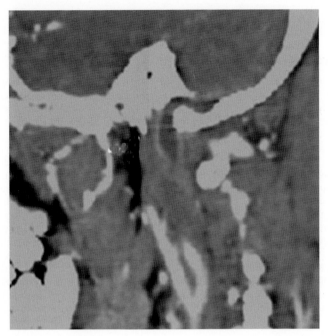

Figure 136-1

HISTORY: A patient's headache and pain in the left occipital region prompts enhanced computed tomographic scanning of the head and neck.

1. Which of the following should be included in the differential diagnosis? (Choose all that apply.)
   A. Glomus jugulare
   B. Thrombophlebitis
   C. Septic aneurysm
   D. Skull base abscess

2. In which space is this lesion localized (see Figure 136-1)?
   A. Masticator space
   B. Prestyloid parapharyngeal space
   C. Poststyloid parapharyngeal space
   D. Retropharyngeal space

3. What is the least common cause of inflammatory disease of the carotid space?
   A. Epiglottitis
   B. Internal jugular vein thrombophlebitis
   C. Pharyngitis
   D. Lymphadenitis

4. In what ways are the signal intensity characteristics of thromboses of the blood vessels different from those of intraparenchymal hematomas?
   A. Hemosiderin deposition is rarely visualized.
   B. Methemoglobin is not visualized.
   C. Enhancement is not visualized.
   D. Dark T2-weighted material is not visualized.

See Supplemental Figures section for additional figures and legends for this case.

CASE 136

Internal Jugular Vein Thrombophlebitis

1. **B.** The diagnosis should include thrombophlebitis. Note that the lesion goes into the internal jugular vein in the figure with a low-density clot. There is no enhancing tumor, and so it would not be glomus jugulare; the lesion also is not in the arterial side or an aneurysm, so it would not be septic aneurysm.

2. **C.** This lesion is localized in the poststyloid parapharyngeal space (also known as the *carotid space*). It is not in the fat-containing spaces (prestyloid parapharyngeal and retropharyngeal spaces) or in the muscular space (masticator). The jugular vein is within the poststyloid parapharyngeal space.

3. **A.** Epiglottitis is a very rare cause of inflammatory disease of the carotid space. Lymphadenitis is a very common cause. Jugular thrombophlebitis usually results from the use of catheters, and internal jugular vein thrombophlebitis from pharyngitis may be the result of Ludwig angina or Lemierre disease.

4. **A.** The signal intensity characteristics of thromboses of the blood vessels are different from those of intraparenchymal hematomas in that clots rarely demonstrate hemosiderin deposition. Both thrombi and hematomas may have no enhancement, dark T2-weighted deoxyhemoglobin, and high-signal T1-weighted methemoglobin. These three characteristics are not differentiators.

Comment

Differential Diagnosis

The usual differential diagnosis of internal jugular vein thrombophlebitis includes neck abscess. In thrombophlebitis, the jugular vein is usually normal or increased in size, and there is a history of catheter insertion, malignancy, hypercoagulable state, leukemia/lymphoma, or drug use with jugular venous injection (Figure S136-1). Slow flow in the jugular vein may cause high-signal intensity on T1-weighted scans and may simulate thrombosis. To avoid this potential pitfall, one should perform magnetic resonance venography (MRV). Unfortunately, hyperintense clot on T1-weighted images may look like flow in the jugular vein on time-of-flight MRV.

Causes of Internal Jugular Vein Thrombophlebitis

In this case, because the clot is emanating from above, its most likely source is otomastoiditis with meningitis. Ludwig angina is an infection of the oral cavity or oropharynx that can obstruct the airway and, in rare cases, also infiltrates the carotid sheath structures (poststyloid parapharyngeal space) after it has spread to the prestyloid parapharyngeal space. In Lemierre syndrome (postanginal sepsis), a peritonsillar abscess with anaerobic bacteria can lead to thrombophlebitis of the jugular vein, bacteremia, and emboli to the lung. Pneumonia may ensue. The thrombophlebitis may spread to the venous sinuses in the brain (as seen in this figure). The most common pathogen is *Fusobacterium necrophorum*.

Reference

Kim BY, Yoon DY, Kim HC, Kim ES, Baek S, Lim KJ, et al. Thrombophlebitis of the internal jugular vein (Lemierre syndrome): clinical and CT findings. *Acta Radiol.* 2013;54(6):622-627.

Cross-Reference

Neuroradiology: The Requisites, 3rd ed, 153-156.

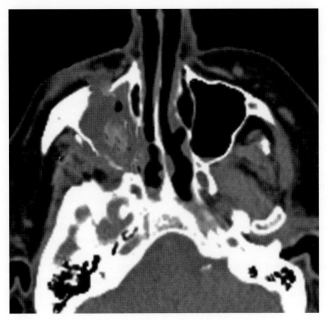

Figure 137-1

HISTORY: A patient with acquired immunodeficiency syndrome (AIDS) presents with facial pain and sinusitis.

1. Which of the following should be included in the differential diagnosis? (Choose all that apply.)
   A. Allergic fungal sinusitis
   B. Invasive fungal sinusitis
   C. Mucocele
   D. Fungus ball

2. Which is true of acute invasive fungal sinusitis?
   A. It is characterized by air-fluid levels.
   B. The survival rate is about 50%.
   C. Surgery does not improve prognosis.
   D. Affected patients with AIDS have a better prognosis than do those with diabetes.

3. How can a sinus filled with fungal sinusitis simulate one with normal aeration on magnetic resonance imaging (MRI)?
   A. Both have air within them.
   B. Fungi, like aeration, may appear dark on T1- and T2-weighted scans.
   C. Fungal calcification from mycetoma simulates aeration.
   D. Hemorrhage looks like air.

4. What is *not* a risk factor for mycetoma?
   A. Recent surgery
   B. Radiotherapy
   C. Alcoholism
   D. Marijuana use

See Supplemental Figures section for additional figures and legends for this case.

CASE 137

Acute Invasive Fungal Sinusitis

1. **B.** Invasive fungal sinusitis is suggested by the extension into soft tissues and the hyperdensity of the sinus contents. Allergic fungal sinusitis and fungus ball are not as aggressive and destructive as what is seen in this case. In addition, the sinus is not expanded which is typically seen in a mucocele; instead, the sinus is eroded.

2. **B.** The rate of survival of acute invasive fungal sinusitis is about 50%. This condition is not characterized by air-fluid levels. Surgery is a positive predictor of better outcome. Affected patients with diabetes tend to do better than those with AIDS but the prognosis, no matter what, is very poor.

3. **B.** Dense, calcified, manganese-encrusted fungi, like aeration, may appear dark on T1- and T2-weighted scans. Fungal calcification from mycetoma does not usually fill the whole sinus, and fungal sinusitis is not hemorrhagic.

4. **C.** There is no relationship between alcoholism and mycetoma. Recent surgery, radiotherapy, and marijuana use are all risk factors for mycetoma.

Comment

Acute and Chronic Invasive Fungal Sinusitis

The computed tomographic scan shows an aggressive infection that is growing through the anterior, medial, and posterior walls of the maxillary sinus into the masticator space (Figure S137-1). Acute invasive fungal sinusitis is classically a disease of immunocompromised hosts and may also aggressively invade the orbit, cavernous sinus, and intracranial compartment. *Acute* invasive fungal sinusitis is defined as an infection that is less than 4 weeks in evolution. Complications include infarcts, cerebritis, meningitis, intracranial granulomas, sinus thrombosis, and pseudoaneurysms. *Chronic* invasive fungal sinusitis, by definition, has a time course longer than 12 weeks. Most affected patients are immunocompetent. In immunosuppressed patients, the erosive nature is more protracted.

Magnetic Resonance Imaging Findings

Fungi and/or inspissated secretions may have a signal void on T2-weighted MRI. Even on T1-weighted gadolinium-enhanced scans, this patient's sinus looked dark. Some authorities believe that this appearance is caused by calcification; others think that it is caused by manganese accumulation in the fungus. Calcifications are certainly visible in aspergillomas, but *Drechslera* fungi grew out of this patient's cultures. *Aspergillus fumigatus* and mucormycosis are pathogens that usually cause intracranial disseminated mycotic infections in immunocompromised individuals (e.g., patients with AIDS, patients taking immunosuppressive drugs, patients with leukemia, patients undergoing dialysis, people who abuse intravenous drugs, transplant recipients). Once the brain is involved, the prognosis is poor, with the potential for abscess, infarcts, and meningeal spread. Mycotic aneurysms and intracranial hematomas may also occur as the fungi cause intraluminal obstruction. Rings of low signal intensity on T2-weighted scans are often seen with *Aspergillus* brain abscesses, just as the sinusitis may appear dark on T2-weighted scans. In the author's experience, the worst cause of fungal infections spreading intracranially have actually been invasive *Mucorales* species, not *Aspergillus*.

Reference

Mossa-Basha M, Ilica AT, Maluf F, et al. The many faces of fungal disease of the paranasal sinuses: CT and MRI findings. *Diagn Interv Radiol*. 2013;19(3):195-200.

Cross-Reference

Neuroradiology: The Requisites, 3rd ed, 425-430.

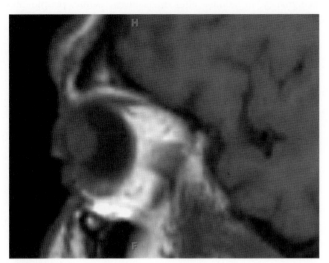

Figure 138-1

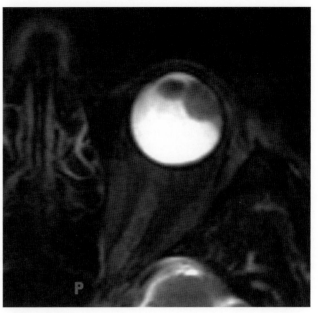

Figure 138-2

HISTORY: A 50-year-old man presents with right-sided visual blurring.

1. Which of the following should be included in the differential diagnosis? (Choose all that apply.)
   A. Retinal detachment
   B. Retinoblastoma
   C. Vitreous hemorrhage
   D. Choroidal melanoma

2. What are the unique signal intensity–related features of melanin-containing melanomas of the orbit?
   A. They appear bright on T2-weighted images.
   B. They exhibit calcification.
   C. Melanin usually appears bright on T1-weighted scans and with intermediate to low intensity on T2-weighted scans.
   D. They usually appear dark on susceptibility-weighted scans.

3. If calcification within an ocular mass is present, what should *not* be included in the differential diagnosis?
   A. Retinoblastoma
   B. Choroidal hemangiomas
   C. Choroidal osteomas
   D. Retinal hemangioblastomas

4. In a child who has a small globe and a lesion that is hyperintense on T1-weighted scans in the globe, what diagnosis should be considered?
   A. Persistent hyperplastic primary vitreous
   B. Retinoblastoma
   C. Retrolental fibroplasia
   D. Retinal hemangioblastoma

See Supplemental Figures section for additional figures and legends for this case.

CASE 138

Choroidal Melanoma

1. **D.** The enhancement suggests choroidal melanoma. The location in the uveal region is not correct for retinal detachment, retinoblastoma (unusual without calcification and in an adult), or vitreous hemorrhage (the shape does not suggest this and the location is far anterior, not to mention the enhancement).

2. **C.** Melanin usually appears bright on T1-weighted scans without contrast and intermediate to low intensity on T2-weighted scans. Melanomas rarely calcify. They do enhance.

3. **D.** Retinal hemangioblastomas do not calcify. Ninety percent of retinoblastomas calcify, and choroidal hemangiomas and osteomas may show calcification or ossification, respectively.

4. **A.** Persistent hyperplastic primary vitreous should be considered in a child who has a small globe and a lesion that is hyperintense on T1-weighted scans in the globe. The globe is usually normal in size with retinoblastoma, and retrolental fibroplasia (retinopathy of prematurity) and retinal hemangioblastoma do not appear bright on T1-weighted scans.

Comment

Incidence of Melanomas

Ocular melanomas can be found in the iris (6%), the ciliary body (9%), and the choroid (85%). These three structures constitute the uveal tract, which contains melanocytes, from which these tumors develop (Figures S138-1, S138-2, and S138-3). Melanomas are the second most common intraocular malignancy in adults, after metastases. White people are affected more than eight times more frequently than African Americans. Melanomas may grow along the optic nerve, into the subarachnoid space, or outside the uveal tract and globe (10% to 15% of cases). This finding has dramatic prognostic implications; the rate of 5-year survival drops to 40%. Magnetic resonance imaging is more sensitive and specific than high-frequency ultrasonography in detecting extraocular growth. Hematogenous dissemination most commonly leads to liver metastases.

Treatment of Melanomas

Treatment of ocular melanoma is similar to that of retinoblastoma in that it depends on tumor size. Options include laser therapy, photocoagulation, transpupillary thermotherapy (TTT), brachytherapy, local excision, or enucleation. Poor prognosis is associated with older age of the patient, larger tumor size, extraocular extension, and metastases. Mixed or epithelioid histologic features confer a worse prognosis than do necrotic histologic features.

Reference

Lemke AJ, Hosten N, Bornfeld N, Bechrakis NE, Schüler A, Richter M, et al. Uveal melanoma: correlation of histopathologic and radiologic findings by using thin-section MR imaging with a surface coil. *Radiology.* 1999;210(3):775-783.

Cross-Reference

Neuroradiology: The Requisites, 3rd ed, 328-329.

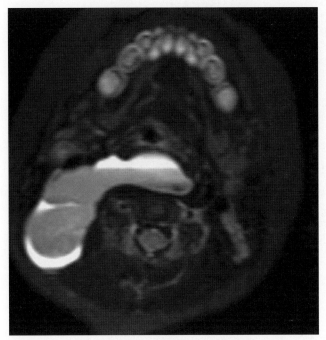

Figure 139-1

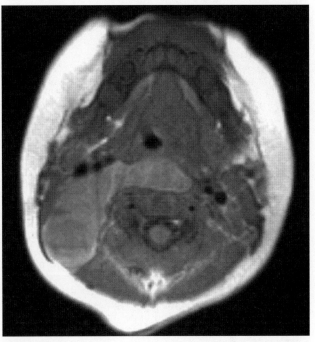

Figure 139-2

HISTORY: This patient presents with right-sided neck swelling.

1. Which of the following should be included in the differential diagnosis? (Choose all that apply.)
   A. Branchial cleft cyst
   B. Lymphatic malformation
   C. Hemangioma
   D. Venous vascular malformation (VVM)

2. Which feature is suggestive of lymphatic malformations?
   A. Absence of enhancement
   B. Blood-fluid levels
   C. Phleboliths
   D. Late, slow enhancement

3. What are the most common locations in the head and neck for cystic hygromas?
   A. Posterior triangle and axilla
   B. Orbit and oral cavity
   C. Carotid sheath and subcutaneous tissue
   D. Visceral space and upper mediastinum

4. What percentage of lymphatic malformations are found in the neck?
   A. 0% to 20%
   B. 21% to 40%
   C. 41% to 60%
   D. >60%

See Supplemental Figures section for additional figures and legends for this case.

CASE 139

Lymphangioma: Lymphatic Vascular Malformation

1. **B.** The diagnosis should include lymphatic malformation due to the age of the patient and location of the malformation. This is not the correct appearance or location for a branchial cleft cyst. There is no enhancement, and so the lesion is not likely to be a hemangioma or VVM.

2. **B.** Blood-fluid levels are classical, reliable evidence of lymphatic malformations (although they are also reported in some VVMs and in aneurysmal bone cysts). Phleboliths are more indicative of VVMs. Neither late, slow enhancement or absence of enhancement provides enough evidence to diagnose lymphatic malformations.

3. **A.** The most common locations in the head and neck for cystic hygromas are the posterior triangle and axilla. They uncommonly develop in the orbit and oral cavity. They rarely appear in the carotid sheath and subcutaneous tissue or in the visceral space and upper mediastinum.

4. **D.** Of all lymphatic malformations, 70% to 80% are found in the neck.

Comment

Classification of Lymphatic Malformations

Lymphatic malformations are classified as low-flow malformations. The overwhelming majority occur in the neck and have a predilection for the posterior triangle of the neck and the axilla. Lymphatic malformations are subclassified into microcystic and macrocystic varieties. The macrocystic malformations are more commonly associated with intralesional hemorrhage and have large cystic spaces that are multiloculated and can manifest as neck masses. The microcystic malformations are characterized by cyst sizes of 2 mm or less.

Imaging Findings

Unless venous components are associated with them, most lymphatic malformations do not enhance on imaging (Figures S139-1, S139-2, and S139-3). However, VVMs are often part of them. Lymphatic malformations are often septated lesions that cross the usual fascia-defined spaces of the head and neck. Hyperintensity on T1-weighted images may be indicative of blood, chylous material, or just hyperproteinaceous contents.

Associations with Lymphatic Malformations

Associations include Turner syndrome, Down syndrome, Noonan syndrome, and Klippel-Trenaunay-Weber syndrome. Cowchock Wapner Kurtz syndrome is characterized by cystic hygroma, lymphedema, and cleft palate. Treatment options include surgical excision, injection sclerotherapy, and laser therapy.

Reference

Flors L, Leiva-Salinas C, Maged M, Norton PT, Matsumoto AH, Angle JF, et al. MR Imaging of soft-tissue vascular malformations: diagnosis, classification, and therapy follow-up. *Radiographics*. 2011;31(5): 1321-1340; discussion, *Radiographics*. 2011;31(5):1340-1341.

Cross-Reference

Neuroradiology: The Requisites, 3rd ed, 445-446, 503.

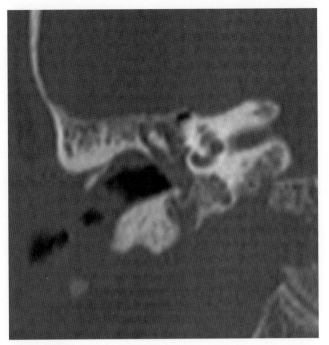

Figure 140-1

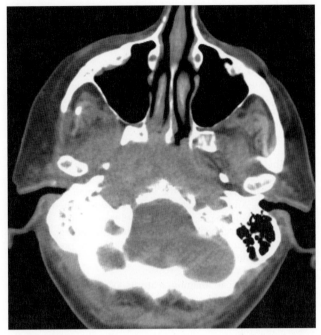

Figure 140-2

HISTORY: An elderly patient presents with hearing loss and pain on the right side of the head.

1. Which of the following should be included in the differential diagnosis? (Choose all that apply.)
   A. Nasopharyngeal carcinoma
   B. Ear cancer spreading down the eustachian tube
   C. Malignant otitis externa (MOE)
   D. Necrotizing otitis externa

2. Which of the following best describes the classical patient with the lesion shown in Figure 140-1?
   A. An elderly diabetic patient with external ear granulation who has recently had the ear irrigated
   B. A patient with human immunodeficiency virus (HIV) infection and otitis media
   C. Young cold-water swimmer with "swimmer's ear"
   D. Patient with nasopharyngeal carcinoma who has undergone radiation treatment

3. What are the classic imaging features of MOE?
   A. Middle ear thickening or mass, cortical bone erosion in the external auditory canal (EAC), and a nasopharyngeal mass
   B. Internal auditory canal thickening or mass, cortical bone erosion in the internal auditory canal, and a soft tissue mass at the skull base
   C. EAC thickening or mass, cortical bone erosion in the EAC, and a soft tissue mass at the skull base
   D. EAC hyperostosis, cortical bone erosion in the ossicles, and a soft tissue mass at the skull base

4. What is the pathway of spread from the EAC to skull base with MOE?
   A. Vidian canal
   B. Fissures of Santorini
   C. Eustachian tube
   D. Canals of Schlemm

See Supplemental Figures section for additional figures and legends for this case.

CASE 140

Malignant Otitis Externa

1. **B, C, and D.** The diagnosis should include ear cancer spreading down the eustachian tube (squamous cell carcinoma could lead to this), MOE (typical of this infection), and necrotizing otitis externa (another name for MOE). Nasopharyngeal carcinoma does not usually extend to the external auditory canal.

2. **A.** This lesion classically occurs in elderly diabetic patients with external ear granulation who have recently had the ear irrigated. This is not the typical presentation for swimmer's ear. An HIV-infected patient with otitis media would be more likely to present with middle ear disease. A patient with nasopharyngeal carcinoma who has undergone radiation treatment would be more likely to present with osteoradionecrosis.

3. **C.** The classical imaging features of MOE include EAC thickening or mass, cortical bone erosion in the EAC, and a soft tissue mass at the skull base. Erosion or sclerosis is visible at the skull base on computed tomography (CT) and fatty marrow replacement or enhancement on magnetic resonance imaging (MRI).

4. **B.** The routes of spread from EAC to skull base are the fissures of Santorini. They course inferomedially from the junction of the bony and cartilaginous portions of the EAC to the parapharyngeal space. The eustachian tubes lead to the middle ear, not the EAC. Canals of Schlemm are in the globe. The Vidian canal is not a route from the EAC.

Comment

Imaging Findings

On CT, the classic imaging features of MOE include a soft tissue mass in the EAC, cortical bone erosion of the walls of the EAC, and a soft tissue inflammatory process at the skull base (Figures S140-1 and S140-2). In this case, CT shows opacification of the external ear, middle ear, and mastoid air cells with erosion of the walls of the EAC. It also reveals obliteration of the fat planes at the base of the skull and parapharyngeal space with erosions of the anterior mastoid bone. There may be subtle sclerosis or erosion of the clivus or occipital condyle.

On MRI, the granulation tissue of MOE classically has low intensity on T1- and T2-weighted scans, like a fungal infection, although MOE is caused by *Pseudomonas aeruginosa*. Affected patients may have symptoms of cranial nerve disease because of the involvement of the jugular foramen (and hence involvement of cranial nerves IX through XI) or the facial nerve in the temporal bone. One must remember that resolution of findings of MOE on CT and MRI can be greatly delayed in comparison with clinical response. In fact, the erosive bony changes may persist indefinitely. Clinicians tend to rely on sedimentation rates and patients' symptoms to confirm eradication of the *P. aeruginosa* infection. If an imaging study is used to monitor MOE, a gallium scan is recommended because it reflects disease activity better than does CT or MRI.

Epidemiology of Malignant Otitis Externa

Although this condition is classically a disease of elderly diabetic men, immunosuppressed individuals—those with human immunodeficiency virus (HIV) infection/acquired immunodeficiency syndrome (AIDS), those undergoing chemotherapy or external beam radiation therapy—are also susceptible to malignant otitis externa. Treatment is with aggressive systemic antibiotics, but complications may include temporomandibular joint/clivus osteomyelitis, sigmoid sinus thrombosis, and meningitis. This condition was traditionally termed *malignant* because until the 1970s, mortality rates were as high as 70%.

Reference

Okpala NC, Siraj QH, Nilssen E, Pringle M. Radiological and radionuclide investigation of malignant otitis externa. *J Laryngol Otol.* 2005;119(1):71-75.

Cross-Reference

Neuroradiology: The Requisites, 3rd ed, 386-387.

Acknowledgment

Thank you to Carolina Paulazo, MD, for providing the figures for this case.

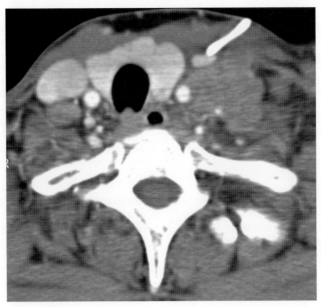

Figure 141-1

HISTORY: This patient has lower neck discomfort for 2 weeks.

1. Which of the following should be included in the differential diagnosis? (Choose all that apply.)
   A. Thyroid cancer
   B. Hodgkin disease
   C. Non-Hodgkin lymphoma
   D. Third branchial cleft cyst

2. Which vessel shows tumoral encasement: the carotid, vertebral, or branch vessel?
   A. Vertebral
   B. Carotid
   C. Branch
   D. Both carotid and branch

3. What is the most accurate criterion for diagnosing vascular invasion by tumor?
   A. Luminal ingrowth
   B. 180 degrees of circumferential involvement
   C. 270 degrees of circumferential involvement
   D. Effaced fat adjacent to the vessel

4. At which T stage of the American Joint Commission on Cancer (AJCC) TNM staging system is carotid invasion classified?
   A. T3
   B. T4a
   C. T4b
   D. T4c

See Supplemental Figures section for additional figures and legends for this case.

CASE 141

Vascular Encasement by Lymphoma

1. **B and C.** The supraclavicular fossa and lower neck are correct locations for Hodgkin disease, and a nodal mass could represent non-Hodgkin lymphoma. The mass is separate from the thyroid gland and thus unlikely to be thyroid cancer. In addition, it is a solid mass, and so it is unlikely to be a cyst. Squamous cell carcinomas should also be considered in the differential diagnosis.

2. **C.** The branch vessel is encased.

3. **C.** The most accurate criterion for diagnosing vascular invasion by tumor is 270 degrees of circumferential involvement because this is a sensitive and specific finding. Luminal ingrowth is a specific but not sensitive finding, and effaced fat adjacent to the vessel is a sensitive but not specific finding. The finding of 180-degree circumferential involvement is less specific than 270-degree circumferential involvement.

4. **C.** Carotid invasion is classified as T4b, insofar as this represents far advanced disease. T3 and T4a classifications do not address carotid involvement or invasion.

Comment

Criteria for Vascular Encasement

Circumferential involvement of a vessel of 270 degrees or more is the criterion for unresectability of the tumor; this characteristic also yields a near 100% accuracy for diagnosing squamous cell carcinoma (Figure S141-1) vascular invasion. This finding combines excellent sensitivity and specificity, whereas such findings as tumor abutting the vessel or effacing adjacent fat yield far too many false-positive scans. Luminal involvement has high positive predictive value, but in very few cases of unresectable disease does imaging actually show such far advanced findings of luminal encroachment. Some tumors, however, even with 360 degrees of circumferential involvement, can be stripped from the vessel without sacrificing that vessel. Such tumors include chordomas, which are relatively gelatinous and easily aspirated, and some meningiomas that can be peeled from the vessel.

Treating Vascular Encasement by Lymphoma

When metastatic disease involves carotid arteries, surgery does not appear to change the long-term survival. There are reports that the rate of *1-year* survival with far advanced T4b disease is between 0% and 44%. Among patients with more than and less than 180 degrees of circumferential tumor encasement of the artery, overall survival rates of 8% and 33%, respectively, have been reported. If resection of the carotid artery is an option, a temporary balloon occlusion test or a test of perfusion to the brain during temporary balloon occlusion may be helpful. The surgeon may try to preserve the artery in what is called a *carotid peel*: separating the tumor from the vessel in the subadventitial plane. A carotid peel leaves residual microscopic disease that must be addressed thereafter by radiation therapy. Carotid rupture is then a major risk to the compromised vessel.

Subtypes of Lymphoma

Hodgkin lymphoma affects the supraclavicular lymph nodes at a higher rate (80% to 90%) than does non-Hodgkin lymphoma. It has an orderly progression of spread from one nodal chain to the next, but it may spread to the mediastinum or up the neck. Subtypes include the following:

- Nodular sclerosis Hodgkin lymphoma
- Mixed-cellularity Hodgkin lymphoma
- Lymphocyte-depleted Hodgkin lymphoma (worst prognosis)
- Lymphocyte-rich classical Hodgkin lymphoma (best prognosis)

Stages of Lymphoma

Involvement of a single lymph node region (mostly the cervical region) is considered stage I; stage Ie is involvement of a single extralymphatic site. Involvement of two or more lymph node regions on the same side of the diaphragm is considered stage II; stage IIe is involvement of one lymph node region and a contiguous extralymphatic site. Stage III is involvement of lymph node regions on both sides of the diaphragm, which may include the spleen (stage IIIs) and/or limited areas of a contiguous extralymphatic organ (stage IIIe) or site (stage IIIes). Stage IV is disseminated involvement of one or more extralymphatic organs. Fortunately, current treatment strategies with radiation, chemotherapy, and stem cell therapy have yielded very high cure rates. Surgery would not be contemplated in this case because lymphoma is primarily a medical condition, not a surgical one, even with vascular encasement.

Reference

Yousem DM, Gad K, Tufano RP. Resectability issues with head and neck cancer. *AJNR Am J Neuroradiol.* 2006;27(10):2024-2036.

Cross-Reference

Neuroradiology: The Requisites, 3rd ed, 568-569.

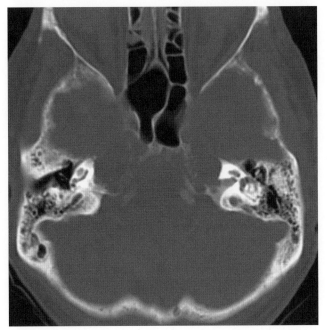

Figure 142-1

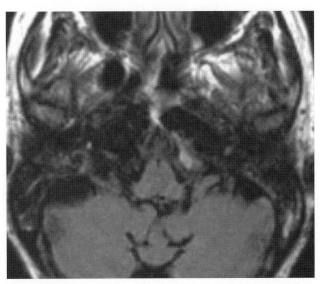

Figure 142-2

HISTORY: A patient presents with what appeared to be cerebrospinal fluid (CSF) rhinorrhea; the side of origin is unclear.

1. Which of the following should be included in the differential diagnosis? (Choose all that apply.)
   A. Arachnoid cysts
   B. Meningocele
   C. Cholesterol granuloma
   D. Petrous apicitis

2. What common causes of meningoceles affect the tegmen tympani?
   A. Congenital
   B. Traumatic
   C. Postoperative
   D. All of the above
   E. None of the above

3. How often is the jugular bulb congenitally dehiscent?
   A. <10%
   B. 11% to 20%
   C. 21% to 40%
   D. >40%

4. How often is the cribriform plate macroscopically dehiscent?
   A. <10%
   B. 11% to 20%
   C. 21% to 40%
   D. >40%

See Supplemental Figures section for additional figures and legends for this case.

CASE 142

Petrous Apex Meningocele

1. **A and B.** The diagnosis should include arachnoid cysts and meningocele. The diagnosis would not include cholesterol granuloma or petrous apicitis when there is CSF signal on fluid-attenuated inversion recovery (FLAIR) imaging (cholesterol granuloma appears bright) and an expanded nature to the lesion (petrous apicitis does not expand the petrous apex).

2. **D.** The common causes of meningoceles that affect the tegmen tympani include congenital, traumatic, and postoperative entities. Postinflammatory causes could also affect the tegmen tympani after otomastoiditis.

3. **A.** In approximately 8% of cases, the jugular bulb is dehiscent. However, in 15% of cases, it is high riding: that is, in a position above the lower level of internal auditory canal.

4. **A.** In approximately 3% of cases, the cribriform plate is congenitally widely dehiscent. This characteristic, too, could cause CSF rhinorrhea.

Comment

Differential Diagnosis

Petrous apex meningoceles may arise from herniation from the posterolateral portion of the Meckel cave into the petrous apex (Figures S142-1 and S142-2). Some authorities have called these *arachnoid cysts* and others have called them *meningoceles*. They may be associated with trigeminal neuralgia, headaches, or CSF leakage. Thirty percent are bilateral. Of importance is that this is *not* a cholesterol granuloma, which would typically have magnetic resonance imaging (MRI) features of blood or high protein. This lesion has FLAIR signal that is identical to that of CSF. That would also be atypical for epidermoids (although diffusion-weighted imaging would assist with that diagnosis), lytic metastatic bone lesions, or petrous apex mucoceles.

Imaging Findings

At the author's institution, lesions such as this are called *cephaloceles* because it is not always clear whether the defect that is identified on imaging contains brain tissue, meninges, or both. In this case, it looks as if only the meninges and CSF are herniating through the skull defect.

Most acquired cephaloceles occur along the cribriform plate in association with trauma or postoperative defects. Computed tomography should be used to demonstrate the bony dehiscence, and MRI should be used to demonstrate the contents of the cephalocele, to best characterize the lesion for the neurosurgeon or endoscopic sinus surgeon who repairs it. Three-dimensional computed tomography is particularly elegant in demonstrating the location and extent of the holes that must be patched. With temporal or sphenoid bone cephaloceles, the site of dehiscence may be at the sphenopetrosal suture or the foramen lacerum. Those cephaloceles manifest later because the defect is not visible, and often the presenting symptom is seizure or CSF leak. Heterotopic brain tissue may also be seen in either the pterygopalatine fossa or the orbit.

References

Moore KR, Fischbein NJ, Harnsberger HR, Shelton C, Glastonbury CM, White DK, et al. Petrous apex cephaloceles. *AJNR Am J Neuroradiol.* 2001;22(10):1867-1871.

Atmaca S, Elmali M, Kucuk H. High and dehiscent jugular bulb: clear and present danger during middle ear surgery. *Surg Radiol Anat.* 2014;36(4):369-374.

Cross-Reference

Neuroradiology: The Requisites, 3rd ed, 380.

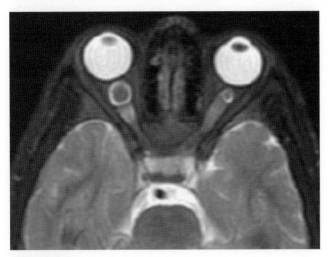

Figure 143-1

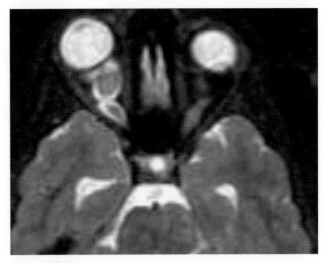

Figure 143-2

HISTORY: A pediatric patient presents with mild right proptosis and mild visual acuity loss.

1. Which of the following should be included in the differential diagnosis? (Choose all that apply.)
   A. Optic neuritis
   B. Optic nerve meningioma
   C. Optic glioma
   D. Sarcoidosis

2. What is arachnoid hyperplasia (gliomatosis), and with what is it associated?
   A. Thickening of the optic nerve sheath meninges, in association with optic nerve gliomas, especially in patients with neurofibromatosis
   B. Thickening of the internal auditory canal meninges, in association with vestibular schwannomas, especially in patients with neurofibromatosis type 2
   C. Thickening of the optic nerve, in association with neurofibromatosis
   D. Thickening of the olfactory nerve meninges, in association with Kallmann syndrome

3. Which of the following affects vision the latest?
   A. Meningiomas
   B. Optic neuritis
   C. Optic nerve glioma
   D. Sarcoidosis

4. What bone dysplasia typically accompanies neurofibromatosis type 1 (NF-1) of the orbit?
   A. Absence or hypoplasia of the greater sphenoid wing
   B. Absence or hypoplasia of the lesser sphenoid wing
   C. Absence or hypoplasia of the optic canal
   D. Absence or hypoplasia of the lateral orbital wall

See Supplemental Figures section for additional figures and legends for this case.

CASE 143

Optic Nerve Glioma

1. **C.** The enlarged nerves seen in Figures S143-1 and S143-2 indicate optic glioma. This enlargement does not indicate optic neuritis or sarcoidosis. Optic nerve meningioma is a lesion of the sheath, not the nerve. Of these lesions, the one seen most commonly in a child is optic glioma.

2. **A.** Arachnoid hyperplasia (gliomatosis) is thickening of the optic nerve sheath meninges in association with optic nerve gliomas, especially in patients with neurofibromatosis type 1.

3. **C.** Optic nerve gliomas manifest with changes in visual acuity late in their course. Meningiomas and sarcoidosis cause visual blurring symptoms earlier in the course of disease than do optic gliomas.

4. **A.** Absence or hypoplasia of the greater sphenoid wing typically accompanies NF-1 of the orbit. Dural ectasias, tibial bowing and pseudarthrosis, and posterior scalloping of the vertebrae may also occur as osseous anomalies, in addition to neural foraminal enlargement.

Comment

Criteria for Diagnosis of Neurofibromatosis Type 1

Head and neck manifestation (excluding intracranial lesions) occur in 14% to 22% of individuals with NF-1. The chief complaints, most often cosmetic deformities, are usually related to pigmentary changes, neurofibromas, and bony dysplasias. Optic nerve gliomas manifest late in their course because the visual disturbance is initially minor or it is present when the child is too young to recognize the abnormality. However, an orbital mass affecting vision or hearing can also be a primary manifestation in children with NF-1. The seven criteria for diagnosing NF-1 are six or more café au lait spots, plexiform neurofibromas, axillary or inguinal freckling, optic pathway glioma, two or more Lisch nodules, an osseous lesion, and a first-degree relative with the disease. Optic gliomas are usually low-grade astrocytomas and therefore are not really neuronal in origin. Nine percent of all individuals with neurofibromas have NF-1 (originally known as *von Recklinghausen disease*), and most neurofibromas are solitary. Neurofibromas are far less common than schwannomas.

Symptoms of Neurofibromatosis Type 1 with Optic Nerve Gliomas

Of 14 children reported with optic nerve glioma and NF-1 in one study cited below, 11 had no symptoms, and the median age at discovery was just over 4 years. Patients with both conditions showed very little or slow progression of their lesions. Patients with optic nerve glioma alone more often had involvement of the chiasm and showed visual changes than those with optic glioma and NF-1. The median age at diagnosis was the same for both groups. Enhancement was present in only 4 patients with optic nerve glioma and NF-1 but in 10 of 13 without NF-1.

Reference

Chateil JF, Soussotte C, Pédespan JM, Brun M, Le Manh C, Diard F. MRI and clinical differences between optic pathway tumours in children with and without neurofibromatosis. *Br J Radiol.* 2001; 74(877):24-31.

Cross-Reference

Neuroradiology: The Requisites, 3rd ed, 347-348.

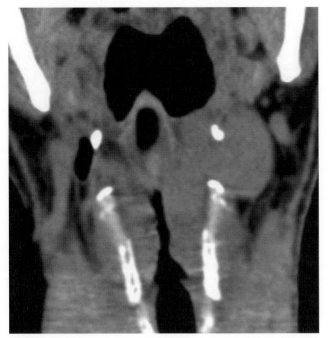

Figure 144-1

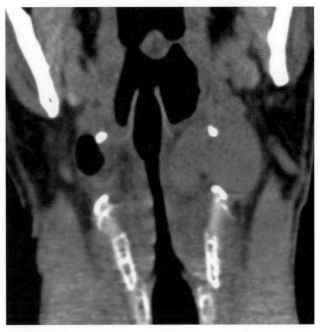

Figure 144-2

HISTORY: A patient is being evaluated for hoarseness.

1. Which of the following should be included in the differential diagnosis? (Choose all that apply.)
   A. Air-filled laryngocele
   B. External laryngocele
   C. Fluid-filled laryngocele
   D. Mixed laryngocele

2. Who is most likely to develop laryngoceles?
   A. People who chew tobacco, chew betel nuts, or work in saw mills
   B. Glass blowers, people who play wind instruments, people with chronic cough, and people with chronic sneezing
   C. People who smoke, sex workers, and people who use illicit drugs
   D. Alcoholic patients, obese patients, and diabetic patients

3. Which classification of laryngocele is a misnomer?
   A. "Internal laryngocele"
   B. "External laryngocele"
   C. "Mixed laryngocele"
   D. "Pyolaryngocele"

4. What maneuvers will cause a laryngocele to become distended?
   A. Puffing the cheek
   B. Trendelenburg position
   C. Reversed Trendelenburg position
   D. Modified Valsalva maneuver

See Supplemental Figures section for additional figures and legends for this case.

CASE 144

Bilateral Laryngoceles

1. **A, B, C, and D.** The diagnosis should include fluid-filled and mixed laryngocele, as seen in Figure S144-1. It should also include air-filled and external laryngocele, as seen in Figures S144-2 and S144-3.

2. **B.** Laryngoceles develop typically in glass blowers, people who play wind instruments, people with chronic cough, and people with chronic sneezing. Chewing tobacco, smoking, and alcoholism do not increase the risk for developing laryngoceles.

3. **B.** "External laryngocele" is a misnomer because these lesions extend out of the larynx, through the thyrohyoid membrane. By definition, all lesions communicate with the laryngeal saccule; therefore, all "external laryngoceles" are truly mixed lesions, having an internal component attached to the saccule.

4. **D.** A modified Valsalva maneuver will cause a laryngocele to become distended. Trendelenburg and reversed Trendelenburg positions have no effect on a laryngocele, and puffing a cheek distends a laryngocele only if accompanied by the Valsalva maneuver.

Comment

Types of Laryngoceles

Laryngoceles are air- or fluid-filled outpouchings of the saccule of the laryngeal ventricle (sinus of Morgagni). The importance of this finding is to make sure there is no obstructing mass in the ventricle. Laryngoceles are much more common in men than in women and in white people than in black people. If the thyrohyoid membrane is not violated, laryngoceles are considered internal; if the thyrohyoid membrane is violated, laryngoceles are considered external; and if a laryngocele has a component that is seen medial/internal to and external to the thyrohyoid membrane (demonstrated in the left in this case), it is considered mixed. The mixed laryngocele is the most common kind. Laryngoceles are bilateral in 32% of cases, and internal ones are twice as common as external ones.

Symptoms of Laryngoceles

Affected patients may complain of hoarseness or respiratory distress. Treatment of isolated internal laryngoceles may be through endoscopic laser therapy, whereas mixed laryngoceles necessitate an external incision. The underlying mass, if there is one, must be dealt with separately. Pharyngoceles (lateral pharyngeal pouches or diverticula) occur in the tonsillar fossa, paraglottic space, and piriform sinus region and along the thyrohyoid membrane.

Reference

Akbas Y, Unal M, Pata YS. Asymptomatic bilateral mixed-type laryngocele and laryngeal carcinoma. *Eur Arch Otorhinolaryngol.* 2004;261(6):307-309.

Cross-Reference

Neuroradiology: The Requisites, 3rd ed, 452.

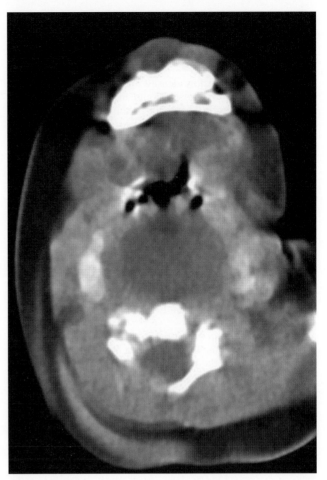

Figure 145-2

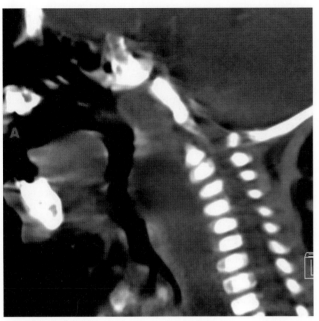

Figure 145-1

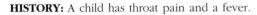

HISTORY: A child has throat pain and a fever.

1. Which of the following should be included in the differential diagnosis? (Choose all that apply.)
   A. Necrotizing adenitis
   B. Retropharyngeal edema
   C. Retropharyngeal abscess
   D. Perivertebral abscess

2. What structure separates the retropharyngeal space from the perivertebral region?
   A. The pharynx
   B. The vertebra
   C. The longus colli musculature
   D. The retropharyngeal fat

3. How far can an inflammatory lesion extend inferiorly from the retropharyngeal space, and to what level does the danger space extend?
   A. C7; T3
   B. T3; T12
   C. T9; T12
   D. L2; S1

4. What is the usual source of a retropharyngeal abscess?
   A. Pharyngitis/tonsillitis
   B. Sinusitis
   C. Dental/odontogenic disease
   D. Epiglottitis/supraglottitis

See Supplemental Figures section for additional figures and legends for this case.

CASE 145

Retropharyngeal Abscess

1. **C.** Because of the low density and mass effect shown in the figures, the diagnosis should include retropharyngeal abscess. The lesion is anterior to the longus musculature, not in the perivertebral space. The size and location (in the midline) do not indicate necrotizing adenitis, and the mass effect is not correct for retropharyngeal edema, although that can accompany the abscess.

2. **C.** The longus colli musculature separates the retropharyngeal space from the perivertebral region. The retropharyngeal space normally contains predominantly fat and lymph nodes.

3. **B.** From the retropharyngeal space, an inflammatory lesion can extend inferiorly to T3, although the danger space can go lower to the diaphragm at T12. This lesion likely has entered the danger space which is a fascial reflection of the retropharyngeal space (a potential space).

4. **A.** The usual source of a retropharyngeal abscess is pharyngitis or tonsillitis. It is unlikely to be dental/odontogenic disease because the mass is too far posterior. Sinusitis and epiglottis/supraglottis are not typical sources of retropharyngeal abscess.

Comment

The Retropharyngeal Space

The retropharyngeal space is bound anteriorly by the buccopharyngeal membrane and part of the middle layer of the deep cervical fascia, laterally by the alar fascia, and posteriorly by the prevertebral fascia. Some authorities believe that the alar and buccopharyngeal fasciae fuse above C3 and below C6, which accounts for the possibility of a localized retropharyngitis between these cervical segments. A reflection of the fascial planes of the retropharyngeal space and alar fascia creates the "danger space." The classical view is that the retropharyngeal space ends at the T3 level but the danger space extends to the diaphragm and therefore can be at the lowest thoracic level. Note how low the collection extends in this case.

Symptoms of Retropharyngeal Abscesses

Retropharyngeal processes usually induce neck pain, limitations in range of movement of the neck, dysphagia, and odynophagia. The differential diagnosis may include tendonitis of the longus colli muscle (usually in association with calcification). The longus colli–longus capitis complex can be displaced surgically to distinguish processes that are retropharyngeal (anterior to these muscles) from those that are perivertebral (posterior to or involving these muscles): Displacement of the muscles posteriorly implies that the lesion is pharyngeal or retropharyngeal. This fact may be of particular use when there are massive skull base lesions that have head and neck components. A lesion that arises in bone (a metastasis, chordoma, or sarcoma) pushes the longus complex anteriorly.

Imaging Findings

When a lesion in the retropharyngeal space has low density on imaging, it may represent pure edema from an adjacent pharyngitis (most common with no mass effect or enhancement), a phlegmon (minimal mass effect and no enhancement), or an abscess (mass effect and often peripheral enhancement) (Figures S145-1, S145-2, S145-3, and S145-4), or it may represent necrotizing adenitis (off midline with round shape in location of expected nodes). An abscess may represent a confluence of multiple suppurative lymph nodes. As criteria for diagnosing a retropharyngeal abscess on computed tomography, low density and enhancing rings have a sensitivity of 43% and a specificity of 63%.

Complications of peritonsillar and retropharyngeal abscesses include septic aneurysms, jugular vein thrombophlebitis, cellulitis, and mediastinitis. Most affected patients can be treated medically with intravenous antibiotics (with or without percutaneous or transoral aspiration). About 25% require surgical drainage.

Reference

Al-Sabah B, Bin Salleen H, Hagr A, Choi-Rosen J, Manoukian JJ, Tewfik TL. Retropharyngeal abscess in children: 10-year study. *J Otolaryngol.* 2004;33(6):352-355.

Cross-Reference

Neuroradiology: The Requisites, 3rd ed, 499-500.

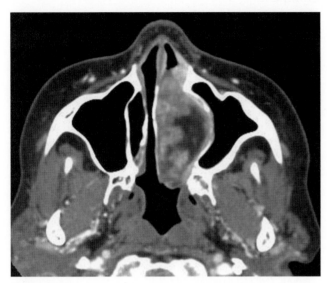

Figure 146-1

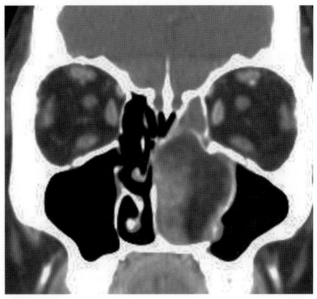

Figure 146-2

HISTORY: A young adult presents with nosebleeds.

1. Which of the following should be included in the differential diagnosis? (Choose all that apply.)
   A. Chondroma
   B. Chondrosarcoma
   C. "Cocaine nose"
   D. Inverted papilloma

2. Which pathogen is least likely to erode the nasal septum?
   A. *Mycobacterium tuberculosis*
   B. *Klebsiella* organisms
   C. *Escherichia coli*
   D. *Mycobacterium leprae*

3. Which syndrome predisposes affected patients to chondroid lesions?
   A. Lupus
   B. Ollier disease
   C. Klippel-Trenaunay-Weber syndrome
   D. Turcot syndrome

4. How often do nasal chondromas show whorls of calcification, typical of most chondroid lesions?
   A. 0% to 25%
   B. 26% to 50%
   C. 51% to 75%
   D. >75%

See Supplemental Figures section for additional figures and legends for this case.

CASE 146

Nasal Chondroma

1. **A, B, and D.** Chondroid lesions and inverted papilloma are the most common and second most common nasal septum masses, respectively. Chondrosarcoma should also be considered in the diagnosis, although this particular lesion does not seem aggressive. "Cocaine nose" is an erosive process, not a mass.

2. **C.** *E. coli* is not known to erode the nasal septum. *M. tuberculosis* is commonly erosive and seen frequently outside the United States. *Klebsiella* organisms and *M. leprae* (which causes leprosy) are also erosive. *Klebsiella* disease is also called *rhinoscleroma*, and leprosy leads to a saddle nose deformity.

3. **B.** Ollier disease predisposes affected patients to chondroid lesions, usually appendicular in location. Lupus, Klippel-Trenaunay-Weber syndrome, and Turcot syndrome are not associated with chondroid lesions.

4. **A.** Unlike most chondroid lesions, only 0% to 25% of nasal chondromas show whorls of calcification. They usually show no matrix.

Comment

Characteristics of Nasal Chondromas

Although the nasal septum contains cartilage, the most common site of sinonasal cartilaginous lesions is the ethmoid sinus (50%); other sites are the maxilla (18%), the nasal septum (17%) (Figures S146-1 and S146-2), the sphenoid sinus (6%), and the alar cartilage (3%). They are lesions of late adolescence and early adulthood. Malignant transformation of chondroid lesions may occur in older patients, in cases of rapid growth, and with invasion of surrounding structures. Elsewhere in the body, chondrosarcomas may also arise from preexisting lesions such as enchondromas or osteochondromas. This is less commonly seen in the head and neck unless the patient has a multiple enchondromas syndrome. Maffucci syndrome and Ollier disease are associated with multiple enchondromas, but usually of the extremities.

Reference

Rahman MZ, Shaifuddin AK, Aliya Shahnaz A, Ghosh PK. Chondroma of the nasal septum—a case report and review of literature [case report]. *Pak J Otolaryngol* 2012;28:97-99.

Cross-Reference

Neuroradiology: The Requisites, 3rd ed, 568-569.

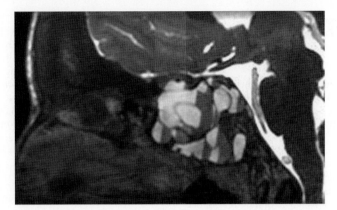

Figure 147-1

HISTORY: An 18-year-old woman is being evaluated for headache.

1. Which of the following should be included in the differential diagnosis? (Choose all that apply.)
   A. Osteoma
   B. Osteoblastoma
   C. Ewing sarcoma
   D. Aneurysmal bone cyst (ABC)

2. What is the characteristic feature of ABCs?
   A. Lytic lesion
   B. Blastic lesion
   C. Eye-of-the-tiger sign
   D. Blood-fluid levels

3. What is the most common site for pediatric head and neck ABCs?
   A. Skull
   B. Jaws
   C. Sinonasal cavity
   D. Temporal bone

4. What is the typical age group for ABCs?
   A. <20 years old
   B. 20 to 40 years old
   C. 41 to 60 years old
   D. >60 years old

See Supplemental Figures section for additional figures and legends for this case.

CASE 147

Aneurysmal Bone Cyst

1. **D.** The appearance is typical of ABC, although the location is unusual. The fluid levels are not characteristic of osteoblastomas unless they have superimposed ABC, and because the lesion is nonaggressive, it is unlikely to be Ewing sarcoma.

2. **D.** Blood-fluid levels are the characteristic feature of ABCs. Lytic and blastic lesions are not typical or classic features. The eye-of-the-tiger sign is a common feature of Hallervorden-Spatz disease, but it is a magnetic resonance imaging (MRI) feature of the basal ganglia.

3. **B.** The jaws—mandible and maxilla—are the most common site of pediatric head and neck ABCs. The skull is the second most common site. The sinonasal cavity and temporal bone are not common sites.

4. **A.** ABCs typically occur in patients younger than 20 years (median age: 17). However, they manifest in a wide range of ages because they can occur in association with giant cell tumors, nonossifying fibromas, and osteoblastomas.

Comment

Incidence of Aneurysmal Bone Cysts

Only 2% of ABCs occur in the head and neck. Of these, there are more cases in the mandible (most common site), maxilla, and sinonasal cavity (Figure S147-1). Most are lytic but may exhibit the characteristic blood-fluid levels. They are expansile lesions that are sclerotic only in approximately 2% of cases. They typically occur in children and young adults. They may be associated with preexisting lesions such as giant cell tumor, fibrous dysplasia, fibromyxoma, hemangioma, osteoblastoma, osteosarcoma, chondroblastoma, chondromyxoid fibroma, nonossifying fibroma, hemangioendothelioma, unicameral bone cyst, and eosinophilic granuloma. When it is a primary lesion, there may be antecedent trauma. Nonetheless, giant cell tumor is associated with secondary ABC in 39% of these lesions, and in 14% of cases of giant cell tumor, ABC components are evident.

Histopathology of Aneurysmal Bone Cysts

The World Health Organization defines the ABC histopathologically as an "expanding osteolytic lesion consisting of blood-filled spaces of variable size separated by connective tissue septa containing trabeculae of osteoid tissue and osteoclast giant cells." Surgery is the treatment of choice.

Reference

Fennessy BG, Vargas SO, Silvera MV, Ohlms LA, McGill TJ, Healy GB, et al. Paediatric aneurysmal bone cysts of the head and neck. *J Laryngol Otol.* 2009;123(6):635-641.

Cross-Reference

Neuroradiology: The Requisites, 3rd ed, 568-569.

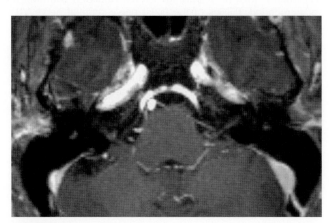

Figure 148-1

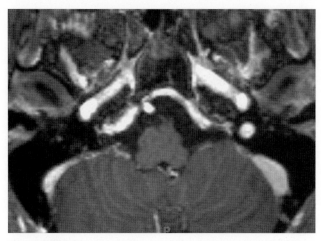

Figure 148-2

HISTORY: A 45-year-old patient has a history of glioblastoma of the high parietal lobe.

1. Which of the following should be included in the differential diagnosis? (Choose all that apply.)
   A. Bell palsy
   B. Ramsay Hunt syndrome
   C. Facial nerve schwannoma
   D. Normal findings

2. In symptom-free individuals, how often does the facial nerve enhance on magnetic resonance imaging (MRI)?
   A. 1% to 25%
   B. 26% to 50%
   C. 51% to 75%
   D. >75%

3. How often is normal facial nerve enhancement asymmetric from side to side?
   A. 1% to 25%
   B. 26% to 50%
   C. 51% to 75%
   D. >75%

4. What cranial nerve is affected most commonly in sarcoidosis?
   A. The facial nerve
   B. The trigeminal nerve
   C. The vestibulocochlear nerve
   D. The vagus nerve (in the neck)

See Supplemental Figures section for additional figures and legends for this case.

CASE 148

Normal Facial Nerve Enhancement

1. **D.** This is normal facial nerve enhancement. The facial nerve may normally enhance in its tympanic and intramastoid descending segments, as well as at the geniculate ganglion.

2. **D.** The facial nerve in the segments described previously enhances on MRI in 75% of symptom-free individuals. Therefore, tympanic and intramastoid facial nerve enhancement should not be considered pathologic.

3. **B.** Normal facial nerve enhancement is asymmetric from side to side in 45% of people. This should not lead to an overdiagnosis of facial nerve schwannoma or neuritis.

4. **A.** The facial nerve is affected most commonly in sarcoidosis. Sarcoidosis may also affect the meninges.

Comment

Determining Normal vs. Abnormal Findings

Gebarski and colleagues (1992) showed that facial nerve enhancement is the norm in most individuals because of the circumneural arteriovenous plexus in the facial nerve's tympanic and intramastoid portions (Figures S148-1, S148-2, and S148-3). Therefore, in a patient with Bell palsy, tympanic or intramastoid facial nerve enhancement is not proof of abnormality, even if the enhancement is asymmetric (seen in 45% of normal patients). Enhancement is abnormal in the intracanalicular or intralabyrinthine portions of the facial nerve. At the geniculate ganglion, enhancement is almost always seen.

When should a patient who has features of Bell palsy (i.e., atypical Bell palsy) undergo imaging? Usually if the patient's symptoms have not resolved by 4 to 8 weeks after onset, or if any other cranial nerves are involved, evaluation with MRI is recommended. Palsies of the facial nerve (cranial nerve VII) can lead to weakness in the bottom eyelid and deficits in upper eyelid closure, but ptosis is a symptom of oculomotor nerve (cranial nerve III) disease. With an oculomotor nerve palsy, the eye can still be shut tightly because of intact facial nerve fibers. A gold weight may be implanted in the eyelid of a person with facial nerve palsy to assist in shutting the eye.

Characteristics of VII Schwannoma

The facial nerve schwannoma may arise in the cerebellopontine angle cistern, the internal auditory canal, the temporal bone, the stylomastoid foramen, the parotid gland, or the face. At the geniculate ganglion, the schwannoma may locally expand the bone, creating a so-called crescent sign. In extracranial schwannoma, the facial nerve is involved less frequently than are the vagus nerve, sympathetic plexus, cervical plexus, and trigeminal nerves. Signal intensity on T2-weighted scans varies according to the ratio of Antoni A and B tissue, the latter being bright and the former dark on scans with long repetition times. On dynamic scanning, persistent uptake in the mass without an early dip in enhancement characterizes schwannomas, as opposed to paragangliomas. On angiography, schwannomas appear much less vascular than do glomus tumors. Gadolinium-enhanced MRI may be even more helpful in planning the surgical approach and in defining the extent of tumor involvement relative to the facial nerve than are intraoperative frozen sections, with which tumor extent is frequently overestimated.

Reference

Gebarski SS, Telian SA, Niparki JK. Enhancement along the normal facial nerve in the facial canal: MR imaging and anatomic correlation. *Radiology.* 1992;183:391-394.

Cross-Reference

Neuroradiology: The Requisites, 3rd ed, 403-405.

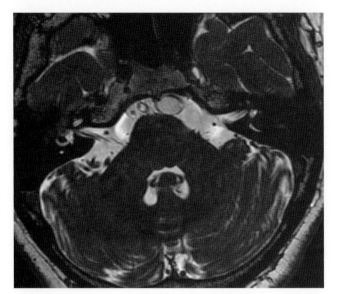

Figure 149-1

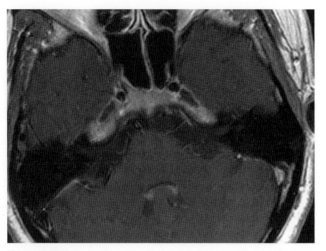

Figure 149-2

HISTORY: The patient has a history of sinusitis (incidental finding).

1. Which of the following should be included in the differential diagnosis? (Choose all that apply.)
   A. Tornwaldt cyst
   B. Ecchordosis physaliphora
   C. Epidermoid
   D. Rathke cleft cyst

2. Which of the following are *not* typical features of ecchordosis physaliphora?
   A. It is attached by a pedicle to the clivus.
   B. It is found in the prepontine cistern.
   C. It is a notochordal remnant.
   D. It causes palsies of cranial nerve V.

3. What imaging feature best distinguishes chordomas from ecchordosis physaliphora?
   A. Chordomas appear bright on T2-weighted images.
   B. Chordomas arise from the clivus.
   C. Chordomas erode bone.
   D. Chordomas enhance on imaging.

4. Which is true regarding ecchordosis physaliphora versus chordoma?
   A. Both are intradural.
   B. Both are extradural.
   C. Ecchordosis physaliphora is intradural, and chordoma is almost always extradural.
   D. Ecchordosis physaliphora is extradural, and chordoma is intradural.

See Supplemental Figures section for additional figures and legends for this case.

CASE 149

Ecchordosis Physaliphora

1. **B.** Ecchordosis physaliphora is visible as a lesion off the clivus without enhancement. Tornwaldt cyst occurs in the nasopharynx. Epidermoids do not have the same intensity as cerebrospinal fluid on constructive interference in steady state (CISS) studies; they look more solid. Rathke cleft cysts do not occur in this location.

2. **D.** Palsies of cranial nerve V are not typical features of ecchordosis physaliphora.

3. **D.** Most chordomas enhance on imaging, but ecchordosis physaliphora does not; thus enhancement is the best way to distinguish the two. Both appear bright on T2-weighted imaging, arise from or near the clivus, and erode bone.

4. **C.** Ecchordosis physaliphora is intradural, and chordoma is almost always extradural. In rare cases, chordomas are intradural. Chordomas are tumors, whereas ecchordosis physaliphora is a remnant that should be left alone.

Comment

Manifestation of Ecchordosis Physaliphora

Ecchordosis physaliphora is a notochordal remnant that can manifest as a retroclival mass. The ascending notochord crosses the clivus in three places: the posterior clivus, the pharyngeal surface, and the dorsum sellae. These may be the sites of ecchordosis physaliphora (Figures S149-1, S149-2, and S149-3). This lesion is present in approximately 2% of autopsy cases, which means that this lesion is seriously underdiagnosed at MRI; it may be mistaken for cerebrospinal fluid pulsation artifacts. It usually has a pedicle to the clivus but manifests as an intradural lesion. It is asymptomatic; chordomas, in contrast, usually manifest with headaches and/or palsies of cranial nerve VI because they irritate the nerve as it runs through the Dorello canal.

Imaging Findings

Notochordal remnants may be found anywhere from the sacrum to the clivus as the notochord ascends and contributes embryologically to tissue of the central nervous system. This accounts for why chordomas can arise in the sacrum, in the intervertebral disks, in the cervical spine, and in the clivus. The pathologic distinction between ecchordosis physaliphora and chordoma is very difficult. Imaging features of aggressive bone destruction, enhancement, rapid growth, and/or calcified matrix help distinguish chordoma from ecchordosis physaliphora. Patients' symptoms may also suggest chordoma.

Reference

Mehnert F, Beschorner R, Küker W, Hahn U, Nägele T. Retroclival ecchordosis physaliphora: MR imaging and review of the literature. *AJNR Am J Neuroradiol.* 2004;25(10):1851-1855.

Cross-Reference

Neuroradiology: The Requisites, 3rd ed, 383-384.

Acknowledgment

Thank you to Gul Moonis, MD, for providing the figures for this case.

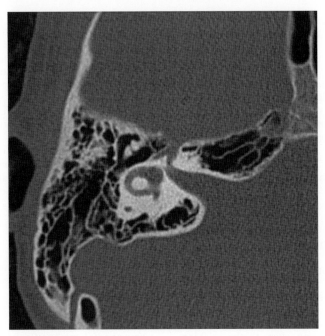

Figure 150-1

HISTORY: A patient presented with right-sided hearing loss.

1. Which of the following should be included in the differential diagnosis? (Choose all that apply.)
   A. Congenital aural atresia
   B. Congenital malleus bar
   C. Tympanosclerosis
   D. Otosclerosis

2. Which of the following are *not* classifications of congenital ossicular anomalies?
   A. Malleoincudal fixations
   B. Stapes fixations
   C. Incudostapedial disconnections
   D. Enlarged vestibular aqueduct syndrome (EVAS)

3. What type of hearing loss is found with a malleus bar?
   A. Sensorineural
   B. Combined conductive and sensorineural
   C. Conductive
   D. None

4. What entity causes stapes fixation most commonly?
   A. Malleus bar
   B. Otospongiosis
   C. Tympanosclerosis
   D. EVAS

See Supplemental Figures section for additional figures and legends for this case.

CASE 150

Malleus Bar

1. **B and C.** The point of fixation to the anterior malleus indicates a congenital malleus bar. Tympanosclerosis should also be considered in the diagnosis because of the ligamentous calcification. Congenital aural atresia is not apparent in this case, and the calcification shown would not cause otosclerosis.

2. **D.** EVAS is not considered an ossicular anomaly. In malleoincudal fixations, the malleus head and incus body are fixed to the epitympanic wall by a fibrous band or bony bar. Stapes fixation is a common anomaly. Incudostapedial disconnections can occur as absence of the incus long process and/or stapes superstructure.

3. **C.** The hearing loss is conductive because the malleus cannot move. The vibrations cannot be transmitted. This would not lead to sensorineural hearing loss.

4. **B.** Otospongiosis occurs at the fissula ante fenestram, just anterior to the oval window and close to the cochlea. Retrofenestral varieties of otospongiosis may affect the whole circumference of the cochlea. Malleus bar, tympanosclerosis, and EVAS do not affect the stapes.

Comment

Causes of Ossicular Fixation

Several entities cause ossicular fixation, some of which are congenital (such as this malleus bar, which is occasionally present in congenital aural atresia; Figure S150-1) and some developmental or inflammatory. Congenital causes that demonstrate normal bone tissue are thought to be due to either failure of the head of the malleus to separate from the walls of the epitympanum during embryogenesis or bone spurs that fuse to the malleus. Otospongiosis causes fixation of the stapes footplate at the oval window by means of new bone growth at the fissula ante fenestram. Tympanosclerosis may cause ligamentous/tendinous calcification or ossification, which can fix an ossicle to the side of the tympanic cavity. This is usually a complication of chronic otitis media. After trauma, hemotympanum may calcify, which can lead to fixation of ossicles. Thus there are three histopathologic types of malleus head fixations: those with normal bone tissue, those with nontympanosclerotic bone remodeling, and those with tympanosclerotic foci in the tympanic cavity.

Reference

Carfrae MJ, Jahrsdoerfer RA, Kesser BW. Malleus bar: an unusual ossicular abnormality in the setting of congenital aural atresia. *Otol Neurotol.* 2010;31(3):415-418.

Cross-Reference

Neuroradiology: The Requisites, 3rd ed, 394-398.

Acknowledgment

Thank you to Gul Moonis, MD, for providing the figures for this case.

Challenge

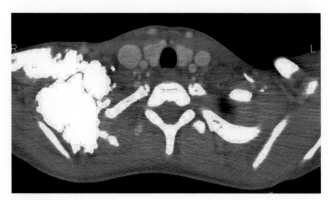

Figure 151-1

HISTORY: A 19-year-old woman presents with a hard, supra-clavicular, right-sided neck mass.

1. Which of the following should be included in the differential diagnosis (Choose all that apply.)
   A. Myositis ossificans
   B. Soft tissue sarcoma
   C. Tumoral calcinosis
   D. Neurofibrosarcoma

2. What age group is most affected by tumoral calcinosis?
   A. <20 years
   B. 21 to 40 years
   C. 41 to 60 years
   D. >60 years

3. Which ethnic group is disproportionately affected by tumoral calcinosis?
   A. Asians
   B. African Americans
   C. Native Americans
   D. People of Nordic ancestry

4. Which of the following are characteristic of tumoral calcinosis?
   A. Pain, periarticular
   B. Painless, periarticular
   C. Pain, mucosal
   D. Painless, mucosal

See Supplemental Figures section for additional figures and legends for this case.

CASE 151

Tumoral Calcinosis

1. **A, B, and C.** The diagnosis should include tumoral calcinosis. It should also include myositis ossificans, although myositis ossificans looks more sheet-like as opposed to the globular appearance of tumoral calcinosis. The differential diagnosis also includes soft tissue sarcomas such as paraosteal osteosarcoma, although there is little mass besides the matrix. Neurofibrosarcoma does not calcify like the lesion in the figure.

2. **A.** Tumoral calcinosis affects primarily people younger than 20 years. This is a disease of the first two decades of life.

3. **B.** African Americans are affected disproportionately by tumoral calcinosis. The reasons are unknown but probably genetic.

4. **B.** Tumoral calcinosis is painless and periarticular. The hip is affected most commonly.

Comment

Nonneoplastic Calcified Soft Tissue Lesions

Soft tissue lesions that have calcified matrix may have a variety of causes. Dystrophic calcification may be secondary to calcium phosphate dysmetabolism syndromes such as hyperparathyroidism and its many "pseudo" and non-"pseudo" variants. Trauma may elicit an unusually proliferative process that leads to soft tissue ossification that may be self-perpetuating. This occurs more aggressively and quickly than tumoral calcinosis, an entity that has autosomal dominant and autosomal recessive forms of inheritance. Tumoral calcinosis (Figure S151-1), like myositis ossificans, can occur secondary to a periarticular infection or traumatic injury with hemorrhage.

Tumors in the Soft Tissues

Tumors that can occur in the soft tissues with matrix include nonosseous but periarticular osteosarcomas, as well as chondrosarcomas and fibrosarcomas. The proliferative nature of this matrix is more indicative of a chondrosarcoma, but little mass is separate from the calcification. Synovial sarcomas, despite their names, may also occur in the soft tissue away from a joint and be characterized by hemorrhage, calcification, or both. Around a joint, consider loose fragments within the joint ("joint mice"), synovial chondromatosis, and pigmented villonodular synovitis. The last entity may be characterized pathologically by excessive hemosiderin staining.

Reference

Olsen KM, Chew FS. Tumoral calcinosis: pearls, polemics, and alternative possibilities. *Radiographics*. 2006;26(3):871-885.

Cross-Reference

Neuroradiology: The Requisites, 3rd ed, 90b, 596.

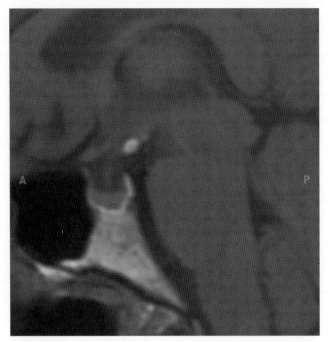

Figure 152-1

HISTORY: A teenager has a lifelong history of multiple hormonal deficiencies.

1. Which of the following should be included in the differential diagnosis? (Choose all that apply.)
   A. Hemorrhagic pituitary adenoma
   B. Dermoid
   C. Lipoma
   D. Ectopic posterior pituitary gland

2. Levels of what hormone are most commonly affected by stalk interruption?
   A. Antidiuretic hormone
   B. Growth hormone
   C. Prolactin
   D. Vasopressin

3. In pituitary stalk transection, what happens to the anterior pituitary gland?
   A. It is unaffected and normal in appearance.
   B. It enlarges.
   C. It is small in size.
   D. It exhibits a Rathke cleft cyst.

4. What hormonal abnormality is most common when the pituitary stalk cannot be visualized on imaging?
   A. Multiple hormonal deficiencies
   B. Isolated growth hormone deficiency
   C. Syndrome of inappropriate antidiuretic hormone secretion (SIAHS)
   D. Elevated prolactin level

See Supplemental Figures section for additional figures and legends for this case.

CASE 152

Undescended Pituitary Stalk

1. **B, C, and D.** The bright lesion in the suprasellar region probably represents an ectopic posterior pituitary gland. Dermoid and lipoma are also possibilities, but only in the presence of a normal posterior pituitary gland. The lesion is separate from the pituitary gland, and so the diagnosis would not include hemorrhagic pituitary adenoma.

2. **B.** Growth hormone is the hormone whose levels are most commonly affected by stalk interruption. Antidiuretic hormone deficiency is not as common as growth hormone deficiency with stalk transection, and prolactin and vasopressin issues are rare with this entity.

3. **C.** In pituitary stalk transection, the anterior pituitary gland is small in size. This may be a result of supportive hormone decline. It is very rare for pituitary stalk transection to coincide with Rathke cleft cyst.

4. **A.** Multiple hormonal deficiencies are present in 73% of patients in whom the pituitary stalk cannot be visualized.

Comment

Differential Diagnosis

An undescended posterior pituitary gland may be secondary to pituitary stalk transection as a result of trauma at birth, or it may be a congenital phenomenon that manifests as ectopic pituitary gland. In such cases, the posterior pituitary gland shows high signal in the midline at the hypothalamus median eminence on imaging (Figure S152-1). The differential diagnosis, which can be addressed with fat-suppressed imaging, includes lipoma and dermoid, both of which should appear bright on T1-weighted scans associated with a normal posterior pituitary gland. One should check for the presence of a thrombosed basilar tip aneurysm or cavernoma in the differential diagnosis.

Growth Hormone Deficiencies

Hormonal abnormalities may be manifold. Growth hormone deficiency is most common with undescended pituitary stalk, but multiple hormones may be affected. Of patients with growth hormone deficiency, 70% have a hypoplastic adenohypophysis and an ectopic posterior pituitary gland. If the pituitary stalk is not seen at all, multiple hormones are usually involved, but if the patient has only growth hormone deficiency, nonvisualization of the pituitary stalk is uncommon. The posterior pituitary tissue, even if ectopic, usually secretes antidiuretic hormone normally, as paradoxical as that may seem. When the high signal is *not* present, diabetes insipidus is a possibility.

Reference

van der Linden AS, van Es HW. Case 112: pituitary stalk transection syndrome with ectopic posterior pituitary gland. *Radiology.* 2007;243(2):594-597.

Cross-Reference

Neuroradiology: The Requisites, 3rd ed, 293.

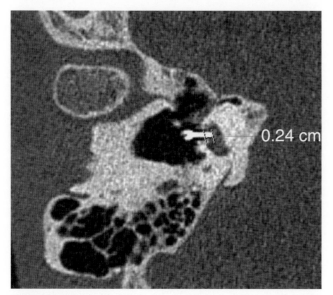

0.24 cm

Figure 153-1

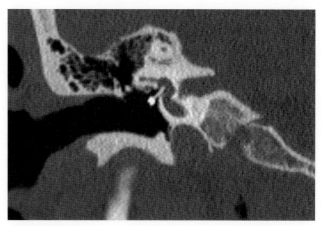

Figure 153-2

HISTORY: Despite previous stapes implantation, a patient had recurrent hearing loss.

1. Which of the following should be included in the differential diagnosis? (Choose all that apply.)
   A. Stapes implant, normal
   B. Stapes implant, migration
   C. Incudostapedial implant, normal
   D. Metallic foreign body

2. What is the maximum depth of a McGee stapes prosthesis in the vestibule?
   A. <2 mm
   B. <3 mm
   C. <4 mm
   D. <5 mm

3. What is the most common reason for a stapes prosthesis insertion?
   A. Presbycusis
   B. Trauma
   C. Cholesteatoma
   D. Otospongiosis/otosclerosis

4. What remains present in a partial ossicular replacement prosthesis (PORP) as opposed to a total ossicular replacement prosthesis (TORP)?
   A. Malleus
   B. Incus
   C. Scutum
   D. The PORP is attached to the stapes capitulum, whereas the TORP is attached to the stapes footplate/oval window.

See Supplemental Figures section for additional figures and legends for this case.

CASE 153

Stapes Implant

1. **B.** The diagnosis is stapes implant migration because the implant is too far into the vestibule. No incus implant is present, and there is no metallic foreign body.

2. **A.** The maximum depth of a McGee stapes prosthesis in the vestibule is less than 2 mm. It is slightly greater for the Smart piston.

3. **D.** Otospongiosis/otosclerosis is the most common reason for a stapes prosthesis insertion because either disease causes stapes footplate fixation. This leads to conductive hearing loss.

4. **D.** The PORP is attached to the stapes capitulum, whereas the TORP is attached to the stapes footplate/oval window. The capitulum is preserved with a PORP.

Comment

Complications with Stapes Implants

Many things can potentially go wrong with a stapes implant. Incus erosion and necrosis from a foreign body reaction and granulation tissue are fairly frequent findings at revision surgery, but prosthesis malposition is also a major issue. The prosthesis can dissociate from the incus despite the little hook that is supposed to keep it fastened; it can dislodge from the oval window; or, in rare situations (as in this case), it can penetrate the oval window too far (Figures S153-1 and S153-2). When this happens, hearing loss and vertigo usually result.

Stapedotomy

Most ossicular prosthesis replacements are performed because of the complications of chronic otitis media/cholesteatoma and trauma and congenital deformities. Because cholesteatomas most commonly affect the more proximal ossicles rather than the stapes, the malleus and incus are more likely to be replaced than the stapes, which is more remote from the middle ear, not derived from the first branchial apparatus, and less affected by trauma. The stapes, however, is directly involved with otospongiosis. In a stapedotomy, the stapes superstructure/capitulum is resected, but the footplate is preserved. Then a small hole is drilled in the footplate, and a Teflon wire piston is advanced through the opening into the oval window, thereby connecting the native ossicular chain to the oval window.

Incidence of Complications

When ossicular replacement prostheses dislodge or become malpositioned, the result, as would be expected, is usually conductive hearing loss (conduction from the tympanic membrane to the oval window). The stapes prosthesis becomes dislodged and migrates posteriorly and inferiorly more commonly (50% to 60% of complications) than is driven deeply into the vestibule (2%), as in this case. Perilymphatic fistulas represent 10% of complications.

Reference

Stone JA, Mukherji SK, Jewett BS, Carrasco VN, Castillo M. CT evaluation of prosthetic ossicular reconstruction procedures: what the otologist needs to know. *Radiographics*. 2000;20(3):593-605.

Cross-Reference

Neuroradiology: The Requisites, 3rd ed, 101-103.

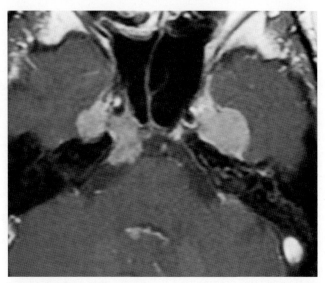

Figure 154-1

HISTORY: On follow-up examination of a patient with previously treated germinoma in the pineal region, new cranial neuropathies were detected.

1. Which of the following should be included in the differential diagnosis? (Choose all that apply.)
   A. Metastasis
   B. Post–radiation therapy meningiomas
   C. Infection in immunocompromised host after chemotherapy
   D. Multiple sclerosis

2. What is median age at diagnosis of germinomas of the pineal region?
   A. 6 years
   B. 2 years
   C. 12 years
   D. 22 years

3. Which of the following is true about the gender ratio with pineal and suprasellar germinomas?
   A. Patients with pineal and suprasellar germinomas are overwhelmingly female.
   B. Patients with pineal and suprasellar germinomas are overwhelmingly male.
   C. Patients with pineal germinomas are overwhelmingly male, but suprasellar germinomas occur in equal numbers of male and female patients.
   D. Patients with pineal germinomas are overwhelmingly male, but those with suprasellar germinomas are mostly female.

4. How often are pineal region germinomas characterized by subarachnoid space dissemination?
   A. 0% to 15%
   B. 16% to 30%
   C. 31% to 45%
   D. >45%

See Supplemental Figures section for additional figures and legends for this case.

CASE 154

Germinoma Metastases

1. **A, B, and C.** Metastasis may be caused by dural spread of tumor with seeding (Figure S154-1). In addition, there could be multiple meningiomas after radiation therapy or infection (such as tuberculosis or fungus) in an immunocompromised host after chemotherapy.

2. **C.** The median age at diagnosis of germinomas of the pineal region is 12 years. The mean age is 17, and fewer than 5% of cases are diagnosed after the age of 27.

3. **C.** Pineal germinomas occur overwhelmingly in male patients, but suprasellar germinomas occur in equal numbers of male and female patients.

4. **A.** Subarachnoid space dissemination occurs with 0% to 15% of pineal region germinomas. Despite this occurrence, responses to radiation therapy are excellent.

Comment

Incidence and Treatment of Germinomas

Germinomas represent more than 50% of all pineal region masses. Germ cell tumors also include teratomas, embryonic cell carcinomas, yolk sac tumors, and choriocarcinoma. Germinomas are extremely radiosensitive, and the prognosis for 5-year survival is greater than 80%. With the addition of combined chemotherapy and radiation therapy, the cure rate is higher than 90%. Age is a poor prognostic factor in central nervous system germinoma of the pineal gland: Patients presenting after age 30 have a 2.2 times higher rate of mortality. Race and extent of surgical resection do not affect outcomes. The tumors are more common in Asians.

Tumor Markers

Tumor markers are useful for diagnosing germ cell tumors:

TUMOR MARKER PROFILE FOR GERM CELL TUMORS

Tumor	AFP	Cytokeratin	HCG	PLAP
Germinoma			+*	+
Choriocarcinoma		+	++	+/−
Embryonal carcinoma		+		+
Endodermal sinus tumors	++	+		+/−
Malignant teratoma	+/−	+		

From Göbel U, Schneider DT, Calaminus G, Haas RJ, Schmidt P, Harms D. Germ-cell tumors in childhood and adolescence. GPOH MAKEI and the MAHO study groups. *Ann Oncol.* 2000;11(3):263-271.
*Positive in special cases in which syncytiotrophoblastic giant cells are present.
+, Cases are positive; +/−, some cases are positive and some cases are negative; ++, prominent immunohistochemistry appearance.
AFP, α-fetoprotein; HCG, β-chorionic gonadotropin; PLAP, placental alkaline phosphatase.

Reference

Göbel U, Schneider DT, Calaminus G, Haas RJ, Schmidt P, Harms D. Germ-cell tumors in childhood and adolescence. GPOH MAKEI and the MAHO study groups. *Ann Oncol.* 2000;11(3):263-271.

Cross-Reference

Neuroradiology: The Requisites, 3rd ed, 96, 377.

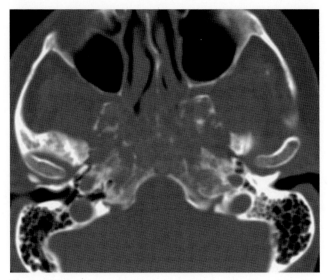

Figure 155-1

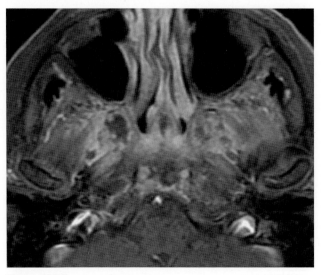

Figure 155-2

HISTORY: A patient with previously treated nasopharyngeal carcinoma had a deep, boring headache.

1. Which of the following should be included in the differential diagnosis? (Choose all that apply.)
   A. Myeloma
   B. Chordoma
   C. Nasopharyngeal carcinoma
   D. Radiation necrosis

2. What of the following is the tumor for which treatment most commonly causes radiation necrosis of the skull base?
   A. Sinonasal cancer
   B. Nasopharyngeal carcinoma
   C. Glioblastoma
   D. Retinoblastoma

3. Which is the strongest risk factor for nasopharyngeal carcinoma?
   A. Smoking
   B. Human papilloma virus
   C. Epstein-Barr virus
   D. Alcohol

4. What is first line of therapy for nasopharyngeal cancer?
   A. Surgery
   B. Chemoradiation
   C. Brachytherapy
   D. Laser

See Supplemental Figures section for additional figures and legends for this case.

CASE 155

Radiation Necrosis

1. **C and D.** Radiation necrosis may destroy bone, and nasopharyngeal carcinoma can grow through bone. The pattern of destruction and location are not correct for myeloma or chordoma.

2. **B.** Nasopharyngeal carcinoma is the tumor for which treatment most commonly causes radiation necrosis of the skull base. There may also be radiation changes and/or necrosis in the temporal lobes. The retinoblastoma gene may also cause sarcomas. Sinonasal cancer and glioblastoma very rarely erode the clivus.

3. **C.** The Epstein-Barr virus is the strongest risk factor for nasopharyngeal carcinoma, along with Southeast Asian ancestry. Smoking and alcohol (wine, in particular) cause a slight risk.

4. **B.** Chemoradiation is first line of therapy for nasopharyngeal cancer. Brachytherapy is sometimes used for recurrence.

Comment

Differential Diagnosis

The permeative and diffuse pattern of destruction of the skull base and surrounding tissues, including the adjacent musculature, is typical of radiation necrosis (Figures S155-1 and S155-2). The other possible diagnosis is malignant otitis externa with *Pseudomonas* infection, osteomyelitis, and myositis. There really is very little mass in this case; it is more a destructive tissue-limited process and hence suggestive of radiation necrosis.

Treatment of Nasopharyngeal Carcinoma

For nasopharyngeal carcinoma, radiation therapy is often the primary mode of ablation. Recurrence or residual disease may be treated with second-line treatment regimens such as brachytherapy, inasmuch as surgery is not an option. Chemotherapy is often used concomitantly. After multiple treatments, the risk of radiation necrosis increases. Intensity-modulated radiotherapy with doses of up to 70 Gy for recurrent nasopharyngeal carcinoma leads to temporal lobe necrosis in 6% to 19% of patients. Osteoradionecrosis occurs in 10% of cases of successfully treated nasopharyngeal carcinoma; if pharyngeal mucosa necrosis is evident endoscopically, the rate of osteoradionecrosis is as high as 56%.

Imaging Findings

If this bone destruction pattern is accompanied by white matter changes bilaterally and symmetrically in the temporal lobes or, worse, by areas of peripheral enhancement in the temporal lobes with extreme vasogenic edema, radiation injury to the brain has probably occurred as well. These features suggest this diagnosis, as opposed to nasopharyngeal carcinoma, which could also aggressively destroy the skull base or grow intracranially, or both. Usually the intracranial growth is via skull base foramina or the cavernous sinus.

Reference

Chen MY, Mai HQ, Sun R, Guo X, Zhao C, Hong MH, et al. Clinical findings and imaging features of 67 nasopharyngeal carcinoma patients with postradiation nasopharyngeal necrosis. *Chin J Cancer.* 2013;32(10):533-538.

Cross-Reference

Neuroradiology: The Requisites, 3rd ed, 101-103.

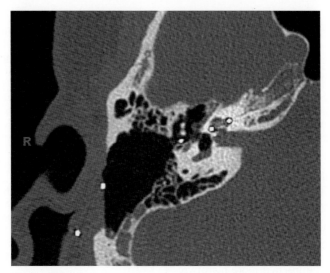

Figure 156-1

HISTORY: Right-sided hearing loss is present after cholesteatoma treatment in a young adult.

1. Which of the following should be included in the differential diagnosis? (Choose all that apply.)
   A. Postoperative changes after mastoidectomy
   B. Postoperative changes after cochlear implantation
   C. Pneumolabyrinth
   D. Otospongiosis

2. Which of the following is true about pneumolabyrinth?
   A. It may occur in cases of sinusitis.
   B. It may result from barotrauma.
   C. It results from a congenital dehiscence.
   D. It frequently accompanies pneumocephalus by virtue of two-way communication between the cochlea and vestibular aqueduct.

3. What symptoms are derived most commonly from pneumolabyrinth?
   A. Hearing loss more than imbalance
   B. Both hearing loss and imbalance
   C. Imbalance more than hearing loss
   D. Neither hearing loss nor imbalance

4. How far into the cochlea should a cochlear implant be inserted?
   A. One-half turn
   B. One turn
   C. Two turns
   D. More than two turns

See Supplemental Figures section for additional figures and legends for this case.

CASE 156

Pneumolabyrinth

1. **A, B, and C.** Postoperative changes after mastoidectomy are visualized as the air gap in the mastoid bone, and cochlear implantation is depicted by the metal in the cochlea. Pneumolabyrinth is visualized as the air in the vestibule, an expected postoperative finding. There is no evidence of otospongiosis.

2. **B.** Pneumolabyrinth may result from barotrauma and may lead to air in the inner ear. The most common cause is trauma, with or without temporal bone fracture.

3. **C.** Pneumolabyrinth is more likely to cause imbalance than to cause hearing loss, but only to a small degree.

4. **D.** A cochlear implant should be inserted more than two turns into the cochlea. It should optimally be inserted the full length of the cochlea.

Comment

Causes of Pneumolabyrinth

Pneumolabyrinth is most common in cases of barotrauma or in the postoperative setting (Figure S156-1), but it may result from aggressive infections, presumably via a labyrinthine fistula. This is a rare phenomenon with infections because the membranes preventing such breaches are usually resistant, but aggressive or air-producing organisms presumably could cause the introduction of air into the inner ear. In this case, the pneumolabyrinth was a postoperative phenomenon after cochlear implant surgery. This may resolve spontaneously. If a fracture breaches the inner ear structures and also communicates with an air-filled space—such as the mastoid air cells, middle ear, or aerated petrous bone—a pneumolabyrinth may occur.

Cochlear Implants

Cochlear implants are inserted via a canal wall–up mastoidectomy. The implant is placed into the basal turn of the cochlea via the round window. From there, the goal is to insert the implant along the full $2\frac{3}{4}$ turns of the cochlea, from basal turn to middle turn to apical turn. The further in it is inserted, the better the hearing output is.

Reference

Wolansky LJ, Desai NS, Chandrasekhar SS, Lee HJ, Pramanik BK, Finden SG. Computed tomography of bilateral pneumolabyrinth. *Emerg Radiol.* 1998;9/10:356-358.

Cross-Reference

Neuroradiology: The Requisites, 3rd ed, 414-416.

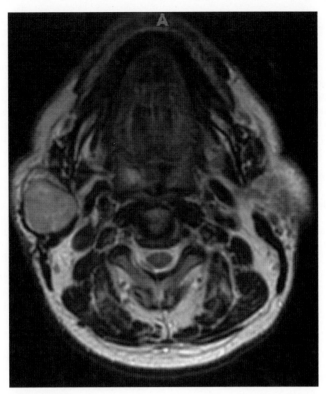

Figure 157-1

HISTORY: A 70-year-old male patient has a complaint of right ear swelling, and a palpable mass was present.

1. Which of the following should be included in the differential diagnosis? (Choose all that apply.)
   A. Warthin tumor
   B. First branchial cleft cyst
   C. Pleomorphic adenoma
   D. Myoepithelioma

2. Which one of the following is *not* a "monomorphic adenoma"?
   A. Myoepithelioma
   B. Oncocytic adenoma
   C. Canalicular adenoma
   D. Pleomorphic adenoma

3. What best describes the features of Warthin tumor?
   A. It occurs primarily in elderly men; it occurs in the tail of the parotid gland.
   B. It occurs primarily in middle-aged women; it occurs in the superficial lobe of the parotid gland.
   C. It occurs primarily in elderly men; it occurs in the deep lobe of the parotid gland.
   D. It occurs primarily in young men; it occurs in the deep lobe of the parotid gland.

4. Why are Warthin tumors electively removed at the patient's option?
   A. On resection, the rate of facial nerve paralysis is high, and so surgeons are reluctant to remove them.
   B. They respond very well to chemotherapy and radiation therapy.
   C. They seed the operative bed.
   D. They have no malignant potential.

See Supplemental Figures section for additional figures and legends for this case.

CASE 157

Parotid Myoepithelioma

1. **A, C, and D.** Because of the location, the diagnosis is most likely a Warthin tumor. The diagnosis should also include pleomorphic adenoma because it is the most common parotid mass. The actual pathologic diagnosis was myoepithelioma. The T2-weighted image suggests a solid mass, and so a first branchial cleft cyst should not be considered.

2. **D.** Pleomorphic adenoma is not a "monomorphic adenoma." Myoepitheliomas, oncocytic adenomas, and canalicular adenomas are the three classic monomorphic adenomas.

3. **A.** Warthin tumors are often seen in older men. They are seen in the tail of the parotid gland near the angle of the mandible.

4. **D.** Warthin tumors have no malignant potential, and so their removal is the patient's choice.

Comment
Features of a Warthin Tumor

Although this case histologically proved to be a myoepithelioma, it had the classical features of a Warthin tumor:
- It occurred in a man.
- The man was elderly.

- The lesion was in the tail of the parotid gland.
- It appeared heterogeneous on T2-weighted images, with darker areas in it (Figure S157-1).

Features of Myoepitheliomas

Myoepitheliomas are varieties of monomorphic adenomas characterized by a variable course. The parotid glands are the locations in 45% of the cases; however, in all salivary glands, pleomorphic adenomas are the most common benign salivary tumors. Monomorphic adenoma masses usually are well-defined and enhance avidly. However, there are malignant varieties of salivary gland myoepithelial tumors and 39% have aggressive features.

Site of Parotid Tumors

With regard to sites of tumors, the most common tumor of the superficial and deep lobes of the parotid gland is the pleomorphic adenoma. The tail of the parotid gland near the angle of the mandible is the only location where Warthin tumor predominates.

Reference

Khademi B, Kazemi T, Bayat A, Bahranifard H, Daneshbod Y, Mohammadianpanah M. Salivary gland myoepithelial neoplasms: a clinical and cytopathologic study of 15 cases and review of the literature. *Acta Cytol.* 2010;54(6):1111-1117.

Cross-Reference

Neuroradiology: The Requisites, 3rd ed, 482-484, 487.

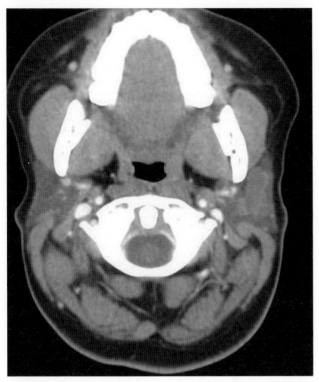

Figure 158-1

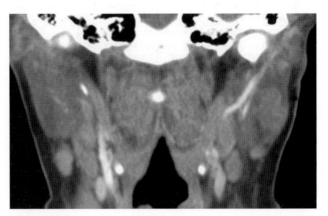

Figure 158-2

HISTORY: A 72-year-old patient has a palpable left-sided neck mass.

1. Which of the following should be included in the differential diagnosis? (Choose all that apply.)
   A. Pleomorphic adenoma
   B. Mucoepidermoid carcinoma
   C. Warthin tumor
   D. Acinic cell carcinoma

2. What two cranial nerves are susceptible to perineural spread from a parotid space malignancy?
   A. X and XII
   B. V and VII
   C. V and XI
   D. VII and XI

3. What is the most common salivary gland malignancy in children?
   A. Pleomorphic adenoma
   B. Mucoepidermoid carcinoma
   C. Adenocarcinoma
   D. Acinic cell carcinoma

4. What is the most common multifocal primary malignancy of the parotid gland?
   A. Adenocarcinoma
   B. Mucoepidermoid carcinoma
   C. Squamous cell carcinoma
   D. Acinic cell carcinoma

See Supplemental Figures section for additional figures and legends for this case.

CASE 158

Acinic Cell Carcinoma

1. **A, B, C, and D.** Pleomorphic adenomas are very common in the parotid gland, and Warthin tumors are common in the tail of the parotid gland. Mucoepidermoid carcinoma is a common malignancy. Acinic cell carcinoma is the correct diagnosis for this particular case.

2. **B.** Cranial nerves V and VII are susceptible to perineural spread from a parotid space malignancy because both have branches in the parotid space.

3. **B.** Mucoepidermoid carcinoma is the most common salivary gland malignancy in children. Acinic cell carcinoma is the second most common, and both arise most commonly in the parotid gland.

4. **D.** Acinic cell carcinoma is the most common multifocal primary malignancy of the parotid gland, occurring in 3% of cases. Mucoepidermoid carcinoma is a common malignancy but rarely multiple.

Comment

Features of Acinic Cell Carcinomas

Although acinic cell carcinoma is a rare parotid malignancy, it is the one that is most commonly multifocal or bilateral (Figures S158-1 and S158-2). This is the malignant equivalent of a Warthin tumor. Like Warthin tumor of the parotid gland, acinic cell carcinoma is rarely seen in the other salivary glands. It carries an intermediate prognosis. Its appearance could represent any number of tumors; the slightly irregular borders may be the only clue that it is not a pleomorphic adenoma.

Pediatric Salivary Gland Tumors

Benign and malignant tumors occur with near equal prevalence in the pediatric age group, whereas in adults, far more tumors are benign (dominated by pleomorphic adenomas). In children, pleomorphic adenomas are still histologically the most common of glandular tumors, and mucoepidermoid carcinoma is the most common malignancy, followed by acinic cell carcinoma. The malignant and benign tumors are most common in the parotid gland.

Reference

da Cruz Perez DE, Pires FR, Alves FA, Almeida OP, Kowalski LP. Salivary gland tumors in children and adolescents: a clinicopathologic and immunohistochemical study of fifty-three cases. *Int J Pediatr Otorhinolaryngol.* 2004;68(7):895-902.

Cross-Reference

Neuroradiology: The Requisites, 3rd ed, 338, 486.

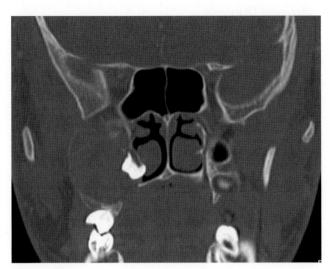

Figure 159-1

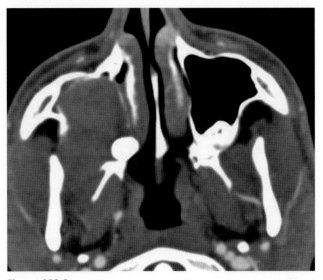

Figure 159-2

HISTORY: A child with sinus congestion is being evaluated before endoscopic surgery.

1. Which of the following should be included in the differential diagnosis? (Choose all that apply.)
   A. Odontogenic cyst
   B. Ameloblastoma
   C. Odontogenic keratocyst
   D. Juvenile ossifying fibroma

2. How often are ameloblastomas in the mandible, as opposed to the maxilla?
   A. They occur more often in the mandible by a ratio of 4:1.
   B. They occur more often in the mandible by a ratio of 2:1.
   C. They occur more often in the maxilla by a ratio of 2:1.
   D. They occur more often in the maxilla by a ratio of 4:1.

3. What percentage of ameloblastomas are associated with an unerupted tooth or dentigerous cyst?
   A. 0% to 25%
   B. 26% to 50%
   C. 51% to 75%
   D. 76% to 100%

4. What imaging features are characteristic of giant cell reparative granulomas of the maxilla?
   A. Neoplastic tissue that is associated with onion skinning
   B. Cystic degeneration and aneurysmal bone cyst features
   C. Unilocular lesion without enhancement
   D. Osteoid production and hemorrhagic components

See Supplemental Figures section for additional figures and legends for this case.

CASE 159

Juvenile Ossifying Fibroma

1. **B and D.** Juvenile ossifying fibroma could account for the dark signal on T2-weighted images. An odontogenic lesion that enhances on magnetic resonance imaging (MRI) may be an ameloblastoma. In view of the dark T2-weighted signal, this is probably not a cyst. The solid enhancement also indicates that this is probably not an odontogenic keratocyst (keratogenic odontogenic tumor).

2. **A.** Ameloblastomas occur more often in the mandible by a ratio of 4:1. Nonetheless, they are common primary odontogenic neoplasms of the maxilla as well.

3. **A.** Ameloblastomas are associated with an unerupted tooth or dentigerous cyst in 20% of cases. However, they are associated with solid tissue and therefore should not be confused with odontogenic cysts.

4. **D.** Osteoid production and hemorrhagic components are characteristic of giant cell reparative granulomas of the maxilla. These are common lesions of the maxilla and mandible.

Comment

Imaging Findings

This lesion is unique in that it produces such dark signal on T2-weighted images and enhances in a solid manner (Figures S159-1, S159-2, S159-3, and S159-4). That characteristic is unusual for all dental lesions, but it can be seen with juvenile ossifying fibromas. These lesions typically are located in the mandible (10%) and maxilla (80% to 90%), arising from the periodontal ligament, and develop in the first two decades of life. They may be aggressive lesions that infiltrate bone widely. They have a high rate of recurrence and differ from conventional ossifying fibromas by their rapid growth cycle. Usually their edges are surrounded by a thin bone shell, and they may have internal calcifications.

Differential Diagnosis

The differential diagnosis includes the desmoplastic variety of ameloblastomas. These are lesions dominated by their fibrous content and hence produce a dark signal on T2-weighted images. Most ameloblastomas produce a higher signal on T2-weighted images and have a cystic component. Ameloblastomas are tumors that occur more often in the mandible than in the maxilla by a 4:1 ratio. They may be unilocular (37.5%) or multilocular (62.5%); the latter have a high rate of recurrence (60% to 80%). In 20% of cases, they may be associated with an unerupted tooth and/or a dentigerous cyst.

Types of Odontogenic Tumors

Odontomas are more common dental tumors than ameloblastomas. With the reclassification of odontogenic keratocysts as neoplasms referred to as *keratocystic odontogenic tumors,* ameloblastomas are the third most common odontogenic tumors. The thickness of the solid component of enhancement in ameloblastomas is much increased in comparison with odontogenic keratocysts. Giant cell reparative granulomas are nonneoplastic lesions that occur in the maxillomandibular region, as well as in the extremities. They occur more often in women than in men, and 80% are found in patients younger than 30 years. They are often partially cystic and have hemorrhagic elements. Myxomas, also included in the differential diagnosis, characteristically appear bright on T2-weighted MRI and usually have only a peripheral rim of enhancement.

References

Keles B, Duran M, Uyar Y, Azimov A, Demirkan A, Esen HH. Juvenile ossifying fibroma of the mandible: a case report. *J Oral Maxillofac Res.* 2010;1(2):e5.

Asaumi J, Hisatomi M, Yanagi Y, Matsuzaki H, Choi YS, Kawai N, et al. Assessment of ameloblastomas using MRI and dynamic contrast-enhanced MRI. *Eur J Radiol.* 2005;56(1):25-30.

Cross-Reference

Neuroradiology: The Requisites, 3rd ed, 456, 492.

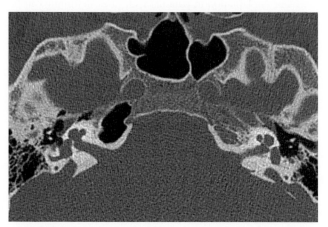

Figure 160-1

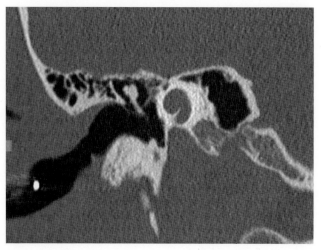

Figure 160-2

HISTORY: This patient presents with long-standing bilateral sensorineural hearing loss.

1. Which of the following should be included in the differential diagnosis? (Choose all that apply.)
   A. Michel deformity
   B. Cock deformity/common cavity
   C. Otospongiosis
   D. Incomplete partition type II (IP-II)

2. Which of the following is *not* present in this case?
   A. Incomplete partition of the semicircular canals
   B. Bilaterally enlarged vestibular aqueducts
   C. Incomplete development of the turns of the cochlea
   D. Pneumatized right petrous apex

3. Which anatomic parts are involved in Pendred syndrome?
   A. Temporal bone and orbits
   B. Temporal bone and thyroid gland
   C. Orbits and thyroid gland
   D. Temporal bone and gastrointestinal tract

4. Which is the correct order of the following syndromes by earliest to latest occurrence in gestation?
   A. Mondini malformation, Michel deformity, Cock deformity
   B. Michel deformity, Mondini malformation, Cock deformity
   C. Michel deformity, Cock deformity, Mondini malformation
   D. Cock deformity, Michel deformity, Mondini malformation

See Supplemental Figures section for additional figures and legends for this case.

CASE 160

Incomplete Partition II

1. **D.** The deficient modiolus of the cochlea indicates IP-II. The cochlea and vestibule are present and separate, and so Michel deformity and Cock deformity/common cavity should not be included in the diagnosis. Otospongiosis is also not included because the bone around the optic capsule is normal.

2. **A.** Incomplete partition of the semicircular canals is not present. The visualized semicircular canals are normal.

3. **B.** The temporal bone and thyroid gland are involved in Pendred syndrome. The thyroid gland is usually enlarged. The orbits and gastrointestinal tract are not affected or involved.

4. **C.** Michel deformity is the defect that occurs earliest in gestation, and the Mondini malformation occurs latest, but inner ear development is completed during the first trimester.

Comment

Features of Cock Deformity

In 1838, Edward Cock described an abnormality in inner ears in which the communication between the cochlea and the vestibule was excessively wide; this Cock deformity is also known as the *common cavity deformity*. This abnormal lack of mature differentiation between the cochlea and the vestibule occurs later in gestation than the abnormality that leads to Michel complete labyrinthine aplasia, in which no cochlea or vestibule is formed. In the Cock deformity, the cochlear spiralization is abnormal, often with only a single turn. Cochlear implantation in patients with Cock deformity can be performed, albeit with a higher risk of poor outcome, cerebrospinal fluid gushers, facial nerve injuries, and meningitis.

Features of Incomplete Partitions

This case is an example of IP-II, formerly referred to as Mondini malformation (Figures S160-1 and S160-2). From earliest in gestation to latest in gestation the deformities one can see are labyrinthine aplasia, cochlear aplasia, common cavity deformities, cystic cochleovestibular malformations (incomplete partition type I [IP-I]), cochleovestibular hypoplasia, and IP-II. In IP-II, the cochlea is cystic, with incomplete spiralization and generally with mild enlargement of the vestibule (which distinguishes it from IP-I, in which there is cystic dilatation of the vestibule). Typically, there are only 1.5 turns to the cochlea in IP-II. Enlargement of the vestibular aqueduct coexists frequently with IP-II, as in this case, but it may exist in isolation or in association with other late-event inner ear dysplasias. Because the facial nerve is in an aberrant location in about 25% of patients with cochleovestibular malformations, it is more likely to be injured at surgery. IP-II is nearly three times more common than IP-I. Many patients with either variety undergo a trial of cochlear implantation with modest results. The risk of cerebrospinal fluid gushers is lower with IP-II. IP-I is only rarely accompanied by enlargement of the vestibular aqueduct.

Reference

Huang BY, Zdanski C, Castillo M. Pediatric sensorineural hearing loss, part 1: practical aspects for neuroradiologists. *AJNR Am J Neuroradiol.* 2012;33(2):211-217.

Cross-Reference

Neuroradiology: The Requisites, 3rd ed, 405.

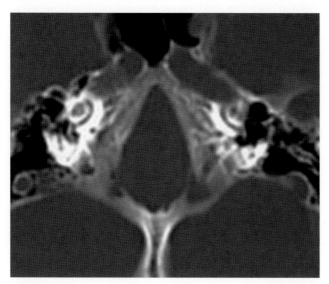

Figure 161-1

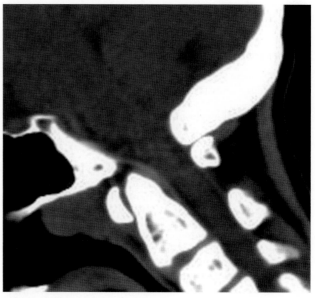

Figure 161-2

HISTORY: This patient has complaints of headaches.

1. Which of the following should be included in the differential diagnosis? (Choose all that apply.)
   A. Dandy-Walker syndrome
   B. Arnold-Chiari malformation
   C. Achondroplasia
   D. Multiple epiphyseal dysplasia

2. Which of the following is not associated with achondroplasia?
   A. Klippel-Feil syndrome
   B. Posterior scalloping
   C. Spinal stenosis
   D. Obstructive sleep apnea

3. What is the most common ear, nose, and throat (ENT) disorder faced by patients with achondroplasia?
   A. Laryngitis
   B. Pharyngitis with tonsillar hypertrophy
   C. Otomastoiditis
   D. Sinusitis

4. What is the normal anteroposterior diameter of the foramen magnum in an adult?
   A. 10 to 20 mm
   B. 20 to 30 mm
   C. 30 to 40 mm
   D. 40 to 50 mm

See Supplemental Figures section for additional figures and legends for this case.

CASE 161

Achondroplasia

1. **C.** The small foramen magnum indicates achondroplasia. This causes cranial neuropathies and headaches.

2. **A.** Klippel-Feil syndrome is not associated with achondroplasia. Spinal stenosis is the source of many issues with chronic pain in patients with achondroplasia.

3. **C.** Otomastoiditis is the most common ENT disorder faced by patients with achondroplasia. Pharyngitis with tonsillar hypertrophy is the second most common manifestation. Obstructive sleep apnea may also be an issue.

4. **C.** The normal anteroposterior diameter of the foramen magnum in adults ranges from 30 to 40 mm. The average anteroposterior width is 33.3 mm, and the average transverse width is 27.9 mm.

Comment

Complications of Achondroplasia

Many potential dangers face patients with achondroplasia. The narrowing of the airway is analogous to that associated with sleep apnea; it can lead to respiratory difficulties, with the inherent long-term effect on cardiovascular health. The severe stenosis of the foramen magnum seen in affected patients (Figures S161-1 and S161-2) can also lead to cardiorespiratory arrest under relatively minor traumatic events. Hydrocephalus often occurs as a result of the obstruction to the flow of cerebrospinal fluid at the foramen magnum. Affected patients also suffer from spinal stenosis, which leads to sensorimotor neuropathies in the extremities.

Causes of Achondroplasia

Achondroplasia is caused by mutations in the fibroblast growth factor receptor 3 (FGFR3) gene on chromosome 4P, which lead to impairment of bone growth. Twenty percent of cases are hereditary, transmitted as an autosomal dominant disorder, and 80% are sporadic. Achondroplasia is the most common form of dwarfism. Despite all of the skeletal manifestations of achondroplasia, it is the mundane otomastoiditis that is the most common manifestation of ENT symptoms in patients with this disorder.

Reference

Collins WO, Choi SS. Otolaryngologic manifestations of achondroplasia. *Arch Otolaryngol Head Neck Surg.* 2007;133(3):237-244.

Cross-Reference

Neuroradiology: The Requisites, 3rd ed, 279, 300, 408.

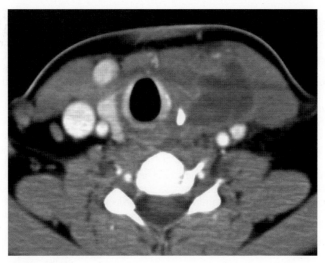

Figure 162-1

HISTORY: A patient has fever, neck pain, and thyroid storm.

1. What is included in the differential diagnosis of this cystic lesion? (Choose all that apply.)
   A. First branchial cleft cyst (BCC)
   B. Second BCC
   C. Third BCC
   D. Thyroglossal duct cyst
   E. Lymphangioma

2. Why is thyroiditis associated with some BCCs?
   A. BCCs occur in the thyroid gland.
   B. BCCs may be accompanied by an inflamed fistula through the thyroid gland.
   C. BCCs irritate the thyroglossal duct.
   D. BCCs are accompanied by a fistula to the palatine tonsil.

3. What is the approximate ratio of second BCCs to third BCCs?
   A. 1:1
   B. 5:1
   C. 15:1
   D. >15:1

4. Which branchial apparatus is responsible for the ultimobranchial bodies?
   A. First
   B. Second
   C. Third
   D. Fourth

See Supplemental Figures section for additional figures and legends for this case.

CASE 162

Third Branchial Cleft Cyst/Fistula

1. **C.** The location and presentation of the cystic lesion indicates third BCC. First BCC is usually found in the parotid gland, and second BCC is usually higher in the neck. Thyroglossal duct cysts are usually midline and not as irregularly shaped. Lymphangiomas are usually located in the posterior triangle.

2. **B.** Some third or fourth branchial cleft cysts may be accompanied by a fistula through the thyroid gland, which may cause thyroiditis. An opening may also be in the piriform sinus of the hypopharynx.

3. **D.** The ratio of second to third BCCs is 20:1.

4. **D.** The fourth branchial apparatus is responsible for the ultimobranchial bodies. This creates the parathyroid tissue and calcitonin-secreting tissue.

Comment

Types of Branchial Cleft Cysts

Cysts in the lower neck may be secondary, third, or fourth BCCs, thyroglossal duct cysts, thymic cysts, and lymphoceles. Thyroglossal duct cysts are the ones that occur most commonly in the midline, along with dermoids and epidermoids. Lymphatic vascular malformations are usually in the posterior triangle or the axilla, and 90% occur in patients younger than 2 years. Thymic cysts are often asymptomatic and occur more commonly on the left side than on the right.

Manifestation of Branchial Abnormalities

Third (Figure S162-1) and fourth branchial apparatus abnormalities may manifest as isolated cysts, but they may also have a fistula to the piriform sinus and/or may lead to a thyroiditis as they tract across the gland. A sinus tract may also lead to a skin opening in the lower neck, and this abnormality is more common on the left side than on the right. Complete excision of the cyst and the tract prevents recurrences. The differential diagnosis includes necrotic cystic lymph nodes, from either squamous cell carcinomas or thyroid cancers. Tuberculosis and actinomycosis are infections that may cause fistula formation.

Reference

Goff CJ, Allred C, Glade RS. Current management of congenital branchial cleft cysts, sinuses, and fistulae. *Curr Opin Otolaryngol Head Neck Surg.* 2012;20(6):533-539.

Cross-Reference

Neuroradiology: The Requisites, 3rd ed, 445, 487, 495.

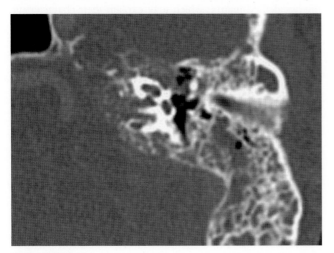

Figure 163-1

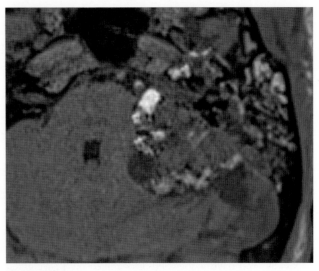

Figure 163-2

HISTORY: A patient has left-sided hearing loss after nephrectomy for renal cell carcinoma.

1. Because this is a hypervascular lesion, what is included in the differential diagnosis? (Choose all that apply.)
   A. Renal cell carcinoma metastasis
   B. Chondrosarcoma
   C. Chordoma
   D. Paraganglioma
   E. Endolymphatic sac tumor

2. With what syndrome are endolymphatic sac tumors (ELST) associated?
   A. Neurofibromatosis
   B. Tuberous sclerosis
   C. Gorlin syndrome
   D. von Hippel–Lindau (VHL) disease

3. What is the characteristic magnetic resonance imaging feature of ELST that distinguishes it from glomus tumors?
   A. Flow voids
   B. Enhancement
   C. Hyperintensity on T1-weighted images
   D. Hyperintensity on T2-weighted images

4. What percentage of ELSTs are associated with VHL disease?
   A. <10%
   B. 11% to 25%
   C. 26% to 50%
   D. >50%

See Supplemental Figures section for additional figures and legends for this case.

CASE 163

Endolymphatic Sac Tumor

1. **A, D, and E.** A hypervascular lesion may represent renal cell carcinoma metastasis or endolymphatic sac tumor (ELST). Renal cell carcinoma metastasis is also destructive. The location best characterizes ELST. The lesion could also be a paraganglioma, although such tumors have a predilection for the jugular foramen. Chondrosarcomas are not hypervascular, and chordomas are not found in this location and are not hypervascular.

2. **D.** VHL disease is associated with hemangioblastomas and ELSTs.

3. **C.** Hyperintensity on T1-weighted images distinguishes ELST from glomus tumors. Both have flow voids, enhance vividly, and have a speckled appearance on T2-weighted images from flow voids.

4. **B.** Twenty percent of ELSTs are associated with VHL disease. Of patients with VHL disease, 11% have an ELST.

Comment

Imaging Findings

ELSTs arise in the temporal bone along the plane of the endolymphatic sac and vestibular aqueduct. They are oriented obliquely and are destructive-looking lesions that may have finely calcified matrix, which may explain their characteristic hyperintense appearance on T1-weighted images (Figures S163-1 and S163-2). They are associated with VHL disease in approximately 20% of cases, and 11% of patients with VHL disease have an ELST. In the presence of a renal cell carcinoma, metastases to the temporal bone should also be considered because both would be hypervascular. ELSTs are bilateral in 33% of patients with VHL disease.

Clinical Findings

The most common clinical finding is hearing loss in the third decade of life, which may be the presenting symptom of VHL disease. Tinnitus and vertigo may plague affected patients as well. The hearing loss is sensorineural, and its onset may be progressive or sudden.

Reference

Manski TJ, Heffner DK, Glenn GM, Patronas NJ, Pikus AT, Katz D, et al. Endolymphatic sac tumors. A source of morbid hearing loss in von Hippel–Lindau disease. *JAMA*. 1997;277(18):1461-1466.

Cross-Reference

Neuroradiology: The Requisites, 3rd ed, 385-416, 596.

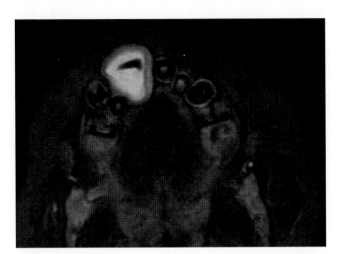

Figure 164-1

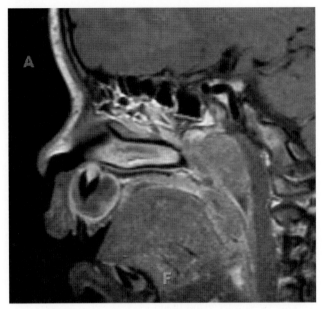

Figure 164-2

HISTORY: Pain in the right maxilla is the presenting symptom for this young man.

1. In view of the location of this lesion, what is included in the differential diagnosis? (Choose all that apply.)
   A. Radicular cyst
   B. Incisive canal cyst
   C. Globulomaxillary cyst
   D. Foramen cecum cyst
   E. Endolymphatic sac tumor

2. What are the typical locations of a globulomaxillary cyst and a nasolabial cyst?
   A. Between medial incisors for both
   B. Between medial and lateral incisors for globulomaxillary cyst and between lateral incisor and canine tooth for nasolabial cyst
   C. Between lateral incisor and canine tooth for globulomaxillary cyst and in the premaxilla for nasolabial cyst
   D. Between canine and premolar teeth for globulomaxillary cyst and in the premaxilla between medial incisors for nasolabial cyst
   E. None of the above

3. What is the typical location of a lateral periodontal cyst?
   A. Between molar teeth
   B. Between premolar teeth
   C. Between lateral incisor and canine tooth
   D. Between canine and premolar teeth
   E. None of the above

4. What is the typical location of a Stafne bone cyst?
   A. Along incisor teeth
   B. Between premolar teeth
   C. Between lateral incisor and canine tooth
   D. Between canine and premolar teeth
   E. None of the above

See Supplemental Figures section for additional figures and legends for this case.

Dental Cyst

1. **C.** The typical location of a globulomaxillary cyst is between lateral incisor and canine tooth. The other lesions do not occur here. Endolymphatic sac tumors arise in the temporal bone, and the foramen cecum is in the base of the tongue.

2. **C.** The typical location of a globulomaxillary cyst is between lateral incisor and canine tooth, and the nasolabial cyst occurs in the premaxillary region along the nasolabial fold. The nasolabial cyst appears as a nodule deforming the skin.

3. **B.** The typical location of a lateral periodontal cyst is between premolar teeth. This is an epithelial rest that does not usually affect the vitality of affected teeth.

4. **E.** The typical location of a Stafne bone cyst is along the lingual surface of the mandible below the inferior alveolar canal in the molar region. It is caused by remodeling of bone by salivary gland tissue.

Comment

Features of Globulomaxillary Cysts

The globulomaxillary cyst was originally described as a fissural cyst between the medial nasal and maxillary plates that interrupted fusion (Figures S164-1, S164-2, and S164-3). It affects exclusively the maxillary teeth, classically between the roots of the lateral incisor and the canine tooth. More evidence suggests that this lesion is of odontogenic origin, inasmuch as the cyst may be associated with unerupted teeth or in a periapical location. Classical descriptions are of an inverted pear shape, as displayed on the coronal scan. These lesions may become infected and may lead to divergence of neighboring teeth.

Features of Nasolabial Cysts

The nasolabial cyst arises at the junction of the medial nasal processes, lateral nasal process, and maxillary process. It is thought to arise from the termination of the nasolacrimal duct. They usually grow submucosally and are more common in women and in adulthood. They appear as pure cysts on magnetic resonance imaging with no enhancement and have the intensity of cerebrospinal fluid. They are situated most often at the base of the nostril and extend to the upper lip. Ten percent of these cysts are bilateral. Treatment is excision.

Features of Lateral Periodontal Cysts

Lateral periodontal cysts arise between premolar teeth and represent another type of fissural cyst. They are unilocular and cause the roots of premolar teeth to splay. Lateral periodontal cysts occur in adults and are more common in the mandible.

Features of Stafne Cysts

A Stafne cyst is an ovoid indentation made by the submandibular gland along the inner cortex of the mandible below the inferior alveolar canal and therefore below the roots of the teeth. It is usually identified at the mandibular molar region posteriorly. It was initially thought to be a pathologic process, but it is now recognized as a normal variant of thinned bone.

Reference

Yoshiura K, Weber AL, Runnels S, Scrivani SJ. Cystic lesions of the mandible and maxilla. *Neuroimaging Clin North Am.* 2003;13(3): 485-494.

Cross-Reference

Neuroradiology: The Requisites, 3rd ed, 450-451.

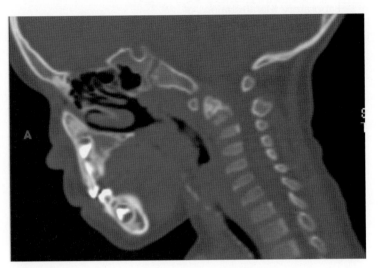

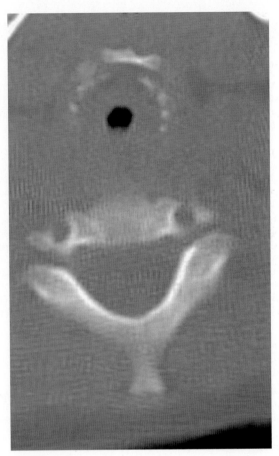

Figure 165-1

Figure 165-2

HISTORY: A patient presents with dwarfism.

1. Which of the following should be included in the differential diagnosis? (Choose all that apply.)
   A. Chondrodysplasia punctata
   B. Chondroectodermal dysplasia
   C. Enchondromatosis
   D. Campomelic dwarfism

2. Which of the following statements is true?
   A. Chondroectodermal dysplasia occurs in Amish populations and is associated with wormian bones in the skull.
   B. Chondroectodermal dysplasia occurs in Ashkenazi Jewish populations and is associated with stenosis at the foramen magnum.
   C. Chondroectodermal dysplasia occurs sporadically and is associated with subependymal nodules and astrocytomas.
   D. Chondroectodermal dysplasia occurs in Southeast Asian populations and is associated with craniosynostosis of the skull.

3. Chondrodysplasia punctata has which of the following characteristics?
   A. High incidence of cleft palate
   B. Multiple stippled epiphyses
   C. Foci of hyperdensity in respiratory cartilage (on imaging)
   D. Dwarfism
   E. All of the above

4. What is the rate of sarcomatous transformation in Ollier disease?
   A. 0% to 20%
   B. 21% to 40%
   C. 41% to 60%
   D. 61% to 80%
   E. >80%

See Supplemental Figures section for additional figures and legends for this case.

CASE 165

Chondrodysplasia Punctata

1. **A.** The correct diagnosis is chondrodysplasia punctata. Chondroectodermal dysplasia does not cause tracheal punctuate hyperdensities. No enchondromas or tracheal lesions are shown.

2. **A.** Chondroectodermal dysplasia is also known as Ellis–van Creveld syndrome. It occurs in Amish populations and is associated with wormian bones in the skull. It is also associated with high rates of polydactyly, congenital heart defects, and short limbs.

3. **E.** The characteristics of chondrodysplasia punctata include a high incidence of cleft palate, multiple stippled epiphyses, foci of hyperdensity in respiratory cartilage (on imaging), and dwarfism.

4. **B.** The rate of sarcomatous transformation in Ollier disease is 21% to 40%. As expected, these tumors are typically chondrosarcomas.

Comment

Features of Chondrodysplasia Punctata

Chondrodysplasia punctata is also known as *congenital stippled epiphyseal syndrome,* and it is associated with rhizomelic dwarfism. It is most commonly an autosomal recessive disorder accompanied by congenital heart defects, cleft palate, distal phalangeal hypoplasia, midface hypoplasia, mental retardation, and death before the age of 2. On imaging, multiple punctuate hyperdensities are visible in the epiphyses of the extremities and axial skeleton; moreover, these same fine calcifications are also visible in the trachea and bronchi (Figures S165-1, S165-2, and S165-3). Clefts in the vertebral bodies are also characteristic. The most common manifestation of the disorder is cataract, occurring in more than 70% of cases, and ichthyosis is also prevalent. Tracheal stenosis, as in this case, is another reported complication of the disease. Flat facies, well demonstrated in the sagittal reconstruction, is another feature of the disorder.

Laboratory Manifestations of Chondrodysplasia Punctata

A defect in the *PEX7* gene, which encodes the receptor for a subset of peroxisomal matrix enzymes affecting vitamin K–dependent arylsulfatase, is associated with chondrodysplasia punctata and has been mapped to chromosome 6. Levels of red cell plasmalogens are depressed, but phytanic acid progressively accumulates.

Reference

Mundinger GS, Weiss C, Fishman EK. Severe tracheobronchial stenosis and cervical vertebral subluxation in X-linked recessive chondrodysplasia punctata. *Pediatr Radiol.* 2009;39(6):625-628.

Cross-Reference

Neuroradiology: The Requisites, 3rd ed, 370.

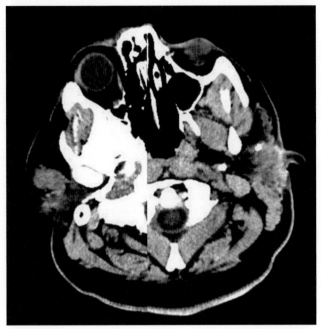

Figure 166-1

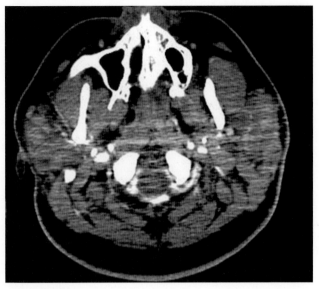

Figure 166-2

HISTORY: Figures 166-1 and 166-2 depict bilateral nodular parotid enlargement in two Japanese patients.

1. Which of the following is included in the differential diagnosis of multiple solid masses in parotid glands? (Choose all that apply.)
   A. Warthin tumors
   B. Lymph nodes
   C. Human immunodeficiency virus (HIV)–related lymphoepithelial lesions
   D. Oncocytomas
   E. None of the above

2. What is the most common inflammatory condition of the parotid space in adults?
   A. Sialadenitis
   B. Sialolithiasis
   C. Abscess
   D. Pleomorphic adenoma

3. What is Kikuchi disease?
   A. An inflammatory adenitis that is common in Japan
   B. A parotitis caused by a type of nematode
   C. Sialadenitis that mimics a neoplasm by its masslike infiltration
   D. Sialolithiasis with ductal obstruction
   E. None of the above

4. What is Kimura disease?
   A. An inflammatory adenitis associated with sialadenitis that is common in Japan
   B. A parotitis caused by a type of nematode
   C. Sialadenitis that mimics a neoplasm by its masslike infiltration
   D. Sialolithiasis with ductal obstruction
   E. None of the above

See Supplemental Figures section for additional figures and legends for this case.

CASE 166

Kimura Disease

1. **A, B, and C.** The differential diagnosis of multiple parotid masses includes Warthin tumors, lymph nodes, and HIV-related lymphoepithelial lesions.

2. **B.** The most common inflammatory condition in the parotid space in adults is sialolithiasis. In this location, stones are more common than infections in adults. Stones can certainly cause secondary glandular inflammation.

3. **A.** Kikuchi disease is an inflammatory adenitis that is common in Japan. Affected patients have fever, enlarged necrotic nodes, rash, and headaches.

4. **A.** Kimura disease is a chronic inflammatory process with associated diffuse hypervascular adenopathy in the cervical chains. It affects the submental and submandibular regions, produces eosinophilia, and has a predilection for Asian men aged 10 to 30. The salivary glands may be swollen and tender.

Comment

Features of Kimura Disease

Kimura disease is a rare inflammatory disease that usually affects Asian patients and is more common in Japan and China than in the United States. It is characterized by swelling of the salivary glands, especially the parotid glands (Figures S166-1 and S166-2), and by neck nodes with a diffuse hypervascular adenopathy in the cervical chains that affects the submental and submandibular regions; it is also characterized by eosinophilia and a predilection for men aged 10 to 30. The immunoglobulin E level is elevated, and the lymph nodes themselves may have eosinophilic infiltration as well. The adenopathy is painless. Rashes may occur. The pathogen for this disease has not been isolated, but it may be related to a parasite or an autoimmune reaction.

Affected Anatomy

The subcutaneous tissues of the head and neck are involved most commonly in Kimura disease, and the lesions evolve from poorly circumscribed to hard. The submandibular glands may be affected more severely than the parotid glands. On computed tomography, the nodes enhance, and the salivary glands appear enlarged. The lesion is hot on positron emission tomography.

Kikuchi disease is a histiocytic necrotizing lymphadenitis presenting with cervical lymphadenopathy and fever. There are cutaneous lesions in 40%.

Reference

Sun QF, Xu DZ, Pan SH, Ding JG, Xue ZQ, Miao CS, et al. Kimura disease: review of the literature. *Intern Med J*. 2008;38(8):668-672.

Cross-Reference

Neuroradiology: The Requisites, 3rd ed, 448.

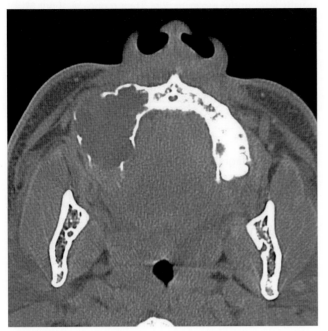

Figure 167-1

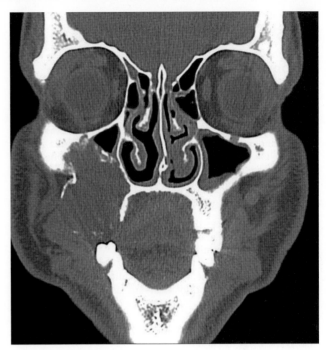

Figure 167-2

HISTORY: A young man had had a right-sided toothache for 4 months, so he arrives at the emergency department.

1. Which of the following are the possible causes of the bone lesion in this patient, in view of the history provided? (Choose all that apply.)
   A. Pathologic fracture resulting from steroid administration
   B. Radicular cyst
   C. Osteonecrosis resulting from bisphosphonate administration
   D. Osteomyelitis resulting from immunocompromised state
   E. Myxoma

2. Which of the following is correct in regard to giant cell tumors of the maxilla?
   A. They may arise from a reparative granuloma.
   B. They are associated with fluorinated water.
   C. They are more common in patients with chronic lymphocytic leukemia.
   D. They metastasize in 20% to 40% of cases.
   E. None of the above.

3. Which of the following is *not* correct in regard to myxomas?
   A. Maxillary myxomas are more common than mandibular myxomas.
   B. They are usually cystic.
   C. They are associated with tiny supernumerary teeth.
   D. They are not associated with plasma cell dyscrasias.
   E. All of the above.

4. What is the rate of invasion of the maxillary sinus by an odontogenic myxoma?
   A. 0% to 20%
   B. 21% to 40%
   C. 41% to 60%
   D. 60% to 80%
   E. >80%

See Supplemental Figures section for additional figures and legends for this case.

Myxoma of the Maxilla

1. **E.** Myxoma is a possible cause of the bone lesion in this patient, in view of the history provided. Pathologic fracture resulting from steroid administration does not cause a cystic lesion. The shape of the lesion is not correct for radicular cyst, especially without demonstration of a carious tooth. Osteonecrosis from bisphosphonate administration is unlikely to manifest as a cyst. There is no periosteal reaction to suggest osteomyelitis in an immunocompromised state.

2. **A.** Giant cell tumors of the maxilla may arise from a reparative granuloma. They also occur with aneurysmal bone cysts and osteoblastomas.

3. **C.** Myxomas are not associated with tiny supernumerary teeth. Compound odontomas are associated with such teeth.

4. **D.** The rate of invasion of the maxillary sinus by an odontogenic myxoma is 60% to 80%.

Comment

Features of Myxomas

Odontogenic myxomas are mesenchymal tumors that occur slightly more often in the maxilla than in the mandible and usually arise in the molar region. They represent about 5% of all odontogenic tumors. Of odontogenic tumors, myxomas are much less common than ameloblastomas and odontomas, and they are also less common than nonodontogenic neoplasms that affect the mandible and maxilla. They frequently invade the maxillary sinus (Figures S167-1 and S167-2). They appear as scalloping lesions that are usually multilocular, with ill-defined borders. Teeth may be displaced, but the roots of the teeth are not resorbed. Treatment options include block/segmental resection and partial or total maxillectomy or mandibulectomy.

Differential Diagnosis

Growing numbers of pediatric cases of myxomas have been reported, but this is usually a tumor of young adulthood. It may be an asymptomatic finding on screening sinus computed tomography. The differential diagnosis includes ameloblastoma, giant cell reparative granulomas, and giant cell tumors. It often has a bubbly shape with lesser enhancement than ameloblastoma. It appears very bright on T2-weighted images.

Reference

Li TJ, Sun LS, Luo HY. Odontogenic myxoma: a clinicopathologic study of 25 cases. *Arch Pathol Lab Med.* 2006;130(12):1799-1806.

Cross-Reference

Neuroradiology: The Requisites, 3rd ed, 62.

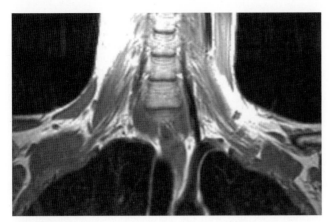

Figure 168-1

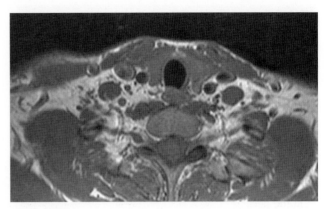

Figure 168-2

HISTORY: Thoracic outlet syndrome affects a patient's right upper extremity with weakness and paresthesias.

1. Which of the following should be included in the differential diagnosis? (Choose all that apply.)
   A. Lymph node
   B. Accessory trapezius muscle
   C. Accessory sternocleidomastoid muscle
   D. Nodular fasciitis
   E. None of the above

2. Which symptoms may occur with this condition?
   A. Thoracic outlet syndrome
   B. Cervical radiculopathy
   C. Fever and night sweats
   D. Restriction of motion
   E. None of the above

3. Is an accessory trapezius muscle more likely to affect the roots of C8 to T1 or those of C6 to C7?
   A. C6 to C7
   B. C8 to T1
   C. C6 to C7 and C8 to T1 equally
   D. None of the above

4. Which of the following is *not* true of nodular fasciitis?
   A. It is a nonneoplastic, fibroproliferative disorder.
   B. It may arise in the skin, subcutaneous tissue, deep fascia, or muscle as a painful mass.
   C. It may regress on its own, or it may necessitate surgery.
   D. It is best detected on T2-weighted imaging with fat suppression.
   E. It usually does not enhance.

See Supplemental Figures section for additional figures and legends for this case.

CASE 168

Accessory Trapezius Muscle

1. **B.** The most plausible diagnosis is accessory trapezius muscle. The shape is not correct for a lymph node, and because of the lack of inflammatory component in the adjacent fat, the condition is unlikely to be nodular fasciitis.

2. **A.** Painful thoracic outlet syndrome may be caused by an accessory trapezius muscle.

3. **A.** An accessory trapezius muscle is more likely to affect the roots of C6 to C7 because it is situated more superiorly in the neck.

4. **E.** Nodular fasciitis usually enhances. It may have variable signal intensity on T2-weighted imaging.

Comment

Features of Accessory Trapezius Muscles

An accessory trapezius muscle (Figures S168-1 and S168-2) is a well-described source of compression of the roots of C6 to C7 or the upper trunk of the brachial plexus, or both. It is of muscular density and intensity, hence its dark signal on T2-weighted imaging. It is manifested as a muscular slip leading from the occipital region to a tendinous insertion on the clavicle, and it functions like a fibrous band to compress the plexus in the scalene triangle. Other muscular anomalies that can compress the plexus are derived from the levator scapulae muscle and accessory middle scalene muscles.

Imaging Findings of Nodular Fasciitis

Nodular fasciitis appears bright on T2-weighted images, and it typically enhances avidly. It may occur at any layer of the soft tissues of the neck. After the upper extremity, the head and neck region is the second most common site for this fibroproliferative disorder. There is a relatively high rate of recurrence if the lesion is incompletely resected. The lesion is often associated with the sternocleidomastoid muscle and may be initiated by trauma or infection. It may represent malfunction of a repair mechanism.

Reference

Hug U, Burg D, Meyer VE. Cervical outlet syndrome due to an accessory part of the trapezius muscle in the posterior triangle of the neck. *J Hand Surg Br.* 2000;25(3):311-313.

Cross-Reference

Neuroradiology: The Requisites, 3rd ed, 40-41.

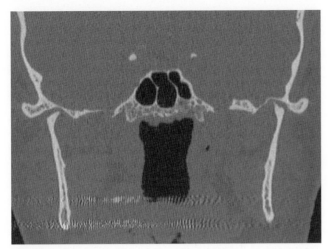

Figure 169-1

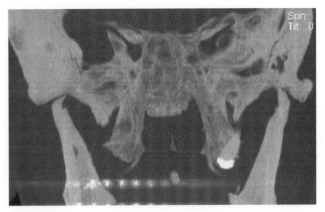

Figure 169-2

HISTORY: A young, athletic woman complains of persistent headaches.

1. Which of the following should be included in the differential diagnosis? (Choose all that apply.)
   A. Osteoradionecrosis
   B. Benign resorption of condyles
   C. Degenerative disease
   D. Gout
   E. Avascular necrosis of the mandibular condyle

2. What is associated with avascular necrosis of the mandibular condyle?
   A. Teflon proplast implant
   B. Caisson disease
   C. Sickle cell disease
   D. Trauma/fracture
   E. All of the above

3. What is associated with mandibular condylar resorption? (Choose all that apply.)
   A. Idiopathic conditions
   B. Osteoarthritis
   C. Avascular necrosis
   D. Collagen vascular disease
   E. All of the above

4. Which of the following is false?
   A. *Cheerleader's syndrome* is another name for idiopathic resorption of the mandibular condyles.
   B. Idiopathic resorption of the mandibular condyles occurs most commonly in teenage girls who participate in sports.
   C. Women are affected more than men by a ratio of more than 6:1.
   D. The abnormality is rare after 20 years of age.
   E. None of the above.

See Supplemental Figures section for additional figures and legends for this case.

CASE 169

Resorption of Mandibular Condyles

1. **B.** The most plausible diagnosis is benign resorption of condyles. The lesion pictured is a bony process, not a joint issue, and so gout and pseudogout would not be included. In addition, there is too much resorption of the mandibles for this to be a degenerative disease. Finally, the patient history does not indicate osteoradionecrosis, which would have a more destructive appearance.

2. **E.** Teflon proplast implant, Caisson disease, sickle cell disease, and trauma/fracture are associated with avascular necrosis of the mandibular condyle.

3. **E.** Trauma, osteoarthritis, avascular necrosis, collagen vascular disease, and idiopathic causes can lead to mandibular condylar resorption.

4. **E.** All of the statements are true. The entity is more common in female patients by a ratio of 9:1 and affects girls who are in their second decade of life, often with a history of subclinical trauma.

Comment

Differential Diagnosis

Cheerleader's syndrome is another name for idiopathic resorption of the mandibular condyles (Figures S169-1 and S169-2). The entity is thought to result from repetitive subclinical trauma to the jaw during sports activities. It affects girls more than boys by a 9:1 ratio, usually in the teen years.

Its occurrence is distinctly uncommon after age 20. The differential diagnosis for mandibular resorption includes trauma, osteoarthritis, avascular necrosis, and collagen vascular disease (including rheumatoid arthritis, lupus, ankylosing spondylitis, scleroderma, psoriatic arthritis). In the idiopathic form, the vertical height of the mandibular condyle decreases, and this results in malocclusion and strain on the meniscus, leading to pain.

Pathogenesis of Resorption of Mandibular Condyles

Because of the demographic variables involved, most oral surgeons believe this entity is associated with estrogen hormone effects, similar to meniscal abnormalities of the temporomandibular joint. The same hormones that may produce ligamentous laxity of the retrodiskal tissues may lead to resorption of the bone and to shrinkage.

Treatment of Resorption of Mandibular Condyles

Conservative treatment, entailing splinting, is often ineffective. Surgical treatment is directed at removing hyperplastic synovial tissue, repositioning the meniscus if necessary, and orthognathic correction of mandibular malposition to improve the bite.

Reference

Wolford LM. Idiopathic condylar resorption of the temporomandibular joint in teenage girls (cheerleaders syndrome). *Proc (Bayl Univ Med Cent)*. 2001;14(3):246-252.

Cross-Reference

Neuroradiology: The Requisites, 3rd ed, 324-327, 341-342, 426.

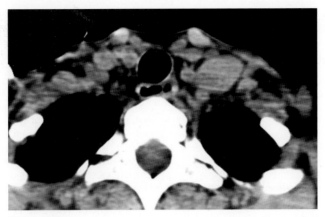

Figure 170-1

HISTORY: A left-sided neck mass is shown to be cystic on ultrasonography, although it produces a few internal echoes. A CT scan is requested for further follow-up.

1. Which of the following should be included in the differential diagnosis? (Choose all that apply.)
   A. Reactive node
   B. Neoplastic node
   C. Thyroid mass
   D. Thyroglossal duct cyst
   E. Thymic cyst

2. Which of the following is *not* true?
   A. A thoracic duct lymphocele manifests more commonly de novo than as a complication of surgery.
   B. A thoracic duct lymphocele is more commonly left-sided.
   C. A thoracic duct lymphocele is also often called a *jugular lymphatic sac*.
   D. None of the above.

3. Which of the following is true of thoracic duct lymphoceles?
   A. They are more commonly solid than cystic.
   B. They may appear bright on T1-weighted images.
   C. They are usually medial to the jugular vein.
   D. They can result in a hemothorax.
   E. None of the above.

4. What characteristic of a lymphocele of the thoracic duct distinguishes it from a node?
   A. Absence of enhancement
   B. Location
   C. Left-sidedness
   D. History of neck dissection
   E. All of the above

See Supplemental Figures section for additional figures and legends for this case.

CASE 170

Thoracic Duct Lymphocele

1. **A and E.** Because of the cystic nature of the lesion, branchial cleft cysts, thymic cysts, lymphoceles, and cystic nodes must be considered.

2. **A.** Most thoracic duct cystic lesions are the result of neck dissections in which the duct is inadvertently injured. These are usually asymptomatic and less than 1 cm large.

3. **B.** Thoracic duct lymphoceles do not result in hemothorax. They arise at the junction of the jugular and subclavian veins, are laterally located, and are more commonly left-sided. They may appear bright on T1-weighted images because of high concentrations of protein and fat.

4. **A.** Absence of enhancement distinguishes a lymphocele of the thoracic duct from a node.

Comment

Causes of Thoracic Duct Lymphocele

Thoracic duct lymphoceles may occur de novo, but in the author's experience, it is more commonly an incidental finding after a neck dissection (reported in 1% to 6% of cases) or a result of blunt trauma. The thoracic duct may be injured because the neck node dissection occurs near the junction of the jugular and subclavian veins.

Imaging Findings

In some cases, a thoracic duct lymphocele may appear as a tiny cyst in the typical location at the junction of the jugular and subclavian veins (Figure S170-1); it may be dismissed as a small lymph node unless contrast is administered. In that case, either magnetic resonance imaging (MRI) or computed tomography demonstrates the cystic nature of the lesion and its probable origin. The lesion may appear bright on T1-weighted MRI without contrast because of the high-protein lymph fluid or fatty chylous material. It always appears bright on T2-weighted images. Aspiration reveals the typical milky white chyle. The lesion is seen far more commonly in the left side of the neck because that is where the main thoracic duct drains; in rare cases, it arises along lymph channels in the right side of the neck. The lesion displaces the carotid sheath structures medially and is typically visible in the supraclavicular fossa. The lesion may expand with Valsalva maneuvers.

Treatment of Thoracic Duct Lymphocele

Treatment, when performed, consists of closed drainage, dietary restriction of fatty substances, and pressure dressings in cases of active gross leakage or chylothorax. Otherwise, in incidental cases, it is best to leave the lesion alone because of its friable wall.

Reference

Nouwen J, Hans S, Halimi P, Laccourreye O. Lymphocele after neck dissection. *Ann Otol Rhinol Laryngol.* 2004;113(1):39-42.

Cross-Reference

Neuroradiology: The Requisites, 3rd ed, 512.

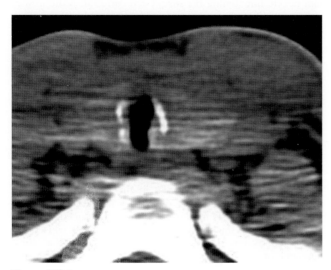

Figure 171-1

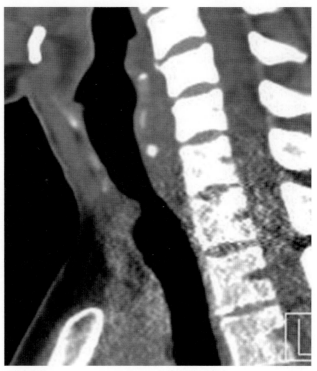

Figure 171-2

HISTORY: This patient has difficulty swallowing and speaking.

1. Which of the following should be included in the differential diagnosis? (Choose all that apply.)
   A. Subglottic squamous cell carcinoma
   B. Papilloma
   C. Posttracheotomy changes
   D. Tracheal stenosis

2. What is the most common cause of tracheal narrowing in an adult?
   A. Goiter
   B. Congenital conditions
   C. Hemangioma
   D. Croup

3. What is the most common cause of tracheal narrowing in a child?
   A. Goiter
   B. Congenital conditions
   C. Hemangioma
   D. Croup

4. Is tracheal narrowing more dangerous in the chest or in the neck?
   A. Equally dangerous in both locations
   B. Chest
   C. Neck
   D. None of the above

See Supplemental Figures section for additional figures and legends for this case.

CASE 171

Tracheal Stenosis

1. **C and D.** The patient had previously undergone tracheotomy, and so the differential diagnosis may include posttracheotomy changes and tracheal stenosis, a complication of tracheostomy. No mass is visible, and so the diagnosis is not subglottic squamous cell carcinoma or papilloma.

2. **A.** Goiters are the most common cause of tracheal narrowing in an adult. Hemangioma and croup do not usually affect adults, and congenital causes of tracheal narrowing are rare.

3. **C.** Hemangioma is the most common cause of tracheal narrowing in a child. It is most common in children, and in this location, it is termed *subglottic*. Croup does not cause permanent narrowing. Goiters do not usually affect children.

4. **B.** Tracheal narrowing is more dangerous in the chest. The airway collapses more readily in the chest. Intrathoracic pressures increase the risk of airway collapse.

Comment

Causes of Tracheal Narrowing

Causes of tracheal narrowing in adults are manifold. The most common cause is a goiter, which, because of its slow growth, can cause severe narrowing and deviation of the trachea before any airway symptoms appear. Once the trachea is narrowed to less than 8 to 10 mm, airway collapse and acute respiratory distress becomes very likely to occur. Another common cause of tracheal narrowing in adults who have

prolonged hospitalizations in intensive care units is posttracheotomy stenosis (Figures S171-1 and S171-2). Granulation tissue that may develop as a result of the tracheotomy can narrow the airway, but the alternative scenario—prolonged intubation with inflammation and/or superimposed infection—is even more dangerous. Tracheitis in an adult is rather uncommon except in such situations. In children, tracheitis can be life-threatening because it can cause an acute airway collapse. Although most causes of laryngotracheitis are viral, *Staphylococcus, Haemophilus,* and *Streptococcus* infections can occur in this location. Thyroid cancers are the malignancies that most commonly infiltrate the trachea in the neck. Lymphoma is a very uncommon cause of tracheal narrowing, and laryngeal cancers usually do not spread so low. Esophageal cancers may invade the trachea but are less common in this location. Primary tracheal cancers are usually squamous cell carcinomas.

Tracheal Procedures

In the emergency setting, procedures to preserve the airway are usually performed in the anterior cricothyroid notch. Tracheotomy tubes for patients in the intensive care unit are usually inserted farther down the trachea. Postintubation tracheal stenosis may result from cuff-induced ischemic damage to the trachea or from stomal injury caused by the tracheostomy. If the injury involves only a short segment of the trachea, treatment is tracheal resection and reconstruction.

Reference

Gaissert HA, Burns J. The compromised airway: tumors, strictures, and tracheomalacia. *Surg Clin North Am.* 2010;90(5):1065-1089.

Cross-Reference

Neuroradiology: The Requisites, 3rd ed, 472.

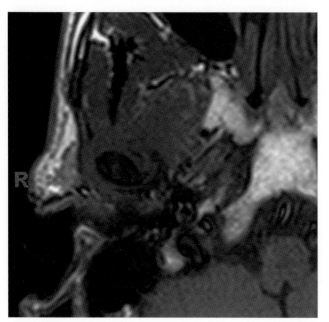

Figure 172-1

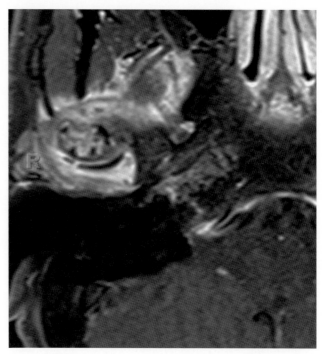

Figure 172-2

HISTORY: A 28-year-old woman complains of pain on chewing.

1. Which of the following should be included in the differential diagnosis? (Choose all that apply.)
   A. Temporomandibular joint (TMJ) synovial sarcoma
   B. TMJ arthritis
   C. Myositis
   D. TMJ effusion

2. Which of the following is *not* a common cause of TMJ arthritis?
   A. Degenerative joint disease
   B. Rheumatoid arthritis
   C. Trauma
   D. Tuberculosis

3. What cranial nerve supplies the pterygoid musculature?
   A. VII
   B. V_1
   C. V_2
   D. V_3

4. What is another name for pseudogout?
   A. Synovial chondromatosis
   B. Calcium pseudogout phosphate deposition disease
   C. Crystalline pyrophosphate disease
   D. Calcium pyrophosphate dihydrate crystal deposition disease

See Supplemental Figures section for additional figures and legends for this case.

CASE 172

Temporomandibular Joint Arthritis and Synovitis

1. **B and C.** The process here is centered on the joint, indicating TMJ arthritis. In addition, the pterygoid muscles are enhancing on postcontrast magnetic resonance imaging (MRI), indicating myositis. The diagnosis would not include TMJ synovial sarcoma because no mass is present. In addition, there is no fluid, which could indicate TMJ effusion (Figures S172-1, S172-2, and S172-3).

2. **D.** Tuberculosis is not a common cause of TMJ arthritis. In addition to the entities specified, one should consider psoriatic arthritis and ankylosing spondylitis, as well as gout and pseudogout.

3. **D.** The V_3 branch (mandibular nerve) supplies the pterygoid musculature. It is a division of the trigeminal cranial nerve.

4. **D.** Pseudogout is also called *calcium pyrophosphate dihydrate (CPPD) crystal deposition disease*. The terms *chondrocalcinosis* and *pyrophosphate arthropathy* are also used.

Comment

Complications of Temporomandibular Joint Arthritis

Like any joint, the TMJ is subject to degeneration, inflammation, and infection. Although degenerative change secondary to malocclusion, meniscal damage, osteoarthritis, and posttraumatic injury are by far the most common causes of TMJ arthritis, there are a multitude of other causes. It is well known that rheumatoid arthritis has a particular predilection for the TMJ, occurring in more than 50% of cases. As elsewhere it can cause erosions, effusions, and alteration of the bony contour. Both juvenile rheumatoid arthritis and juvenile idiopathic arthritis may affect the TMJ. Other collagen vascular diseases also affect the TMJ, although less commonly (especially psoriatic arthritis and ankylosing spondylitis).

Infectious Temporomandibular Joint Arthritis

Of the causes of septic arthritis of the TMJ, staphylococcal species are the most common pathogens. They can affect joints at all ages, usually with trismus, tenderness, and TMJ dislocation. The joint can be destroyed by the pathogen. Usually this infection is acquired via hematogenous dissemination, with rare local spread from otitis media, mastoiditis, parotitis, or a dental infection.

Pseudogout

Pseudogout can cause chondrocalcinosis and joint destruction. The TMJ may be the only joint involved. Gout is less common in this location and affects the TMJ only after other small joints have been affected.

Reference

Gross BD, Williams RB, DiCosimo CT, Williams SV. Gout and pseudogout of the temporomandibular joint. *Oral Surg Oral Med Oral Pathol.* 1987;63(5):551-554.

Cross-Reference

Neuroradiology: The Requisites, 3rd ed, 491.

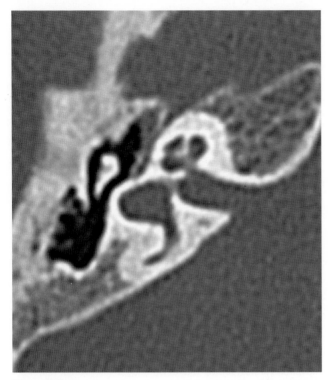

Figure 173-1

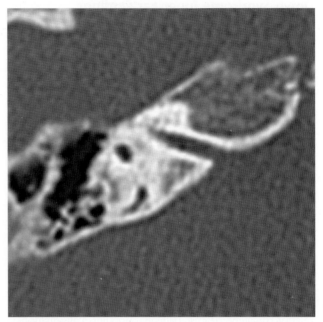

Figure 173-2

HISTORY: These scans show the temporal bones of two children with hearing loss since birth and with the same diagnosis.

1. Which of the following should be included in the differential diagnosis? (Choose all that apply.)
   A. Malignant otitis externa
   B. Mondini malformation
   C. Down syndrome
   D. Labyrinthitis ossificans

2. Which part of the temporal bone is most malformed in Down syndrome?
   A. Squamosal
   B. Inner ear
   C. Middle ear
   D. External ear

3. What is the most common external ear finding in Down syndrome?
   A. External auditory canal (EAC) stenosis
   B. EAC atresia
   C. Osteoma
   D. Epidermoid

4. What is the most common inner ear abnormality in Down syndrome?
   A. Malformed bone islands of the lateral semicircular canal
   B. Cochlear aperture stenosis
   C. Internal auditory canal (IAC) narrowing
   D. Mondini malformation

See Supplemental Figures section for additional figures and legends for this case.

CASE 173

Down Syndrome Inner Ear Findings

1. **C.** The inner ear abnormalities (malformed bone island of the semicircular canal and IAC stenosis) indicate Down syndrome as the diagnosis. There is no erosion of the EAC, which would indicate malignant otitis externa. In addition, there is no evidence of incomplete partition, which would indicate Mondini malformation. Finally, there is no bone replacement of the inner ear structures, which would indicate labyrinthitis ossificans.

2. **D.** The external ear is the part most commonly malformed in Down syndrome.

3. **A.** EAC stenosis is the most common external ear finding in Down syndrome. This occurs in 40% to 50% of cases. EAC atresia is less common than stenosis. Osteoma and epidermoid are uncommon in this patient population.

4. **A.** Malformed bone islands of lateral semicircular canal are the most common inner ear abnormalities in Down syndrome. This occurs in approximately 50% of affected patients. IAC narrowing occurs in approximately 25% of affected patients, and cochlear aperture stenosis occurs in approximately 20% of patients. Mondini malformation is very uncommon.

Comment

External and Middle Ear Complications in Down Syndrome

Many patients with Down syndrome suffer from hearing loss from a variety of reasons. The typical pharyngeal and oral cavity anatomy predisposes them to pharyngitis and to obstructive sleep apnea. Because the eustachian tubes are often obstructed when patients with Down syndrome have upper respiratory infections, middle ear effusions and mastoid fluid accumulation are common. "Glue ear" is the condition in which mucoid secretion accumulates in the middle ear and restricts the mobility of ossicles. The mucoid material often becomes infected. The second most common issue concerns the EAC, which is stenosed in approximately 40% to 50% of these patients. Such stenosis often hampers removal and clearance of cerumen and its byproducts, which leads to plug formation. The outer ear and middle ear pathologies invariably lead to conductive hearing loss.

Inner Ear Anomalies and Down Syndrome

Patients with Down syndrome also may have inner ear anomalies (Figures S173-1 and S173-2). Of these, malformation of the bone islands of the lateral semicircular canal is most common. This leads to a strange appearance to the usual symmetric nature of the lateral semicircular canals' interior. In addition to this anomaly, IAC stenosis, dehiscence of the superior semicircular canal, and cochlear aperture stenosis may occur. These findings may result in sensorineural hearing loss in affected patients.

Reference

Intrapiromkul J, Aygun N, Tunkel DE, Carone M, Yousem DM. Inner ear anomalies seen on CT images in people with Down syndrome. *Pediatr Radiol.* 2012;42(12):1449-1455.

Cross-Reference

Neuroradiology: The Requisites, 3rd ed, 385-386.

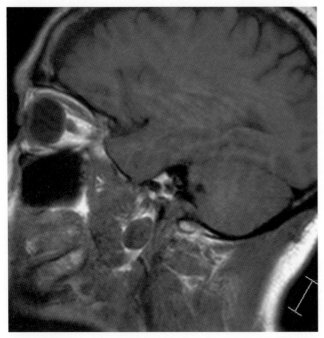

Figure 174-1

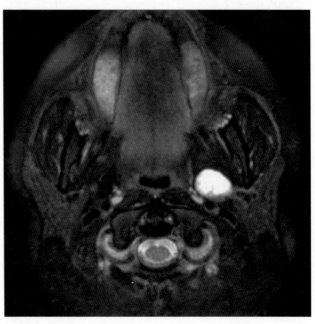

Figure 174-2

HISTORY: A 44-year-old woman has a 6-month history of depression and progressive weakness in the lower extremities. As part of her workup, she underwent brain and cervical spine magnetic resonance imaging (MRI).

1. What is included in the differential diagnosis of a lesion in this location? (Choose all that apply.)
   A. Rhabdomyosarcoma
   B. Pleomorphic adenoma
   C. Schwannoma
   D. Node
   E. Abscess

2. What is the most common lesion to populate the prestyloid parapharyngeal space (PPS)?
   A. Pleomorphic adenoma
   B. Schwannoma
   C. Paraganglioma
   D. Direct spread from primary site of mucosal carcinoma
   E. Nodal metastasis from primary site of squamous cell carcinoma

3. Which of the following is the most common primary site of carcinoma whose metastases invade the PPS?
   A. Parotid gland
   B. Nasopharynx
   C. Oropharynx
   D. Lymphatic system
   E. Paranasal sinuses

4. What percentage of benign prestyloid PPS lesions are pleomorphic adenomas?
   A. 0% to 20%
   B. 21% to 40%
   C. 41% to 60%
   D. 61% to 80%
   E. >80%

See Supplemental Figures section for additional figures and legends for this case.

CASE 174

Parapharyngeal Space Pleomorphic Adenoma

1. **B, C, and D.** Pleomorphic adenoma arise in this location from minor salivary gland rests, not parotid tissue. Schwannoma arises from the branches of cranial nerve V. Nodes can occur in the PPS. Rhabdomyosarcoma does not occur in this location. Abscesses are extremely rare in this location without oropharyngeal infection.

2. **D.** Direct spread from primary site of mucosal carcinoma is the most common lesion to populate the prestyloid PPS. This is the most common malignant tumor of the PPS. Schwannoma is the second most common benign tumor after pleomorphic adenoma, and paraganglioma is the third. Nodal metastasis from primary site of squamous cell carcinoma is the second most common malignant spread after direct spread.

3. **B.** The most common primary site of carcinoma to invade the PPS is the nasopharynx. The oropharynx is the second most common primary site; the parotid gland is the third. Lymphoma and cancers of the paranasal sinuses are rare.

4. **D.** Of benign prestyloid PPS lesions, 61% to 80% are pleomorphic adenomas.

Comment

Identifying Parapharyngeal Space Lesions

Most PPS lesions are discovered incidentally, as in this case. The mass had nothing to do with the patient's lower extremity weakness, but it was discovered on the brain MRI study (Figures S174-1, S174-2, and S174-3). When patients do have complaints, there may be parotid or neck swelling or pain.

Types of Lesions

Although pleomorphic adenomas, derived from minor salivary gland rests in the prestyloid PPS, are the most common primary lesion in the prestyloid PPS, the most common lesion to invade the space is carcinoma from the nasopharynx. When nasopharyngeal carcinoma invades the PPS, the cancer grade is advanced from T1 to T2 (see the following table).

PRIMARY TUMOR (T): NASOPHARYNX

TX	Primary tumor cannot be assessed
T0	No evidence of primary tumor
Tis	Carcinoma in situ
T1	Tumor confined to the nasopharynx, or tumor extends to oropharynx and/or nasal cavity without parapharyngeal extension (e.g., without posterolateral infiltration of tumor)
T2	Tumor with parapharyngeal extension (posterolateral infiltration of tumor)
T3	Tumor involves bony structures of skull base and/or paranasal sinuses
T4	Tumor with intracranial extension and/or involvement of cranial nerves, hypopharynx, or orbit or with extension to the infratemporal fossa/masticator space

Mucosal carcinomas, including oropharyngeal squamous cell carcinomas, invade the PPS from the anteromedial border of the PPS more commonly than do parotid masses spreading from posterolaterally.

Incidence of Pleomorphic Adenomas

In older patients, the pleomorphic adenomas of the PPS can be monitored expectantly because the rate of malignant degeneration is sufficiently low (approximately 5% to 10% in 10 years) that the surgery to remove the adenoma may not be indicated, according to life expectancy statistics. In a younger patient such as this one, however, surgical removal to prevent carcinoma ex pleomorphic adenoma would be advised. Carcinoma ex pleomorphic adenoma represents fewer than 5% of all salivary gland tumors and approximately 10% of malignant parotid masses.

Imaging Findings

Pleomorphic adenomas are characterized by their bright signal intensity on T2-weighted scans and their avid enhancement. The enhancement pattern shows progressive gradual enhancement for up to 10 minutes after injection. The enhancement persists with delayed washout for as long as 20 to 25 minutes.

References

Gangopadhyay M, Bandopadhyay A, Sinha S, Chakroborty S. Clinicopathologic study of parapharyngeal tumors. *J Cytol.* 2012;29(1): 26-29.

Hisatomi M, Asaumi J, Yanagi Y, Konouchi H, Matsuzaki H, Honda Y, et al. Assessment of pleomorphic adenomas using MRI and dynamic contrast enhanced MRI. *Oral Oncol.* 2003;39(6):574-579.

Cross-Reference

Neuroradiology: The Requisites, 3rd ed, 456-457, 482-484, 486-487, 494.

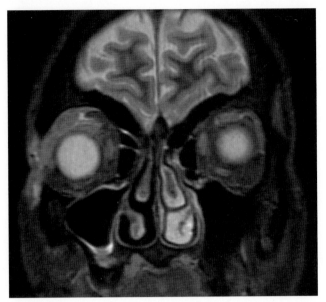

Figure 175-1

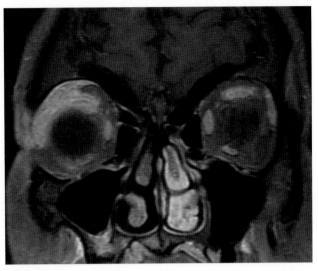

Figure 175-2

HISTORY: A patient complains of right eye irritation.

1. Which of the following should be included in the differential diagnosis? (Choose all that apply.)
   A. Lymphoma
   B. Sarcoidosis
   C. Pseudotumor
   D. Adenoid cystic carcinoma

2. Which of the following diagnoses is least plausible?
   A. Sarcoidosis
   B. Wegener granulomatosis
   C. Sjögren syndrome
   D. Pseudotumor
   E. Dacryoadenitis

3. What is the most common primary epithelial malignancy of the lacrimal gland?
   A. Lymphoma
   B. Adenoid cystic carcinoma
   C. Squamous cell carcinoma
   D. Mucoepidermoid carcinoma

4. How is Mikulicz syndrome different from Sjögren syndrome?
   A. Coexistence of sicca syndrome
   B. Lacrimal gland involvement
   C. Association of Sjögren syndrome with other systemic diseases such as leukemia, lymphoma, or sarcoidosis
   D. Lymphocytic infiltration

See Supplemental Figures section for additional figures and legends for this case.

CASE 175

Orbital Sarcoid

1. **A, B, C, and D.** Lymphoma and sarcoidosis affect orbital adnexal tissues. Pseudotumor can affect any part of the orbit. Adenoid cystic carcinoma is a malignancy of the lacrimal gland.

2. **C.** Sjögren syndrome is the least plausible diagnosis because bilateral involvement of the lacrimal glands is expected in Sjögren syndrome.

3. **B.** Adenoid cystic carcinoma is the most common primary epithelial malignancy of the lacrimal gland. Pleomorphic adenoma is the most common benign epithelial tumor of the lacrimal gland.

4. **C.** Unlike Sjögren syndrome, Mikulicz syndrome is not associated with other systemic diseases. Sjögren syndrome is associated with rheumatoid arthritis, leukemia, and lymphoma. Exclusion of systemic diseases is required for the diagnosis of Mikulicz syndrome.

Comment

Tumors of the Lacrimal Gland

Unilateral lacrimal gland enlargement in an adult can be secondary to a variety of conditions. Imaging cannot provide a specific diagnosis in majority of the cases because most lesions of the lacrimal gland are solid and show some enhancement. About 40% to 50% of the lacrimal gland masses are primary epithelial tumors, and half of those are benign. The most common benign tumor is pleomorphic adenoma, which usually manifests as a painless mass that grows slowly over the course of a year or more. The remaining lacrimal gland primary epithelial tumors are malignant, and the most common malignant tumor is adenoid cystic carcinoma (ACC). The clinical manifestation of ACC is usually of a rapidly enlarging, firm mass. On computed tomography and magnetic resonance imaging (MRI), a soft tissue mass is identified, and it can contain cystic areas. Bone erosion, when present, is relatively characteristic of ACC. ACC has a high tendency for perineural spread, which can be identified on high-resolution MRI.

Complications of Mass Lesions of the Lacrimal Gland

The nonepithelial mass lesions of the lacrimal gland are either inflammatory or lymphoproliferative. Chronic infection (dacryoadenitis) may manifest as a lacrimal gland mass lesion. Involvement of the lacrimal gland by idiopathic orbital inflammation (orbital pseudotumor) is usually indistinguishable on imaging from other mass lesions or inflammatory processes. Painful eye and steroid responsiveness are helpful clinical clues to the diagnosis. Granulomatous inflammatory lesions, such as sarcoidosis and Wegener granulomatosis, are also relatively frequent in the lacrimal gland and can cause unilateral or bilateral uniform enlargement of the glands (Figures S175-1 and S175-2). Sjögren syndrome usually manifests with bilateral involvement of the gland. Lymphoproliferative disorders can manifest as unilateral or bilateral lacrimal gland involvement, which can be limited to the orbit and may be the first sign of the systemic disease or may represent metastasis of known systemic lymphoma.

Reference

Vaidhyanath R, Kirke R, Brown L, Sampath R. Lacrimal fossa lesions: pictorial review of CT and MRI features [Review]. *Orbit*. 2008; 27(6):410-418.

Cross-Reference

Neuroradiology: The Requisites, 3rd ed, 340.

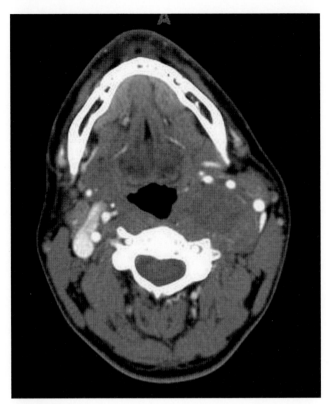

Figure 176-1

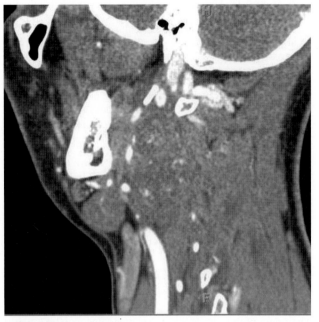

Figure 176-2

HISTORY: Upon workup for possible tonsillectomy, a 34-year-old man with a history of recurrent tonsillitis has a left neck mass that fluctuates in size with episodes of tonsillitis.

1. Which of the following should be included in the differential diagnosis? (Choose all that apply.)
   A. Adenoid cystic carcinoma
   B. Vagus schwannoma
   C. Sympathetic nervous system schwannoma
   D. Paraganglioma
   E. Pleomorphic adenoma

2. Which of the following paragangliomas is most common?
   A. Glomus jugulare
   B. Glomus tympanicum
   C. Carotid body tumor
   D. Glomus vagale
   E. Organ of Zuckerkandl paraganglioma

3. Which nuclear medicine study is the most useful for diagnosing multiple paragangliomas?
   A. Iodine-123–metaiodobenzylguanidine (MIBG) scintigraphy
   B. Technetium-99m scan
   C. Iodine-131 scan
   D. Indium-111 scan
   E. Technetium sestamibi scan

4. From what nerve are most carotid space schwannomas derived?
   A. IX
   B. X
   C. XI
   D. XII
   E. Sympathetic nervous system

See Supplemental Figures section for additional figures and legends for this case.

CASE 176

Schwannoma

1. **B, C, and D.** The lesion is intimately associated with the carotid sheath. Therefore, the most common possibilities are schwannomas—of the cranial nerves IX, XI, and XII and of the sympathetic nervous system (SNS)—and paragangliomas, of which glomus vagale and carotid body tumors would be most likely.

2. **C.** Carotid body tumors, representing 65% of neck paragangliomas, are more common than glomus jugulare tumors followed by glomus vagale and glomus tympanicum tumors.

3. **A.** Iodine-123–MIBG scintigraphy is often used to diagnose catecholamine-secreting tumors, but scans with indium-111–diethylenetriaminepentaacetic acid (DTPA)–pentetreotide may also be useful.

4. **B.** Vagal (X) schwannomas are the most common poststyloid parapharyngeal space (carotid space) masses in the upper neck.

Comment

Features of Schwannoma

The origin of the carotid sheath schwannoma may be inferred from the direction of displacement of the carotid sheath structures. Although vagus nerve schwannomas typically cause the carotid artery and jugular veins to splay apart, SNS schwannomas may not affect these vessels that way (Figures S176-1, S176-2, and S176-3). Both types of schwannoma usually displace the vessels anteriorly. SNS schwannomas have a tendency to displace the vessels laterally as well because there is more SNS tissue along the medial carotid sheath. In rare cases, vagus schwannomas displace the carotid sheath vessels posteriorly; this happens only with a massive SNS schwannoma. In other rare cases, SNS schwannomas cause the internal and external carotid arteries to splay apart, a phenomenon that also occurs with carotid body tumors. Of vagus nerve–associated neoplasms, glomus vagale paragangliomas are more common than vagus schwannomas. An unusual feature of neck schwannomas is that they may be cystic and nonenhancing. This scenario would be very unusual for a paraganglioma.

Reference

Saito DM, Glastonbury CM, El-Sayed IH, Eisele DW. Parapharyngeal space schwannomas: preoperative imaging determination of the nerve of origin. *Arch Otolaryngol Head Neck Surg.* 2007;133(7): 662-667.

Cross-Reference

Neuroradiology: The Requisites, 3rd ed, 62-64, 349-352, 378-380, 399-400, 403, 412, 456, 492, 496, 561-563, 591.

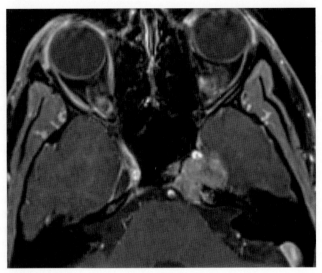

Figure 177-1

HISTORY: A middle-aged man has visual blurring.

1. Which of the following should be included in the differential diagnosis? (Choose all that apply.)
   A. Meningioma
   B. Schwannoma
   C. Chondrosarcoma
   D. Astrocytoma

2. Which of the following is the characteristic appearance of cavernous sinus chondrosarcomas on T2-weighted images?
   A. Predominantly dark because of chondroid matrix
   B. Predominantly isointense
   C. Predominantly bright
   D. Mixed signal intensity because of hemorrhage

3. How are chordomas and chondrosarcomas distinguished traditionally?
   A. Chordomas arise in the clivus, whereas chondrosarcomas arise in the cavernous sinus.
   B. Chordomas arise in the clivus, whereas chondrosarcomas arise at the petroclival junction.
   C. Chordomas arise in the petroclival junction, whereas chondrosarcomas arise at the clivus.
   D. Chordomas arise in the cavernous sinus, whereas chondrosarcomas arise at the clivus.

4. Which cranial nerve is the most medial, and which is the most laterally located in the cavernous sinus?
   A. Cranial nerve VI is most medial; cranial nerve V is most lateral.
   B. Cranial nerve VI is most medial; cranial nerve III is most lateral.
   C. Cranial nerve III is most medial; cranial nerve V is most lateral.
   D. Cranial nerve V is most medial; cranial nerve III is most lateral.

See Supplemental Figures section for additional figures and legends for this case.

CASE 177

Cavernous Sinus Chondrosarcoma

1. **A, B, and C.** Meningioma, schwannoma, and chondrosarcoma should all be included in the diagnosis because what is pictured is a cavernous sinus mass. The location is not correct for astrocytoma.

2. **C.** Cavernous sinus chondrosarcomas appear predominantly bright on T2-weighted images. However, so do chordomas, which is not helpful because the differential diagnosis often includes both.

3. **B.** Chordomas arise in the clivus, whereas chondrosarcomas arise at the petroclival junction.

4. **A.** Cranial nerve VI is the most medial, and cranial nerve V is the most lateral (and inferior).

Comment

Imaging Findings

High-resolution imaging enables identification of the cranial nerves in the cavernous sinus either as outlined by nonenhancing low signal amid the enhancing vascular cavernous sinus or, with high-resolution constructive interference in steady state (CISS) imaging, as dark in signal intensity (Figure S177-1). Cranial nerve VI is most medial and, by virtue of their relationship with the Meckel cave, cranial nerves V$_1$ and V$_2$ are most lateral and inferior (Figure S177-2).

Incidence of Chondrosarcomas

Many different lesions may affect the cavernous sinus; the most common ones are schwannomas and meningiomas, but such malignancies as lymphoma, spread of nasopharyngeal carcinoma, chordomas, and chondrosarcomas should also be considered. Chondrosarcomas confer a better overall prognosis than do chordomas of the cavernous sinus. The rate of chondrosarcoma recurrence is approximately 10% to 20%, whereas that for chordoma recurrence is approximately 20% to 30%. The chondrosarcomas are generally low-grade lesions. The calcified matrix of a chondrosarcoma of the cavernous sinus may be inapparent on magnetic resonance imaging. Only 7% of all head and neck chondrosarcomas are located in the cavernous sinus region. Ollier disease and Maffucci syndrome may predispose to chondrosarcomas by virtue of their association with enchondromas. Of chondrosarcomas of the skull base, 82% are off midline.

Reference

Abdel Razek AAK, Castillo M. Imaging lesions of the cavernous sinus. *AJNR Am J Neuroradiol.* 2009;30:444-452.

Cross-Reference

Neuroradiology: The Requisites, 3rd ed, 380.

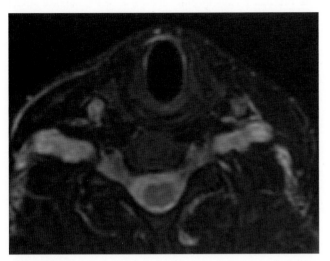

Figure 178-1

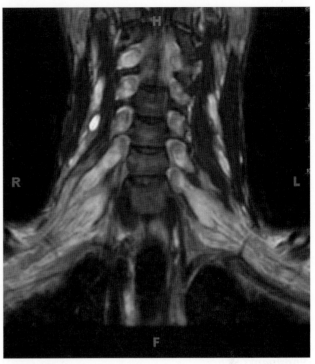

Figure 178-2

HISTORY: A young adult has bilateral neck swelling and discomfort.

1. Which of the following should be included in the differential diagnosis? (Choose all that apply.)
   A. Neurofibromatosis
   B. Chronic inflammatory demyelinating polyneuropathy (CIDP)
   C. Dejerine-Sottas disease
   D. Charcot-Marie-Tooth disease

2. Which of the following is *not* a feature of neurofibromatosis type 2 (NF-2)?
   A. Vestibular schwannoma
   B. Plexiform neurofibroma
   C. Meningiomas
   D. Ependymomas

3. How are Dejerine-Sottas and Charcot-Marie-Tooth diseases classified?
   A. Demyelinating disorders
   B. Hereditary motor and sensory neuropathies (HMSNs)
   C. Glycogen storage diseases
   D. Mitochondrial disorders

4. Which of the following groups correctly lists the parts of the brachial plexus from central to peripheral?
   A. Roots, trunks, cords, divisions, branches
   B. Roots, divisions, trunks, cords, branches
   C. Roots, trunks, branches, cords, divisions
   D. Roots, trunks, divisions, cords, branches

See Supplemental Figures section for additional figures and legends for this case.

Brachial Plexus Neurofibromas (NF-1)

1. **A, B, C, and D.** Neurofibromatosis, CIDP, Dejerine-Sottas disease, and Charcot-Marie-Tooth disease can all account for the bilateral enlargement of the cervical nerves.

2. **B.** Plexiform neurofibroma is a characteristic of neurofibromatosis type 1 (NF-1), not NF-2. Vestibular schwannoma and meningiomas are common tumors in patients with NF-2 (vestibular schwannoma is most common). Ependymomas may occur in the spinal cords of patients with NF-2, whereas astrocytomas of the spinal cord are more common in NF-1.

3. **B.** Dejerine-Sottas and Charcot-Marie-Tooth diseases are HMSNs, types III and I, respectively. HMSN types II, V, and VI are also variants of Charcot-Marie-Tooth disease, and HMSN type IV is also called *Refsum disease*.

4. **D.** From central to peripheral, the parts of the brachial plexus are as follows: roots, trunks, divisions, cords, branches.

Comment

Features of Neurofibromatosis

In the brachial plexus, neurofibromas are more common than schwannomas. Plexiform neurofibromas are more common in patients with NF-1 and increase the potential for malignant tumors of the peripheral nerve sheath. Causes of symmetric bilateral nerve enlargement besides neurofibromatosis include CIDP, HMSN syndromes, multifocal motor neuropathy syndromes, amyloidosis, and lymphomatous infiltration.

Relevant Anatomy

The brachial plexus includes the roots of the cervical spinal segments C5 to T1. From the roots, the neuronal structures evolve into the trunks, divisions, cords, and branches. The brachial plexus passes between the anterior and middle scalene muscles and is intimately associated with the subclavian and axillary arteries (Figures S178-1 and S178-2).

Reference

Reilly MM. Classification and diagnosis of the inherited neuropathies. *Ann Indian Acad Neurol.* 2009;12(2):80-88.

Cross-Reference

Neuroradiology: The Requisites, 3rd ed, 64-65, 306-309, 313-314, 347-348.

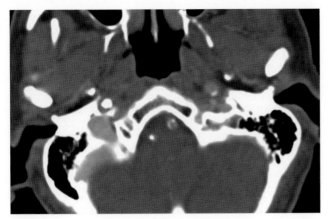

Figure 179-1

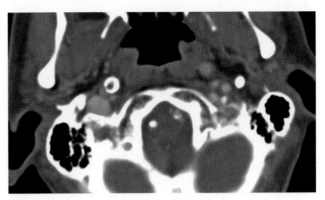

Figure 179-2

HISTORY: A patient with a history of trauma has right-sided Horner syndrome.

1. Which of the following should be included in the differential diagnosis? (Choose all that apply.)
   A. Chondrosarcoma
   B. Atherosclerotic plaque
   C. Chordoma
   D. Calcified pseudoaneurysm of the internal carotid artery (ICA)

2. Why do patients with carotid dissection develop Horner syndrome?
   A. The traumatic event leads to tearing of the branches of the parasympathetic nervous system.
   B. The traumatic event leads to tearing of the branches of the sympathetic nervous system.
   C. The dissection leads to compression of the nerves of the parasympathetic nervous system.
   D. The dissection leads to compression of the nerves of the sympathetic nervous system.

3. What percentage of dissections of the ICA are associated with aneurysms?
   A. <10%
   B. 11% to 20%
   C. 21% to 40%
   D. >40%

4. Besides atherosclerosis and pseudoaneurysm, what is another cause of calcification of the ICA?
   A. Ochronosis
   B. Thorotrast granuloma
   C. Pantopaque
   D. Vitamin D intoxication

See Supplemental Figures section for additional figures and legends for this case.

CASE 179

Calcified Pseudoaneurysm of the Internal Carotid Artery

1. **D.** The diagnosis should include calcified pseudoaneurysm of the ICA. This is a chronic lesion. Chondrosarcoma and chordoma are not tumors of the blood vessels. In addition, this location is not correct for calcified atheromatous plaque, which is usually visible at a bifurcation (Figures S179-1, S179-2, S179-3, and S179-4).

2. **D.** Patients with carotid dissection develop Horner syndrome because the dissection leads to compression of the nerves of the sympathetic nervous system. Rather than shearing, the mass effect compression is what causes the syndrome.

3. **D.** Nearly half of all patients with carotid dissections have an associated aneurysm. However, in one third of these cases, the aneurysm may be on another vessel (potentially because diseases such as fibromuscular dysplasia or Marfan syndrome may predispose to aneurysms and dissections).

4. **B.** Thorotrast is a contrast agent, formerly used in the twentieth century, that can cause vascular calcification.

Comment

Causes of Pseudoaneurysm of the Internal Carotid Artery

Most pseudoaneurysms of the cervical carotid arteries result from traumatic dissection of the vessel. Several syndromic conditions may predispose to the development of dissection and subsequent pseudoaneurysm formation, such as Marfan syndrome, Ehlers-Danlos syndrome, Loeys-Dietz syndrome, and various forms of fibromuscular dysplasia. However, trauma after altercations, stab wounds, or motor vehicular collisions accounts for most cases. The carotid or vertebral arteries may be affected, and there are characteristic locations of dissection for each, including the V_3 segment of the vertebral artery and the upper cervical segment of the ICA. Thorotrast, a contrast agent that was used in the 1930s and 1940s, was employed for direct carotid puncture carotid arteriography. It was the source of many sclerosing calcified granulomas in the neck before the advent of other agents and the Seldinger technique eliminated these complications.

Treatment of Pseudoaneurysm of the Internal Carotid Artery

Calcification of the pseudoaneurysm implies chronicity, but the risk of potential thromboembolism remains if the intima is still traumatized and if thrombogenic wall components are exposed. For this reason, antiplatelet therapy is warranted.

Reference

Touzé E, Randoux B, Méary E, Arquizan C, Meder JF, Mas JL. Aneurysmal forms of cervical artery dissection: associated factors and outcome. *Stroke*. 2001;32:418-423.

Cross-Reference

Neuroradiology: The Requisites, 3rd ed, 495.

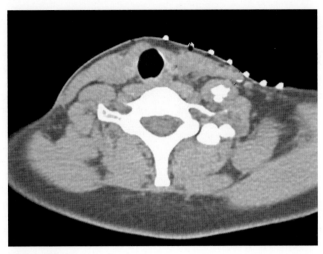

Figure 180-1

HISTORY: A patient presents with numbness, tingling sensation, and weakness in the left arm.

1. What is occurring in which procedure being performed in this case? (Choose all that apply.)
   A. Hematoma has developed in the muscle during a biopsy.
   B. Contrast has been injected into the brachial plexus during administration of a block.
   C. Glue has been injected into an arteriovenous malformation in the lower neck.
   D. An attempt at facet block has failed.
   E. Contrast has been injected into the anterior scalene muscle for a scalene block.

2. What is the purpose of the procedure shown in this case?
   A. To ablate the lesion
   B. To block the brachial plexus
   C. To paralyze the muscle
   D. To determine whether relaxation of the scalene muscles will enlarge the thoracic outlet and relieve symptoms
   E. All of the above

3. What surgical procedures may be performed for thoracic outlet syndrome?
   A. Scalenectomy
   B. Rib resection
   C. Apophysectomy
   D. Band release
   E. All of the above

4. Where is the brachial plexus in relation to the anterior scalene muscle?
   A. Anterior
   B. Posterior
   C. Inferior
   D. Superior
   E. None of the above

See Supplemental Figures section for additional figures and legends for this case.

CASE 180

Scalene Block

1. **E.** The figures and history indicate that contrast has been injected into the anterior scalene muscle as part of a scalene block in the assessment of thoracic outlet syndrome.

2. **D.** This procedure is used to determine whether relaxation of the scalene muscles will enlarge the thoracic outlet and relieve symptoms. The anesthetic injection allows the first rib to descend by causing the scalene muscle to relax and thereby decompress the brachial plexus.

3. **E.** Scalenectomy, rib resection, fibrous band resection, and apophysectomy can be performed for various causes of thoracic outlet syndrome.

4. **B.** The brachial plexus is posterior to the anterior scalene muscle. It is, however, anterior to the middle/posterior scalene muscles.

Comment

Symptoms of Thoracic Outlet Syndrome

Thoracic outlet syndrome may cause numbness and tingling sensation in the upper extremity. Weakness may also be present. Symptoms are worse when the affected arm is raised above the head, after exercise, at night, or when the arm is used for activities such as combing hair or driving a car.

Cause of Thoracic Outlet Syndrome

There are many causes of thoracic outlet syndrome, including cervical ribs, aberrantly large first or second ribs, apophysomegaly, transverse process enlargement, and fibrous bands. The anterior scalene muscle—by virtue of fibrosis, trauma, hematoma, or hypertrophy—may also be a source of compression of either the subclavian artery or the brachial plexus. Pectoralis minor syndrome leads to pain in the anterior chest wall in association with thoracic outlet syndrome. Usually a traumatic event precipitates the onset of pectoralis minor or thoracic outlet syndrome.

Testing for Thoracic Outlet Syndrome

The scalene block is a therapeutic planning prognostic indicator test used to determine whether removal or paralysis of the anterior scalene muscle will benefit the patient (Figure S180-1). The scalene muscle arises from the cervical spine and inserts on the first rib. If, upon administration of anesthetic, the symptoms resolve, it suggests potential benefit from scalenectomy surgery or intramuscular Botox injection. Spread of the anesthetic into the brachial plexus, out of the muscle, can lead to false-positive results of scalene block. This is the reason why contrast material is injected first: to demonstrate lack of extramuscular spread before the anesthetic is injected.

Reference

Mashayekh A, Christo PJ, Yousem DM, Pillai JJ. CT-guided injection of the anterior and middle scalene muscles: technique and complications. *AJNR Am J Neuroradiol.* 2011;32(3):495-500.

Cross-Reference

Neuroradiology: The Requisites, 3rd ed, 503-505.

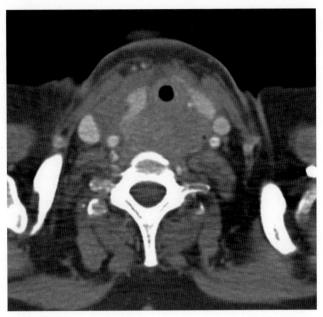

Figure 181-1

HISTORY: An elderly patient presents with a globus sensation and difficulty swallowing.

1. Which of the following sarcomas is most common in the hypopharynx–upper esophagus? (Choose all that apply.)
   A. Osteosarcoma
   B. Rhabdomyosarcoma
   C. Chondrosarcoma
   D. Synovial sarcoma
   E. Fibrosarcoma

2. Which of the following are frequent findings in synovial sarcomas?
   A. Cystic change
   B. Hemorrhage
   C. Calcification
   D. All of the above
   E. None of the above

3. Which of the following best explains why extra-articular synovial sarcomas arise?
   A. Remnant synovial cells are present outside the joint.
   B. They originate from embryologic rests.
   C. Synovial cells are pleuripotential.
   D. The cell of origin is not from the synovium.
   E. They all arise from joints.

4. Where in the aerodigestive system is the most common site of synovial sarcoma?
   A. Sinonasal cavity
   B. Larynx
   C. Nasopharynx
   D. Oropharynx
   E. Hypopharynx

See Supplemental Figures section for additional figures and legends for this case.

CASE 181

Sinus Synovial Sarcoma

1. **D.** Synovial sarcoma is the most common of the sarcomas listed to affect the hypopharynx. Undifferentiated sarcomas may be the next most common. Osteosarcoma is the most common sarcoma to affect the sinonasal cavity.

2. **D.** Cystic change, hemorrhage, and calcification are frequent findings in synovial sarcomas.

3. **D.** "Synovial sarcoma" is a misnomer. The cell of origin is not from the synovium. For that reason, these lesions occur not in joints but in soft tissues.

4. **E.** The hypopharynx is the most common site of synovial sarcoma in the aerodigestive system.

Comment

Location and Incidence of Sinus Synovial Sarcomas

Synovial sarcomas are extremely enigmatic lesions. Most occur in the extremities; only 3% arise in the head and neck. However, they can occur anywhere in the head and neck, most commonly in the parapharyngeal and masticator space, and they have a highly heterogeneous appearance. Cystic, hemorrhagic (40%), and calcific (27%) changes, as well as necrosis, occur. Punctate and coarse calcifications have been described. Twenty percent of these lesions have fluid-fluid levels. Multiloculation and internal septation is the rule. The average age at diagnosis is approximately 30 years. The lesions are usually painful. The rate of 5-year survival is 60%, which is higher than for many other sarcomas. Of patients with synovial sarcomas, 25% develop metastases, usually to the lungs, and the rate of recurrence is high.

Relevant Anatomy

This case shows a highly unusual site of occurrence of synovial sarcoma. They affect the soft tissue more commonly than the mucosal space, and when they affect a mucosal surface, they arise more commonly in the hypopharynx (Figure S181-1). Variants of synovial sarcomas are subclassified into four types: (1) biphasic type with epithelial and spindle cell components, (2) monophasic spindle cell type with little or no evidence of epithelial differentiation, (3) monophasic epithelial type, and (4) poorly differentiated type.

Reference

O'Sullivan PJ, Harris AC, Munk PL. Radiological features of synovial cell sarcoma. *Br J Radiol.* 2008;81(964):346-356.

Cross-Reference

Neuroradiology: The Requisites, 3rd ed, 470, 494.

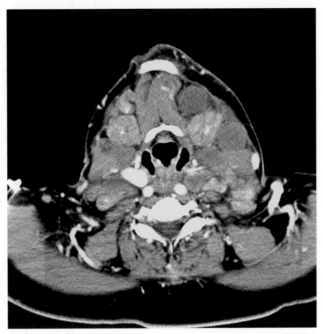

Figure 182-1

HISTORY: A middle-aged adult presents with multiple neck masses.

1. For bilateral nonnecrotic massive lymphadenopathy, which of the following should be included in the differential diagnosis? (Choose all that apply.)
   A. Human immunodeficiency virus (HIV) disease
   B. Lymphoma
   C. Squamous cell carcinoma
   D. Mycobacterial infection
   E. Sinus histiocytosis

2. Which of the following is true of Rosai-Dorfman disease?
   A. It is more common in adults than in children.
   B. It is characterized by massive lymphadenopathy.
   C. It is rarely accompanied by extranodal disease.
   D. It is associated with hypercalcemia.
   E. It is related to Epstein-Barr virus exposure.

3. The incidence of posttransplantation lymphoproliferative disorder (PTLD) is highest after which of the following procedures?
   A. Bone marrow transplantation
   B. Liver transplantation
   C. Lung transplantation
   D. Renal transplantation

4. What is the most common site of extranodal Rosai-Dorfman disease in the head and neck?
   A. Brain
   B. Sinonasal cavity
   C. Salivary glands
   D. Masticator space
   E. Orbit

See Supplemental Figures section for additional figures and legends for this case.

369

CASE 182

Rosai-Dorfman Disease (Sinus Histiocytosis with Massive Lymphadenopathy)

1. **B and E.** Bilateral nonnecrotic massive lymphadenopathy is common in lymphoma and sinus histiocytosis. Necrosis is a feature of squamous cell carcinoma and tuberculous adenitis. HIV nodes are usually not massive.

2. **B.** Rosai-Dorfman disease is characterized by massive lymphadenopathy and is more common in children and adolescents. More than 40% of affected patients have extranodal manifestations.

3. **C.** PTLD has the highest incidence among lung transplant recipients. PTLD after renal transplantation is not as common. The incidence of PTLD after liver transplantation is quoted as 2%.

4. **B.** The most common site of extranodal Rosai-Dorfman disease in the head and neck is the sinonasal cavity. The salivary glands are the second most common sites. The masticator space and orbit are not as commonly affected.

Comment

Differential Diagnosis

Rosai-Dorfman disease is also called *sinus histiocytosis with massive lymphadenopathy*. It is a disease of childhood (80% of affected patients are younger than 20 years, and 67% are younger than 10 years) and causes bilateral massive cervical lymphadenopathy (Figure S182-1). Therefore, it is included in the differential diagnosis with mononucleosis, cat scratch disease, lymphoma, and mastocytosis, which also affect younger patients. Affected patients may have fever, elevated erythrocyte sedimentation rates, and polyclonal hypergammaglobulinemia.

Imaging Findings

Imaging features are that of large, nonnecrotic lymphadenopathy. The nodes are usually hot on gallium scanning and positron emission tomography (PET). Extranodal deposits occur in approximately half of affected patients and may be in the skin, the sinonasal cavity, the salivary glands, the orbits, and the bones. Hypointensity of sinonasal sinus histiocytosis on T2-weighted scans implies a differential diagnosis of lymphoma, sarcoidosis, fungal disease, pseudotumor, and granulomatous infections. The most common manifestation in the orbit is an extraconal mass that causes proptosis.

Relevant Anatomy

Intracranially, Rosai-Dorfman disease may infiltrate the dura of the sella, cavernous sinus, periclival regions, and foramen magnum. The dura around venous sinuses may also be affected.

Treatment of Rosai-Dorfman Disease

Treatment is watchful waiting at first. The disease is often self-limited. However, interferon, steroids, chemotherapy, radiation therapy, or a combination of these may be administered for advanced disease. Surgery is confined to cases of progressive, obstructive disease.

Reference

La Barge DV 3rd, Salzman KL, Harnsberger HR, Ginsberg LE, Hamilton BE, Wiggins RH 3rd, et al. Sinus histiocytosis with massive lymphadenopathy (Rosai-Dorfman disease): imaging manifestations in the head and neck. *AJR Am J Roentgenol.* 2008;191(6): W299-W306.

Cross-Reference

Neuroradiology: The Requisites, 3rd ed, 448.

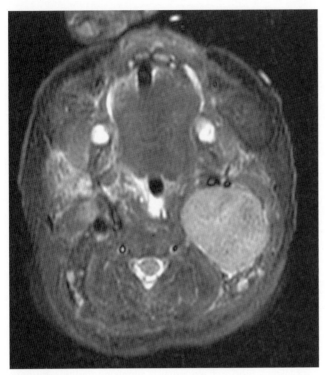

Figure 183-1

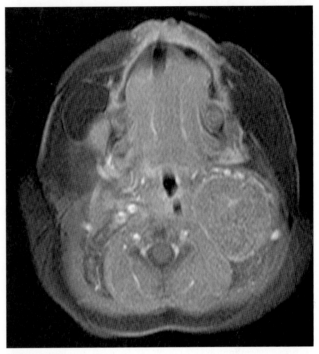

Figure 183-2

HISTORY: This left-sided neck mass, previously identified on ultrasonography in a newborn, is evaluated further on magnetic resonance imaging (MRI).

1. Which of the following should be included in the differential diagnosis of a neonatal neck mass? (Choose all that apply.)
   A. Teratoma
   B. Neuroblastoma
   C. Lymphangioma (lymphatic malformation)
   D. Thyroid carcinoma
   E. Lingual thyroid

2. What is the most common cystic neck mass in the neonatal period?
   A. Thyroglossal duct cyst
   B. Branchial apparatus cysts
   C. Venous malformation/hemangioma
   D. Lymphangioma (lymphatic malformation)
   E. Thymic cyst

3. What is the most common solid tumor in the neck in the neonatal period?
   A. Teratoma
   B. Neuroblastoma
   C. Rhabdomyosarcoma
   D. Adenopathy
   E. Hemangioma

4. Which of the following is true?
   A. Congenital neck neuroblastomas represent metastases from retroperitoneal primary tumors.
   B. Congenital neuroblastomas confer a favorable prognosis.
   C. Neck neuroblastomas are less common than neck ganglioneuromas.
   D. Teratomas of the neck are usually located in the hypopharynx.

See Supplemental Figures section for additional figures and legends for this case.

CASE 183

Cervical Neuroblastoma

1. **A, B, and C.** Teratomas, lymphangiomas, and, less commonly, neuroblastomas are neck masses that may be detected in a neonate. In association with teratomas and neuroblastomas, calcifications may be present. Lymphangiomas may be multiloculated cysts. Thyroid lesions, besides thyroglossal duct cysts, are uncommon in neonates.

2. **A.** Thyroglossal duct cysts are the most common cystic neck mass in the neonatal period. Branchial apparatus cysts are the second most common. Lymphangiomas are located most commonly in the neck, but they are not the most common mass lesions in the neck. Most hemangiomas and venous malformations manifest after the neonatal period, with the exception of congenital hemangiomas, which are not cystic. Thymic cysts are uncommon.

3. **A.** Teratoma is the most common solid tumor in the neck in the neonatal period. Neuroblastoma, although rare, is the second most common solid tumor of the neck in the newborn period and was the actual diagnosis in this case. Rhabdomyosarcoma is the most common primary malignant tumor of the neck in children, but it is rare in newborns. Hemangiomas overall are the most common tumors in the neck, but they rarely manifest in the newborn period (congenital hemangioma). Adenopathy is uncommon in the neonatal period.

4. **B.** Patients with neuroblastomas of the neck have an excellent prognosis. These tumors are located primarily in the neck, and neuroblastomas far outnumber ganglioneuromas and ganglioneuroblastomas in this location.

Comment

Types and Features of Mass Lesions in the Neck

Neuroblastomas that originate in the neck arise from the sympathetic chain in the vicinity of the carotid artery (Figures S183-1 and S183-2), as demonstrated in this case. They are typically posterior to the carotid artery. Horner syndrome is a common finding in patients with primary neck neuroblastomas. Metastatic neuroblastoma in the head and neck can involve lymph nodes, the calvaria, the dura, the sutures, and the orbits, causing bone destruction and spiculated periosteal reaction.

Congenital mass lesions in the neck are often diagnosed on prenatal ultrasonography or at birth. Congenital and neonatal neck masses include the following:

- Thyroglossal cyst
- Branchial cleft cyst
- Hemangioma/vascular malformation
- Thymic cyst
- Dermoid cyst
- Ectopic thymus
- Teratoma
- Neuroblastoma
- Rhabdomyosarcoma
- Adenopathy
- Fibromatosis colli

Associations with Mass Lesions

Of pediatric rhabdomyosarcomas, 40% affect the head and neck, often arising in the subcutaneous soft tissues, nasal cavity, orbit, middle ear, paranasal sinuses, and nasopharynx. Associated bone destruction is common but does not occur in all patients. Confluent inflammatory or infectious cervical lymph nodes can appear masslike, can be solid or necrotic, or may have variable vascularity and no specific imaging characteristics. Fibromatosis colli can clinically mimic true neoplasms, and characteristic ultrasonographic findings include focal thickening of the sternocleidomastoid muscle without associated extramuscular abnormality. Congenital hemangiomas can also mimic other mass lesions because of their highly infiltrative appearance. Macrocystic lymphatic malformation is typically a multilocular fluid-filled mass rather than a purely solid lesion. Microcystic lymphatic malformation contains multiple small cysts that can enhance, similar to a solid mass.

Reference

Abramson SJ, Berdon WE, Ruzal-Shapiro C, Stolar C, Garvin J. Cervical neuroblastoma in eleven infants—a tumor with favorable prognosis. Clinical and radiologic (US, CT, MRI) findings. *Pediatr Radiol.* 1993;23(4):253-257.

Cross-Reference

Neuroradiology: The Requisites, 3rd ed, 438, 566-567.

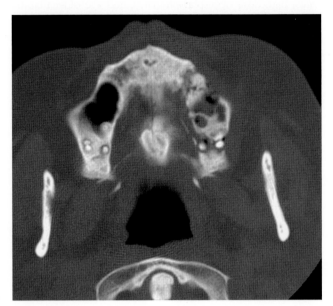

Figure 184-1

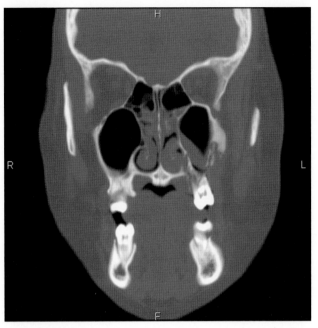

Figure 184-2

HISTORY: A female patient being treated for metastatic breast cancer experiences jaw pain.

1. Which of the following are the possible causes of the bone lesion in this patient, in view of the history provided? (Choose all that apply.)
   A. Pathologic fracture resulting from steroid administration
   B. Metastasis
   C. Osteonecrosis resulting from bisphosphonate administration
   D. Osteomyelitis resulting from immunocompromised state

2. For what conditions are bisphosphonates administered?
   A. Bone metastases from breast cancer
   B. Paget disease
   C. Osteoporosis
   D. Hypercalcemia
   E. All of the above

3. What is the incidence of jaw necrosis in patients with bone metastases who are being treated with bisphosphonates?
   A. <25%
   B. 26% to 50%
   C. 51% to 75%
   D. >76%

4. What is the approximate ratio of involvement of the mandible versus the maxilla in bisphosphonate-induced osteonecrosis?
   A. 10:1 in favor of the mandible
   B. 10:1 in favor of the maxilla
   C. 3:1 in favor of the maxilla
   D. 3:1 in favor of the mandible

See Supplemental Figures section for additional figures and legends for this case.

CASE 184

Bisphosphonate Osteonecrosis

1. **A, B, C, and D.** Metastasis, pathologic fracture resulting from steroid administration, osteonecrosis resulting from bisphosphonate administration, and osteomyelitis resulting from immunocompromised state are all possible causes of the bone lesion in this patient. Because of the treatment with bisphosphonate, the diagnosis of osteonecrosis would be favored.

2. **E.** Bisphosphonates are administered for bone metastases from breast cancer, Paget disease, osteoporosis, myeloma, and hypercalcemia. Patients with compression fractures, those at risk for hip fractures, and those undergoing long-term steroid therapy may also be treated with bisphosphonates.

3. **A.** Jaw necrosis occurs in fewer than 25% of patients with bone metastases who are being treated with bisphosphonates.

4. **D.** The approximate ratio of involvement in bisphosphonate-induced osteonecrosis is 3:1 in favor of the mandible over the maxilla.

Comment

Complications of Bisphosphonate Therapy

Osteonecrosis of the maxilla is one potential complication of the use of bisphosphonates to treat the bone metastases of breast cancer, lung cancer, prostate cancer, and myeloma. These agents are also used to treat hypercalcemia, Paget disease, and generalized osteoporosis. The onset of osteonecrosis occurs sooner (2 to 3 years) after use for cancer treatment than that of osteoporosis (6 years). The risk factors for development of osteonecrosis include female sex, recent dental extractions, intravenous administration of bisphosphonates, high dose of bisphosphonates, and age older than 60 years. This complication of therapy is very difficult to treat, and withdrawal of the agent does not necessarily lead to reversal of the process. Recommendations from the Canadian Association of Oral and Maxillofacial Surgeons are as follows:

- Dental examination and radiographs before the initiation of intravenous bisphosphonate therapy
- Completion of urgent surgical dental procedures before the initiation of high-dose bisphosphonate therapy and completion of nonurgent procedures 3 to 6 months after cessation of bisphosphonate therapy
- Cessation of smoking, limiting of alcohol intake, and maintenance of good oral hygiene
- If osteonecrosis occurs, initiation of supportive care, management of pain, treatment of secondary infection, and removal of necrotic debris and sequestrum

Imaging Findings

Imaging features reveal a mixed pattern of both osteolytic lesions and sclerotic regions in the mandible or maxilla, but lucent lesions predominate on computed tomographic images (Figures S184-1 and S184-2). Periosteal reaction is variable but more commonly seen than not. On T1-weighted magnetic resonance images, the normal marrow signal is replaced with hypointense signal. Enhancement in the cortex and subcortical bone is present, and the enhancement may involve the adjacent muscles of mastication.

Reference

Thumbigere-Math V, Sabino MC, Gopalakrishnan R, Huckabay S, Dudek AZ, Basu S, et al. Bisphosphonate-related osteonecrosis of the jaw: clinical features, risk factors, management, and treatment outcomes of 26 patients. *J Oral Maxillofac Surg.* 2009;67(9): 1904-1913.

Cross-Reference

Neuroradiology: The Requisites, 3rd ed, 101-103.

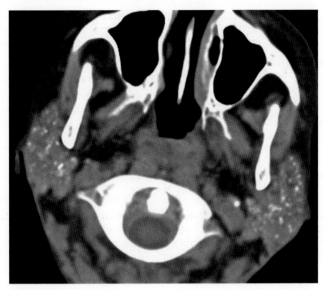

Figure 185-1

HISTORY: A patient with a collagen vascular disorder complains of a sensation of fullness in the jaw.

1. Which of the following should be included in the differential diagnosis? (Choose all that apply.)
   A. Chronic parotitis
   B. Lupus
   C. Hyperparathyroidism
   D. Sjögren syndrome

2. Patients with Sjögren syndrome are susceptible to which of the following tumors?
   A. Mucoepidermoid carcinoma
   B. Kaposi sarcoma
   C. Mucosa-associated lymphoid tissue (MALT) lymphoma
   D. Synovial sarcoma

3. Which of the following is true in regard to sialadenosis?
   A. It is usually painless.
   B. Calcification is common.
   C. It is associated with diabetes insipidus.
   D. It predisposes to cancer.

4. What is the recurrence rate for salivary stones after removal?
   A. 0% to 15%
   B. 16% to 30%
   C. 31% to 45%
   D. 46% to 60%

See Supplemental Figures section for additional figures and legends for this case.

CASE 185

Parotid Calcifications from Lupus

1. **A, B, C, and D.** Chronic parotitis can lead to intraparotid calcifications. Lupus may lead to glandular calcifications. Parotid calcifications (Figure S185-1) can occur with hyperparathyroidism. Sjögren syndrome causes multiple stones.

2. **C.** Patients with Sjögren syndrome are susceptible to MALT lymphoma. A significant predisposition raises the risk factor by more than 10 times.

3. **A.** Sialadenosis is usually painless; enlargement without pain is the hallmark. It is associated with diabetes mellitus, alcoholism, hypothyroidism, obesity, and a variety of medications. Calculi are rare, and it is a benign condition.

4. **B.** The recurrence rate for salivary stones after removal is about 20% to 25%.

Comment

Causes of Parotid Calcifications

There are numerous reasons why patients may have multiple parotid calculi. Stone formation is more common in patients who are starving, who are dehydrated, and who are taking medications that cause thickening of saliva, including antihistamines, antihypertension medications, antidepressants, and psychiatric medications. In addition to Sjögren syndrome and lupus, other connective tissue disorders predispose to glandular calculi.

Associations with Parotid Calcifications

Lupus may be associated as a connective tissue disorder with Sjögren syndrome, or it can occur in isolation. In those instances, multiple fine calcifications may occur in the parotid ductules. However, lupus is also associated with diffuse calcinosis, which can occur within joints or diffusely in the soft tissues as calcinosis universalis. Dermatomyositis more commonly causes this phenomenon than does lupus.

Treatment of Parotid Calcifications

Treatment may include stimulants for saliva production, massage and manual delivery of the stone, incisions to remove the stone, sialoendoscopy with thorough rinsing and plucking of the stone, Stensen ductal dilation, and steroids (injected locally or administered orally) for flares of parotitis. In the worst-case scenario, the duct and gland are removed.

Reference

Hopkins C, Kanegaonkar R, Chevretton EB. Parotid calcification in systemic lupus erythematosis. *J Laryngol Otol.* 2002;116(10): 859-861.

Cross-Reference

Neuroradiology: The Requisites, 3rd ed, 140, 353, 480, 549.

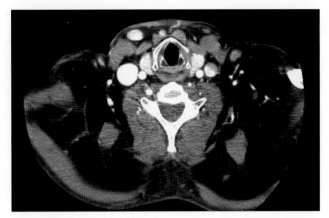

Figure 186-1

HISTORY: A patient presents with bilateral puffiness in the neck.

1. Which of the following should be included in the differential diagnosis? (Choose all that apply.)
   A. Lipoma
   B. Metastasis
   C. Cushing disease
   D. Madelung disease
   E. Liposarcoma

2. Which is *not* a characteristic feature of Madelung disease?
   A. Symmetry
   B. Location in the head and neck
   C. Higher prevalence in men than in women
   D. Increased risk of liposarcoma
   E. None of the above

3. Which of the following is a feature of Madelung disease?
   A. More common in smokers
   B. Painful
   C. More common in Europeans than Americans
   D. Usually avascular
   E. All of the above

4. What clinical feature is typical of Madelung disease?
   A. Headaches
   B. Peripheral neuropathies
   C. Myelopathies
   D. Hypertrophic motor neuropathies
   E. None of the above

See Supplemental Figures section for additional figures and legends for this case.

CASE 186

Madelung Disease

1. **D.** Madelung disease is the most likely diagnosis for this case. There are no soft-tissue masses, which might indicate metastasis, and the fatty proliferation is too masslike to be Cushing disease. The fatty infiltration is too diffuse to be a lipoma or liposarcoma.

2. **D.** The characteristic features of Madelung disease are symmetry and location in the head and neck, and the disease affects men more than women. The risk of liposarcoma degeneration is not increased.

3. **C.** Madelung disease is not painful or avascular. It is common in drinkers and in Europeans more so than Americans.

4. **B.** Most affected patients have no symptoms, but some have peripheral neuropathies. Such patients may complain of a loss of neck mobility and of pain.

Comment

Features of Madelung Disease

Madelung disease is an idiopathic symmetric lipomatosis of the neck (Figure S186-1), also known as Launois-Bensaude adenolipomatosis and first described by Otto Madelung. The fatty infiltration is usually distributed in the neck and across the shoulders ("horse collar" formation) and hips. It is found most commonly in countries bordering the Mediterranean Sea. There is an association with alcoholism, and the disease occurs more commonly in men than in women in a ratio higher than 8:1. Symptoms may result from peripheral neuropathies, but the entity is usually painless. Rapid growth may occur over weeks to months, followed by stabilization of the deformity. Patients with human immunodeficiency virus (HIV) infection who take protease inhibitors may develop a Madelung disease–like condition with diffuse proliferation of the subcutaneous fat. Treatment with liposuction is preferred over dermolipectomy. This is usually performed for the cosmetic deformity rather than for neurologic complaints.

Reference

Ramos S, Pinheiro S, Diogo C, Cabral L, Cruzeiro C. Madelung disease: a not-so-rare disorder. *Ann Plast Surg*. 2010;64(1):122-124.

Cross-Reference

Neuroradiology: The Requisites, 3rd ed, 494.

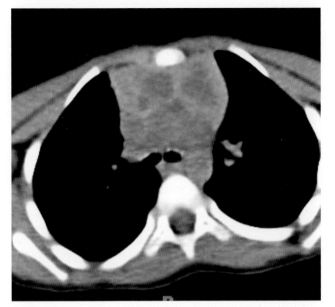

Figure 187-1

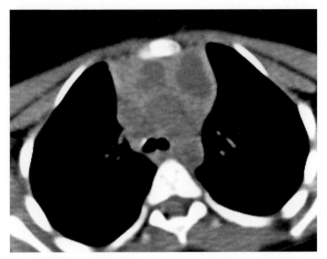

Figure 187-2

HISTORY: A lesion was found in a workup for cervical spine trauma.

1. What is the most likely source of this patient's cysts? (Choose all that apply.)
   A. Branchial cleft
   B. Thymus
   C. Thyroid gland
   D. Lymphatic channels
   E. Thyroglossal duct

2. Which is true of thymic cysts?
   A. Thymic cysts are less commonly infrahyoidal than suprahyoidal.
   B. Thymic cysts are more commonly right-sided.
   C. Thymic cysts are often a result of multinodular goiter.
   D. Thymic cysts are most commonly asymptomatic.
   E. Thymic cysts are thyroidal in anlage.

3. The thymopharyngeal anlage derives from which branchial pouch?
   A. First
   B. Second
   C. Third
   D. Fourth
   E. Fifth and/or sixth

4. What of the following entities predispose to thymic cysts?
   A. Human immunodeficiency virus (HIV)
   B. Rebound phenomenon
   C. Radiation therapy for Hodgkin disease
   D. All of the above
   E. None of the above

See Supplemental Figures section for additional figures and legends for this case.

CASE 187

Thymic Cysts

1. **B.** The source of this patient's cysts is probably the thymus. The site is too low for the source to be the thyroid gland or thyroglossal duct.

2. **D.** Thymic cysts are usually asymptomatic. They may manifest as a painless neck mass. Dyspnea, hoarseness, stridor, and dysphagia are reported in 10% of affected patients.

3. **C.** The thymopharyngeal anlage derives from the third branchial pouch. The thymus descends to the anterior mediastinum along the thymopharyngeal duct.

4. **D.** HIV, rebound phenomenon, and radiation therapy for Hodgkin disease all predispose to thymic cysts. There is no association between small cell carcinoma and thymic cysts. Myasthenia gravis may predispose to hyperplasia but not to cysts.

Comment

Etiology of Thymic Cysts

Multilocularity of thymic cysts (Figures S187-1 and S187-2) implies an inflammatory cause, as opposed to unilocular thymic cysts, which are congenital. Congenital cysts arise from the remnant of the thymopharyngeal duct, a derivative of the third pharyngeal pouch at the sixth week of gestation. The duct eventually separates from pharynx. By the eighth week of gestation, the thymic buds have descended into the mediastinum to create the thymus. Congenital thymic cysts are more common on the left side than on the right. Thymic cysts represent 3% of mediastinal masses.

Associations with Thymic Cysts

Multilocular inflammatory thymic cysts have thicker secretions, and adjacent soft tissue may exhibit reactive changes. These cysts have a higher rate of recurrence than do the congenital ones. They are associated with acquired immunodeficiency syndrome (AIDS), Sjögren's syndrome, myasthenia gravis, and lupus. They must be distinguished from cystic degeneration of a thymoma, which may also occur.

Differential Diagnosis

The differential diagnosis in this location includes necrotic lymph nodes, abscess/phlegmon, thymoma, and teratoma. Hassall corpuscles identified through cyst aspiration are suggestive of the thymic origin. Thymolipomas have fatty density. They may grow very large before detection because they are usually asymptomatic and noncompressing lesions. They are much less common in the neck than in the chest. Thymomas of the anterior mediastinum usually occur in adults and are associated with myasthenia gravis, pure red blood cell aplasia, acquired hypogammaglobulinemia, paraneoplastic syndromes, and collagen vascular diseases.

Reference

Choi YW, McAdams HP, Jeon SC, Hong EK, Kim Y-H, Im J-G, et al. Idiopathic multilocular thymic cyst: CT features with clinical and histopathologic correlation *Am J Roentgenol.* 2001;177: 881-885.

Cross-Reference

Neuroradiology: The Requisites, 3rd ed, 445.

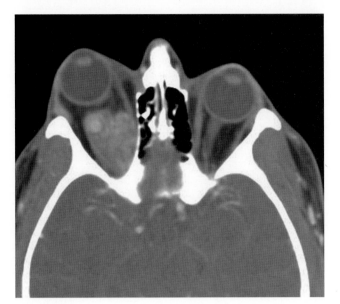

Figure 188-1

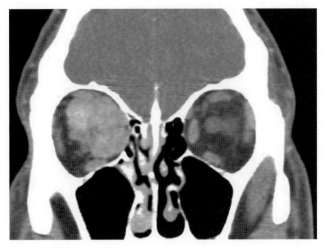

Figure 188-2

HISTORY: A patient presents with right-sided proptosis.

1. Which of the following should be included in the differential diagnosis? (Choose all that apply.)
   A. Hemangioma/venous vascular malformation
   B. Schwannoma
   C. Lymphoma
   D. Venous varix
   E. Fibrous histiocytoma

2. Which of the following is true with regard to orbital fibrous histiocytomas?
   A. They have benign and malignant forms.
   B. They are benign lesions.
   C. They are malignant lesions.
   D. They are nonneoplastic.
   E. None of the above.

3. What is the most common primary mesenchymal tumor of the orbit?
   A. Fibrous histiocytoma
   B. Schwannoma
   C. Hemangioma
   D. Rhabdomyosarcoma
   E. None of the above

4. What cranial nerve is the source of most schwannomas of the orbit?
   A. II
   B. III
   C. IV
   D. V
   E. VI

See Supplemental Figures section for additional figures and legends for this case.

CASE 188

Orbital Fibrous Histiocytoma

1. **A, B, C, and E.** The differential diagnosis should include hemangioma/venous vascular malformation, schwannoma, lymphoma, and fibrous histiocytoma. The findings are not tubular-enhancing, as would a varix.

2. **A.** The orbital fibrous histiocytoma (OFH) is a neoplasm with benign (85%) and malignant (15%) forms. One fourth of malignant OFHs are buccally aggressive.

3. **A.** The most common primary mesenchymal tumor of the orbit is fibrous histiocytoma. Schwannoma and rhabdomyosarcoma are less common. Hemangioma is not considered mesenchymal.

4. **D.** Cranial nerve V (the trigeminal nerve) is the source of most schwannomas of the orbit. Optic nerve tumors are not schwannomas; they are gliomas.

Comment

Features of Orbital Fibrous Histiocytoma

The fibrous lesions of the orbit include orbital fibrous histiocytoma, fibroma, solitary fibrous tumor, fibrosarcoma, fibromatosis, and nodular fasciitis. Fibrous histiocytoma usually occurs in adults and commonly manifests as a mass with proptosis and visual disturbance. The aggressiveness of the tumor varies from completely benign (60%) to locally aggressive (25%) to malignant (15%). It may invade the intracranial space from its origin in the orbit, and metastases have also been described. Recurrence rates also vary, depending on the aggressiveness of the tumor, from 25% (benign) to 64% (malignant). Treatment is surgical. Solitary fibrous tumors of the orbit have a more benign course but can look similar to OFH. They are in the same category of disease.

Imaging Findings

The OFH mass is usually a well-defined process with a predilection for the upper, nasal portion of the orbit (Figures S188-1 and S188-2). Remodeling of the bone in the benign form, as in this case, is common. When benign, the lesion enhances homogeneously. More aggressive features on imaging include bone destruction, inhomogeneous enhancement, spiculated margins, low T2 signal, and perineural spread. Many of these tumors are periocular.

Reference

Font RL, Hidayat AA. Fibrous histiocytoma of the orbit. A clinicopathologic study of 150 cases. *Hum Pathol.* 1982;13(3):199-209.

Cross-Reference

Neuroradiology: The Requisites, 3rd ed, 352.

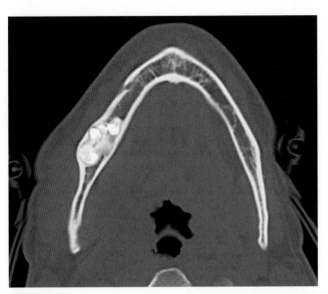

Figure 189-1

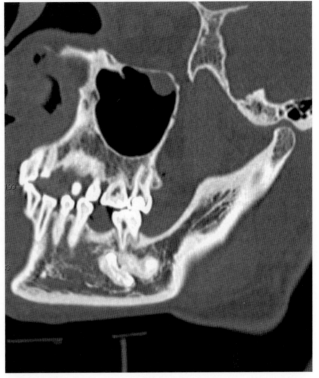

Figure 189-2

HISTORY: A 16-year-old patient presents with left-sided jaw pain.

1. Which of the following should be included in the differential diagnosis? (Choose all that apply.)
   A. Odontogenic keratocyst
   B. Ameloblastoma
   C. Squamous cell carcinoma
   D. Sclerosing osteomyelitis of Garré
   E. Cementoblastoma

2. Besides developmental/congenital lesions, what other category of disease should be considered?
   A. Infection
   B. Neoplastic
   C. Vascular
   D. Degenerative
   E. None of the above

3. What is the best variable for distinguishing Ewing sarcoma of the mandible from osteosarcoma of the mandible?
   A. Age
   B. The presence of systemic symptoms
   C. Biopsy
   D. The soft tissue mass

4. Which of the following is correct with regard to multifocal osteomyelitis?
   A. The diagnosis is usually delayed because of its insidious progressive nature.
   B. It frequently involves the mandible.
   C. Each lesion does not simulate a sarcoma.
   D. All of the above.

See Supplemental Figures section for additional figures and legends for this case.

CASE 189

Cementoblastoma of the Mandible

1. **E.** The differential diagnosis should include cementoblastoma. This lesion is not a cystic bone lesion (odontogenic keratocyst). Ameloblastoma is usually associated with the teeth, is expansile, usually has cystic components, and is more masslike. This lesion is not of mucosal origin and does not grow into the mandible (squamous cell carcinoma). It is also not an inflammatory lesion such as sclerosing osteomyelitis of Garré.

2. **E.** None of the disease categories listed are correct. This is not a joint lesion. The periosteal reaction would not be seen with degenerative lesions unless there has been an associated fracture. No congenital lesions look like this. Avascular necrosis can cause sclerosis, but because of the presence of tooth elements in this mass, it is unlikely to be vascular.

3. **C.** The best variable for distinguishing Ewing sarcoma of the mandible from osteosarcoma of the mandible is biopsy. On imaging, the two are similar in appearance in the mandible.

4. **A.** The diagnosis of multifocal osteomyelitis is usually delayed because of its insidious progressive nature. The long bones are more commonly involved than is the mandible. The lesions may look like a Ewing sarcoma because of the periosteal reaction.

Comment

Patient Presentation

This patient presented with jaw pain on the left, and the face had an inflamed appearance. The initial consideration was an inflammatory process, possibly related to an odontogenic origin around the mandibular molar teeth. The absence of fat stranding and the presence of a true mass led to the recommendation of biopsy, which revealed cementoblastoma (Figures S189-1 and S189-2). Cementoblastomas are seen in the posterior mandible of patients younger than 20 years. They are usually associated with the root of the first molar tooth (to which they may still be attached but are surrounded by a radiolucent perimeter) and are dense/sclerotic (cementum-containing) lesions of the mandible with bone expansion in 73% of cases. The differential diagnosis is usually osteosarcoma or odontoma. The latter, like cementoblastoma, can be associated with multiple teeth, deciduous teeth, or unerupted molars.

Differential Diagnosis

Periapical cemental dysplasia is a disease that affects young adults, African Americans more commonly than Caucasians, and women more commonly than men. It appears predominantly between the mandibular canine teeth and may be purely lytic (25%), sclerotic (20%), or mixed (65%) in density. Osteosarcomas of the head and neck are uncommon, but the mandible is the most common site. These may also develop in the setting of Paget disease with sarcomatous degeneration. That too may occur in the mandible, other facial bones, or the skull. Periosteal reaction may occur in the setting of trauma (including stress fractures) and infection (with or without sclerosis, as in sclerosing osteomyelitis of Garré) and with neoplasms. The neoplasm that most commonly affects the mandible is spread of squamous cell carcinoma from the mucosal surface (gum, gingival, tongue, floor of mouth, alveolus). In rare cases, nodal metastases also spread to the bone.

Reference

Iannaci G, Luise R, Iezzi G, Piattelli A, Salierno A. Multiple cementoblastoma: a rare case report. *Case Rep Dent.* 2013;2013:828373.

Cross-Reference

Neuroradiology: The Requisites, 3rd ed, 450-451.

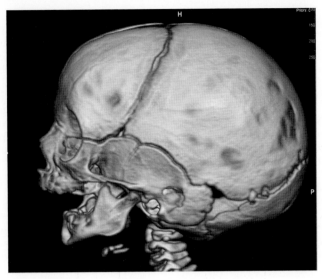

Figure 190-1

HISTORY: A scan was performed to evaluate the unusual facial appearance of this infant with developmental delay.

1. In which of the following is micrognathia a characteristic? (Choose all that apply.)
   A. Pierre Robin syndrome
   B. Crouzon syndrome
   C. Beckwith-Wiedemann syndrome
   D. None of the above

2. What entity is associated with enlargement of the mandible?
   A. Bone metastases
   B. Hurler syndrome
   C. Acromegaly
   D. Beckwith-Wiedemann syndrome
   E. All of the above

3. What is the long-term risk with micrognathia?
   A. Airway obstruction
   B. Poor dentition
   C. Choanal atresia
   D. All of the above

4. Which of the following is *not* seen in Pierre Robin syndrome? (Choose all that apply.)
   A. Microtia
   B. Craniosynostosis
   C. High, arched palate
   D. Craniofacial dysmetria

See Supplemental Figures section for additional figures and legends for this case.

CASE 190

Micrognathia

1. **A and B.** Micrognathia is a characteristic of Pierre Robin syndrome, and Crouzon syndrome.

2. **E.** Bone metastases, Hurler syndrome, acromegaly, and Beckwith-Wiedemann syndrome are all characterized by a large mandible. Beckwith-Wiedemann syndrome is also characterized by exomphalos, macroglossia, and gigantism.

3. **D.** Long-term risks with micrognathia include airway obstruction, poor dentition, and acquired choanal atresia.

4. **B.** Microtia, craniofacial dysmetria, and high, arched palate are characteristic of Pierre Robin syndrome. Craniosynostosis is not part of the syndrome.

Comment

Associations with Micrognathia

Micrognathia is associated with many syndromes, usually as part of a microfacial syndrome (Figure S190-1). Entities with associated abnormal ears include Cornelia de Lange, Goldenhar, Miller, Pierre Robin, Stickler, Treacher-Collins, and velocardiofacial syndromes. Trisomy 13 (Patau syndrome) is also associated with micrognathia, as well as with cleft lip and palate, polydactyly, colobomas, mental retardation, and congenital heart disease. Trisomy 18 (Edwards syndrome) has characteristics similar to those of trisomy 13 in addition to kidney problems, diastatic recti abdominis muscles with omphaloceles, and esophageal atresia, and the rate of micrognathia exceeds 80%. Maxillary hypoplasia is more common in patients with achondroplasia, Down syndrome, and craniosynostosis syndromes. Pierre Robin syndrome is characterized not only by micrognathia but also cleft soft palate and high, arched hard palate. The presence of natal teeth is another feature. Affected patients demonstrate poor eating, recurrent ear infections, and, often, airway compromise. The tongue often collapses backward and may obstruct the airway.

Imaging Findings

Micrognathia may be suggested on prenatal ultrasonography when the jaw index—measured as the anteroposterior mandibular diameter/biparietal diameter × 100—is less than 23. Retrognathia is diagnosed when the frontal nasomental angle is less than 142 degrees. Underdevelopment of the chin predisposes to airway compromise and therefore is an important imaging finding.

Reference

Mueller DT, Callanan VP. Congenital malformations of the oral cavity. *Otolaryngol Clin North Am.* 2007;40(1):141-160.

Cross-Reference

Neuroradiology: The Requisites, 3rd ed, 298-300.

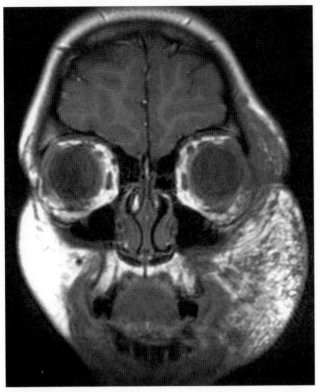

Figure 191-1

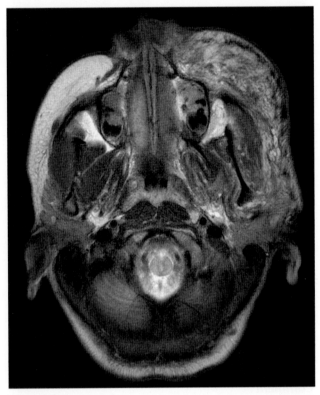

Figure 191-2

HISTORY: A patient presents with left-sided facial enlargement.

1. Which of the following may lead to unilateral facial swelling? (Choose all that apply.)
   A. Klippel-Trenaunay syndrome
   B. Neurofibromatosis
   C. McCune-Albright syndrome
   D. Proteus syndrome
   E. None of the above

2. Which of the following is among the seven criteria for diagnosing neurofibromatosis type 1 (NF-1)?
   A. Two or more schwannomas
   B. Shagreen patch
   C. Dural ectasia
   D. Plexiform neurofibroma
   E. None of the above

3. Which of the following is *not* among the seven criteria for diagnosing NF-1? (Choose all that apply.)
   A. Lisch nodules
   B. Café au lait spots
   C. Bone dysplasia
   D. Optic pathway glioma
   E. None of the above

4. Which cranial nerve is affected most commonly in NF-1 and in neurofibromatosis type 2 (NF-2)?
   A. V in NF-1 and VII in NF-2
   B. VII in NF-1 and VIII in NF-2
   C. VIII in NF-1 and V in NF-2
   D. VII in NF-1 and V in NF-2
   E. None of the above

See Supplemental Figures section for additional figures and legends for this case.

CASE 191

Facial Plexiform Neurofibroma

1. **A, B, C, and D.** Klippel-Trenaunay syndrome, neurofibromatosis, McCune-Albright, and Proteus syndrome may lead to unilateral facial swelling.

2. **D.** Plexiform neurofibroma is a criterion for the diagnosis of NF-1. Lisch nodules, café au lait spots, bone dysplasia, and optic pathway glioma are also criteria.

3. **E.** All of the choices listed are criteria for NF-1, as described in the answer to question 2. The seven criteria are (1) Lisch nodules, (2) six or more café au lait spots, (3) bone dysplasia, (4) optic pathway glioma, (5) two or more typical neurofibromas or one plexiform neurofibroma, (6) first-degree relative with NF-1, and (7) axillary freckling.

4. **E.** Cranial nerve V is affected most commonly in NF-1, and cranial nerve VIII, in NF-2. Criteria for the diagnosis of NF-2 are (1) bilateral vestibular schwannomas or (2) a first-degree relative with NF-2 and a unilateral vestibular schwannoma or (3) a first-degree relative with NF-2 and at least two of the following: meningiomas, gliomas, schwannomas, and juvenile cataracts.

Comment

Criteria for Diagnosing Neurofibromatosis Type 1

Plexiform neurofibroma is one of the seven criteria for diagnosing NF-1. Although the plexiform neurofibroma is conceptualized as infiltrating the distribution of a cranial nerve (most commonly cranial nerve V), it may manifest as a cutaneous and subcutaneous diffusely infiltrating process, as demonstrated in this case (Figures S191-1, S191-2, and S191-3).

Development of Plexiform Neurofibromas

Plexiform neurofibromas can develop into malignant peripheral nerve sheath tumors, which have a potential for metastatic spread. In positron emission tomography (PET), a standard uptake value of 7.0 or higher is correlated with malignant degeneration of a neurofibroma. PET may facilitate diagnosis by directing biopsy to a specific area of degeneration. Whereas plexiform neurofibromas show stability in 80% of affected adults, they may demonstrate significant growth in affected patients in their teens and early 20s. Rapid growth in a patient older than 25 years indicates high risk for malignant transformation. Other authorities have suggested that diffusion-weighted imaging can demonstrate restricted diffusion in areas of plexiform neurofibromas undergoing dedifferentiation. Superficial and deep neurofibromas combined are more common in NF-1 than are just superficial ones. The median number of neurofibromas per patient with NF-1 is 15. Approximately 20% to 40% of affected NF-1 patients develop plexiform neurofibromas.

Reference

Van Meerbeeck SF, Verstraete KL, Janssens S, Mortier G. Whole body MR imaging in neurofibromatosis type 1. *Eur J Radiol.* 2009;69(2): 236-242.

Cross-Reference

Neuroradiology: The Requisites, 3rd ed, 307, 378, 492, 562-563.

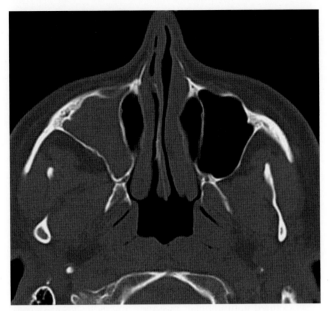

Figure 192-1

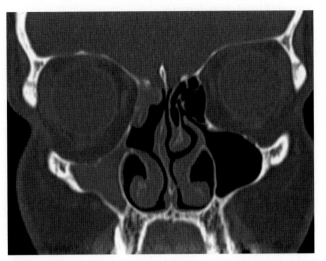

Figure 192-2

HISTORY: A 35-year-old patient presents with enophthalmos.

1. Which of the following should be included in the differential diagnosis? (Choose all that apply.)
   A. Maxillary sinus hypoplasia
   B. Polyps
   C. Silent sinus syndrome (SSS)
   D. Fungus ball

2. What is the presumed cause of SSS?
   A. Decreased pressure, which leads to sinus "atelectasis," pulling the walls of the sinus inward
   B. Increased pressure, which causes bone remodeling
   C. Chronic sinusitis
   D. Obstruction of ostia, which leads to opacification

3. Which of the following is the correct definition of hypoglobus?
   A. Low pressure in orbit
   B. Enophthalmos
   C. Downward displacement of the globe in the orbit
   D. Small globe

4. Which feature is *not* seen with SSS?
   A. Increased fat outside the walls of the sinus
   B. Downward displacement of the orbital floor
   C. Thickened sinus walls/chronic osteitis
   D. Small sinus volume

See Supplemental Figures section for additional figures and legends for this case.

CASE 192

Silent Sinus Syndrome

1. **C.** SSS accounts for this "atelectatic" sinus. Polyps and fungus ball would not be seen as a cause of a small maxillary sinus. This specific case, showing enophthalmos, does not indicate maxillary sinus hypoplasia. Hypoglobus and increased retromaxillary fat are unusual with mere sinus hypoplasia but are seen in SSS.

2. **A.** Negative pressure retraction in SSS causes the walls of the maxillary sinus to be sucked inward. This also leads to the orbital floor depression and hypoglobus.

3. **C.** Hypoglobus is the downward displacement of the globe in the orbit. Low pressure in orbit is called *hypotony*. Inward displacement is *enophthalmos*, and a small globe is *microglobia* or *microphthalmos*. Hypoglobus is a feature of SSS.

4. **C.** Thickened sinus walls/chronic osteitis are not characteristic of SSS. Some features include increased fat outside the walls of the sinus, downward displacement of the orbital floor, and small sinus volume.

Comment

Symptoms and Complications of Silent Sinus Syndrome

As the volume of the affected sinus decreases, the orbital volume has a commensurate increase. This leads to enophthalmos, which is the most common complaint associated with SSS, not the chronic sinusitis, which is the etiologic feature. Because of the depression of the orbital floor into the collapsing maxillary antrum, the globe may also show inferior depression *(hypoglobus)*. Most affected patients have complete opacification of the "atelectatic" sinus and obstruction at the ostium (Figures S192-1 and S192-2). The entity affects the maxillary sinus exclusively, and documented negative pressure within the sinus accounts for the retraction.

Classification of Silent Sinus Syndrome

Why is this not simply maxillary sinus hypoplasia, which is many times more common than SSS? Criteria for diagnosing maxillary sinus hypoplasia include a small maxillary sinus, often with thickened walls; vertical enlargement of the orbit; elevated canine fossa; enlarged superior orbital and pterygopalatine fossa; and lateral position of the infraorbital nerve canal. The uncinate process is usually hypoplastic as well. A classification of maxillary sinus hypoplasia has been developed:

- Type I: normal uncinate process, a well-defined infundibular passage, and mild sinus hypoplasia
- Type II: absent or hypoplastic uncinate process, ill-defined infundibular passage, and soft tissue–density opacification of a significantly hypoplastic sinus
- Type III: absent uncinate process and profoundly hypoplastic, cleftlike sinus

Reference

Hourany R, Aygun N, Della Santina CC, Zinreich SJ. Silent sinus syndrome: an acquired condition. *AJNR Am J Neuroradiol.* 2005;26(9): 2390-2392.

Cross-Reference

Neuroradiology: The Requisites, 3rd ed, 422, 424f.

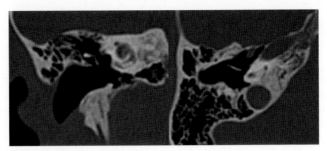

Figure 193-1

HISTORY: A patient presents with unilateral, right-sided sensorineural hearing loss.

1. Which of the following should be included in the differential diagnosis? (Choose all that apply.)
   A. Otosclerosis
   B. Osteogenesis imperfecta
   C. Labyrinthitis ossificans
   D. Paget disease

2. What is the most common source of labyrinthitis ossificans?
   A. Meningitis
   B. External otitis
   C. Otospongiosis
   D. Eustachian tube dysfunction

3. What is the classic location of otosclerosis?
   A. Cochlear aperture
   B. Semicircular canal
   C. Incus
   D. Fissula ante fenestram

4. What does osteogenesis imperfecta simulate in the inner ear?
   A. Ménière syndrome
   B. Labyrinthitis ossificans
   C. Otosclerosis
   D. Tympanosclerosis

See Supplemental Figures section for additional figures and legends for this case.

CASE 193

Labyrinthitis Ossificans

1. **C.** The increased density in the turns of the cochlea indicates labyrinthitis ossificans. Osteogenesis imperfecta causes demineralization, and Paget disease does not affect the cochlear perilymph. Otosclerosis causes demineralization around the cochlea or near the oval window.

2. **A.** Meningitis is a common source of labyrinthitis ossificans. External otitis does not affect inner ear structures, and otospongiosis and eustachian tube dysfunction are unrelated to labyrinthitis ossificans. Bacterial labyrinthitis, chronic otitis media, and barotrauma may be other sources, however.

3. **D.** The fissula ante fenestram is the classical location of otosclerosis. The disorder fixes the stapes footplate from this location, just anterior to the oval window.

4. **C.** Osteogenesis imperfecta simulates otosclerosis in the inner ear. Otosyphilis is also in this differential diagnosis.

Comment

Causes of Labyrinthitis Ossificans

Labyrinthitis ossificans can occur as a sequela to meningitis (which is most commonly associated with bacterial labyrinthitis), otitis media, hemorrhage in the inner ear, or chronic barotrauma. Meningitis may spread to the inner ear via the cochlear aqueduct or the internal auditory canal. Hearing loss associated with meningitis occurs in 5% of patients with meningitis, but it is more common with bacterial varieties.

Imaging Findings and Complications

Labyrinthitis ossificans manifests as increased-density bone formation in the cochlea, vestibule, and/or semicircular canals when it is mature (Figure S193-1). However, it may start out as a fibrous obliteration, which is why some head and neck radiologists prefer constructive interference in steady state (CISS) magnetic resonance imaging (MRI) over computed tomography to make the diagnosis. In that situation, the bright fluid of the perilymph and endolymph is replaced by dark fibrous tissue (or bone) on the heavily T2-weighted sequence. The most common region of cochlear ossification affected is the scala tympani of the basal turn. This ossification is a source of sensorineural hearing loss. Labyrinthitis ossificans may be accompanied by tympanosclerosis, in which the tympanic membrane, tympanic ligaments, and other supporting tissue may calcify or ossify.

Reference

Liu BP, Saito N, Wang JJ, Mian AZ, Sakai O. Labyrinthitis ossificans in a child with sickle cell disease: CT and MRI findings. *Pediatr Radiol.* 2009;39(9):999-1001.

Cross-Reference

Neuroradiology: The Requisites, 3rd ed, 380, 382b, 382f, 412, 567.

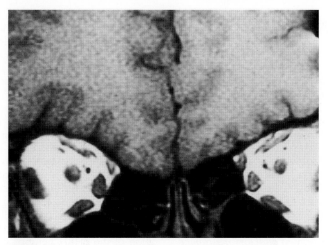

Figure 194-1

HISTORY: The patient has had a poor sense of smell since birth.

1. Which of the following should be included in the differential diagnosis? (Choose all that apply.)
   A. Kallmann syndrome
   B. Holoprosencephaly
   C. Neuronal migrational anomaly
   D. Duane syndrome

2. What is the most common cause of loss of sense of smell?
   A. Trauma
   B. Neoplasm
   C. Idiopathic entity
   D. Upper respiratory tract infection

3. What tumor classically affects the region of the ciliary nerves as they pass to the olfactory bulbs?
   A. Meningioma
   B. Sinonasal undifferentiated carcinoma
   C. Esthesioneuroblastoma
   D. Inverted papilloma

4. What is the mechanism for posttraumatic anosmia?
   A. Temporal lobe hematomas
   B. Shearing at the cribriform plate
   C. Injury to the gyrus rectus (in the frontal lobe)
   D. Sinus hematoma

See Supplemental Figures section for additional figures and legends for this case.

CASE 194

Kallmann Syndrome

1. **A and B.** Kallmann syndrome is a source of congenital anosmia. Congenital anosmia can occur in isolation without a syndrome and in holoprosencephaly (also called *arrhin-encephaly*). In Duane syndrome, cranial nerve VI (the abducens nerve) is absent, and the lateral rectus muscle is innervated by cranial nerve III (the oculomotor nerve).

2. **D.** Upper respiratory tract infections and sinusitis are the most common causes of loss of the sense of smell (upper respiratory tract infections more so than sinusitis). Trauma, neoplasms, and idiopathic entities are not common causes.

3. **C.** Esthesioneuroblastoma, also termed *olfactory neuroblastoma,* is the tumor that classically affects the region of the ciliary nerves as they pass to the olfactory bulbs. Meningioma is a common tumor but not classically in this location. This location is also not typical for inverted papilloma. Sinonasal undifferentiated carcinoma is a rare tumor.

4. **B.** Shearing at the cribriform plate traumatizes the ciliary nerves. Injury to the gyrus rectus and to the olfactory bulb and tract occurs less commonly. Temporal lobe hematomas and sinus hematoma are not very common.

Comment

Features of Kallmann Syndrome

Kallmann syndrome consists of hypogonadotropic hypogonadism in association with anosmia caused by olfactory bulb aplasia. Aureliano Maestre de San Juan described the entity 88 years before Franz Josef Kallmann in 1856. The syndrome is transmitted most frequently as an X-linked disorder characterized by infertility and anosmia. Reported cases of patients with cerebellar dysfunction, gait disturbance, spasticity, visual and extraocular motion abnormalities, and hearing loss suggest that the disease process is multifaceted. Kallmann syndrome may be inherited as an autosomal dominant or recessive trait as well. It is five times more frequent in men than in women. The olfactory sulci may or may not develop along the gyrus rectus region (sulci are not seen in this case in Figure 194). Some authorities believe that patients with Kallmann syndrome have no olfactory neuroepithelium, whereas others believe that the olfactory axons connect intracranially. The hypogonadism of Kallmann syndrome is thought to result either from a lack of cells that can express luteinizing hormone–releasing hormone (LHRH) or from abnormal migration of the LHRH neurons from the olfactory placode in the nose to the hypothalamus. Among individuals with congenital anosmia, olfactory bulb and tract absence (68% to 84%) and hypoplasia (16% to 32%) are common. In this case, the patient had no bulbs, tracts, or "olfactory sulci" (Figure S194-1).

Reference

Yousem DM, Geckle RJ, Bilker W, Mckeown D, Doty RL. MR evaluation of the patients with congenital hyposmia or anosmia. *AJR Am J Roentgenol.* 1996;166:439-444.

Cross-Reference

Neuroradiology: The Requisites, 3rd ed, 189-190.

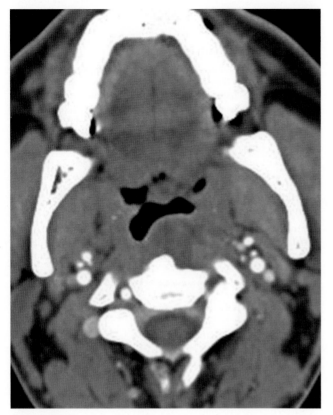

Figure 195-1

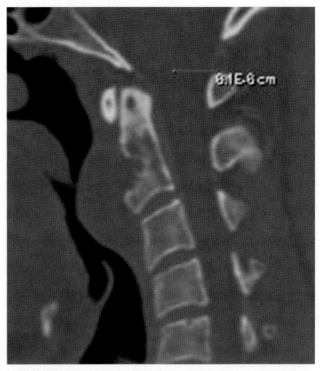

Figure 195-2

HISTORY: A 60-year-old patient presented with neck and head pain.

1. Which of the following should be included in the differential diagnosis? (Choose all that apply.)
   A. Metastasis
   B. Squamous cell carcinoma
   C. Rhabdomyosarcoma
   D. Chordoma

2. What percentage of all chordomas arise from the vertebrae?
   A. 0% to 10%
   B. 11% to 20%
   C. 21% to 30%
   D. >30%

3. What is the most common "submucosal pseudomass" normal variant in the pharynx?
   A. Retropharyngeal carotid artery
   B. Styloid process
   C. Mucous retention cysts
   D. Osteophytes

4. What is the typical signal intensity of chordomas on T2-weighted images?
   A. Mixed intensity because of matrix
   B. Bright
   C. Dark
   D. Isointense

See Supplemental Figures section for additional figures and legends for this case.

CASE 195

Chordoma

1. **A and D.** The lesion shown could be metastasis, inasmuch as it may arise from the cervical spine. It could also be a cervical spine chordoma. It is not mucosa based, so it would not be squamous cell carcinoma. Rhabdomyosarcoma rarely arises in the bone and would be unlikely in a 60-year-old person.

2. **B.** Fifteen percent of all chordomas arise from the vertebrae. Most are in the sacrococcygeal region; the clivus is the second most common site.

3. **D.** Osteophytes are the most common "submucosal pseudomass" normal variants of the pharynx, especially in adults from the cervical spine. The retropharyngeal carotid artery is the second most common. An enlarged styloid process (Eagle syndrome) is not very common, and mucous retention cysts are not seen as submucosal.

4. **B.** The typical signal intensity of chordomas on T2-weighted images is bright, maybe because of their gelatinous nature. They have variable enhancement.

Comment
Imaging Findings

Chordomas usually appear bright on T2-weighted images and dark on T1-weighted images, and their enhancement is variable. Although they may have some internal calcified matrix that is visible on computed tomography (CT), they nonetheless appear overwhelmingly bright on T2-weighted images.

Beyond that matrix, the lesion tends to appear lytic on CT (Figures S195-1 and S195-2).

Locations of Chordomas

Most adult chordomas affect the sacrum (50%) or clivus (35%), but occasionally they arise from the cervical spine (15%). Whereas some may be centered at the intervertebral disk where the notochordal remnants reside, others, like this one, appear as exophytic bone lesions. Thus they may appear as if they are submucosal masses in the aerodigestive system. In children, chordomas are more common in the skull base (63%) than in the vertebrae (16%) or the sacrococcygeal region (12%).

Differentiating Benign Notochordal Cell Tumors from Chordomas

Recently, authors have attempted to distinguish benign notochordal cell tumors from chordomas. Accordingly, the imaging findings that characterize a benign notochordal cell tumor are as follows:
- Being purely intraosseous without an extraosseous component
- Presence of mild bone sclerosis without bone destruction
- Absence of enhancement

Reference

Géhanne C, Delpierre I, Damry N, Devroede B, Brihaye P, Christophe C. Skull base chordoma: CT and MRI features. *JBR-BTR.* 2005;88(6): 325-327.

Cross-Reference

Neuroradiology: The Requisites, 3rd ed, 380, 382b, 382f, 412, 567.

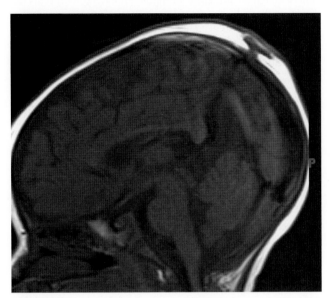

Figure 196-1

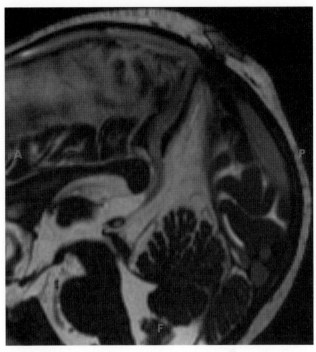

Figure 196-2

HISTORY: A 3-year-old patient has a seizure disorder.

1. Which of the following should be included in the differential diagnosis? (Choose all that apply.)
   A. Agenesis of the corpus callosum with cyst
   B. Caput medusae
   C. Atretic encephalocele
   D. Sinus pericranii

2. What is the most common location for atretic encephaloceles?
   A. Frontal
   B. Temporal
   C. Parietal
   D. Occipital

3. How is the straight sinus oriented in atretic encephaloceles?
   A. It is absent.
   B. It is more horizontal.
   C. It is more vertical.
   D. It faces downward.

4. What constitutes the "spinning top" appearance on imaging in an atretic encephalocele?
   A. Cerebrospinal fluid swirling through the skull defect
   B. High falx-tentorial junction in association with prominence of the subjacent superior cerebellar cistern
   C. Torcula-lambdoid inversion
   D. Sagittal sinus fenestration by the encephalocele

See Supplemental Figures section for additional figures and legends for this case.

CASE 196

Atretic Parietal Encephalocele

1. **C.** The appearance with intracranial and extracranial abnormalities is typical of parietal atretic encephalocele. Agenesis of the corpus callosum with cyst and caput medusae are not present. Sinus pericranii is a vascular process, not present in this case, but it can coexist with an atretic encephalocele.

2. **C.** The most common location for atretic encephaloceles is parietal. The occipital area is next most common.

3. **C.** The straight sinus turns more vertically in atretic encephaloceles.

4. **B.** High falx-tentorial junction associated with prominence of the subjacent superior cerebellar cistern constitutes the "spinning top" appearance in an atretic encephalocele. Cerebrospinal fluid does not swirl through the skull defect. Torcula-lambdoid inversion occurs in Dandy-Walker syndrome. Sagittal sinus fenestration by the encephalocele may be present, but it does not constitute the "spinning top" appearance.

Comment

Imaging Findings

Atretic parietal encephaloceles have a characteristic appearance on sagittal magnetic resonance imaging in which the straight sinus is vertically oriented, fibrous strands run along with the sinus, and there is a defect through the parietal bone above the lambdoid suture through which soft tissue protrudes into the scalp (Figures S196-1, S196-2, and S196-3). The vein of Galen is elongated. Computed tomography reveals the defect in the calvaria. As many as 10% of meningoencephaloceles may be atretic. They usually are not associated with developmental delay.

Associations with Atretic Parietal Encephalocele

Associated anomalies such as dysgenesis of the corpus callosum, interhemispheric cysts, and neuronal migrational anomalies may, however, coexist and lead to symptoms. After the parietal location, the occipital region is the next most common location of atretic encephaloceles. The herniated tissue may contain meninges, rests of glial and/or central nervous system tissues, and even a sinus pericranii, albeit rarely. Walker-Warburg syndrome is present in 25% to 50% of children with atretic encephaloceles.

Treatment of Atretic Parietal Encephalocele

Treatment is usually performed only in the following cases: (1) for cosmetic reasons if the protruding tissue is large, (2) for painful dura, (3) for ulceration of skin, and (4) for persistent meningeal infections or seizures.

Reference

Patterson RJ, Egelhoff JC, Crone KR, Ball WS Jr. Atretic parietal cephaloceles revisited: an enlarging clinical and imaging spectrum? *AJNR Am J Neuroradiol.* 1998;19(4):791-795.

Cross-Reference

Neuroradiology: The Requisites, 3rd ed, 282-290.

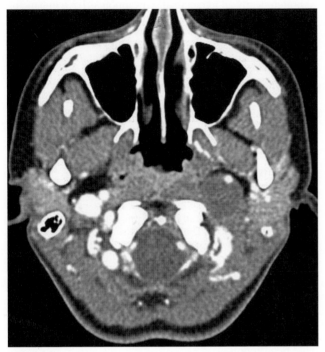

Figure 197-1

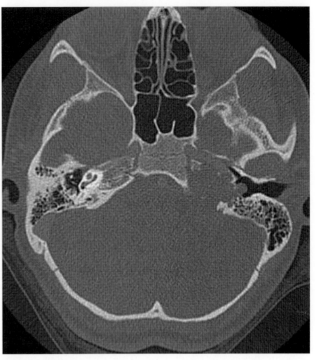

Figure 197-2

HISTORY: A patient presents with hoarseness and a mass at the skull base.

1. Which of the following should be included in the differential diagnosis? (Choose all that apply.)
   A. Schwannoma
   B. Paraganglioma
   C. Neurofibroma
   D. Chondromyxoid fibroma

2. Where are the most common locations for chondromyxoid fibromas in the head and neck?
   A. Mandible and maxilla
   B. Carotid sheath and parapharyngeal space
   C. Paranasal sinuses and nasal cavity
   D. Supraclavicular fossa and brachial plexus

3. What percentage of schwannomas of the head and neck are cystic?
   A. 0% to 25%
   B. 26% to 50%
   C. 51% to 75%
   D. >75%

4. What percentage of chondromyxoid fibromas occur in the head and neck below the skull base?
   A. 0% to 25%
   B. 26% to 50%
   C. 51% to 75%
   D. >75%

See Supplemental Figures section for additional figures and legends for this case.

CASE 197

Carotid Sheath Chondromyxoid Fibroma

1. **A, B, C, and D.** The true diagnosis is chondromyxoid fibroma. Paraganglioma and neurogenic tumors may also be considered but are less likely in this case because it is rare for paragangliomas, schwannomas, and neurofibromas not to enhance.

2. **A.** The most common locations of chondromyxoid fibromas in the head and neck are the mandible and the maxilla. Chondromyxoid fibromas of the paranasal sinuses and nasal cavity have been reported in only 25 cases in recent literature. The carotid sheath and parapharyngeal space are quite uncommon locations, and supraclavicular fossa and brachial plexus have not been reported as sites.

3. **A.** Of schwannomas in the head and neck, 4% to 10% are cystic. This makes the diagnosis difficult, and the differential diagnosis therefore includes branchial cleft cysts, cystic nodes, and other congenital cysts in the neck.

4. **A.** Of chondromyxoid fibromas in the head and neck, 5.4% occur below the skull base. This case is thus a rare occurrence.

Comment
Imaging Findings

When a mass in the carotid sheath does not enhance, one must take a pause. Of masses that do not enhance, paragangliomas would be the least common entity; because of their vascular hyperperfused nature, they almost always enhance.

Although nearly all intracranial schwannomas have enhancing components, a significant subpopulation in the head and neck do *not* enhance. This is more likely to occur on CT than on magnetic resonance imaging, whose contrast resolution is superior to that of CT. Necrotic adenopathy could be a consideration, as could Bailey type 3 second branchial cleft cysts in this specific case (Figures S197-1 and S197-2). Chondroid lesions, as in this case, could have a zebra-stripe pattern of enhancement, but many of them show minor enhancement. Carotid dissection with a clotted pseudoaneurysm, another nonenhancing lesion, would be included in the differential diagnosis, but it is also uncommon.

Symptoms of Carotid Sheath Chondromyxoid Fibroma

Chondromyxoid fibromas rarely (5.4% of cases) occur in the head and neck. When they do, they usually involve the maxilla and mandible. This lesion is usually found in the long bones of the lower extremity, especially the tibia. Even in those locations, they are rare, representing fewer than 5% of all benign bone lesions. They are generally lytic, characterized by bright signal on T2-weighted images. Calcifications in the matrix are present in about 15% of such lesions. For chondromyxoid fibromas at the skull base, the differential diagnosis includes chordoma, chondroid chordoma, and low-grade myxoid chondrosarcoma. Cases isolated to the temporal bone have been reported.

Reference

McClurg SW, Leon M, Teknos TN, Iwenofu OH. Chondromyxoid fibroma of the nasal septum: case report and review of literature. *Head Neck.* 2013;35(1):E1-E5.

Cross-Reference

Neuroradiology: The Requisites, 3rd ed, 496-498.

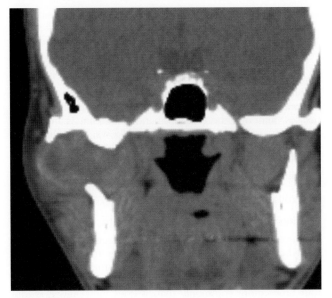

Figure 198-1

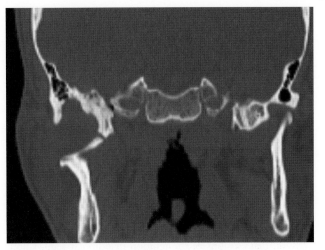

Figure 198-2

HISTORY: A patient presents with pain radiating to the right ear.

1. Which of the following should be included in the differential diagnosis? (Choose all that apply.)
   A. Gout
   B. Synovial chondromatosis
   C. Pigmented villonodular synovitis
   D. Normal

2. What are the imaging features of pigmented villonodular synovitis on magnetic resonance imaging (MRI)?
   A. Hemorrhagic byproducts
   B. Erosive changes of bone and cartilage
   C. Dark signal on T2-weighted scans because of the presence of hemosiderin
   D. All of the above

3. In avascular necrosis of the condylar head, what are the early findings on MRI?
   A. Dark signal intensity on T1-weighted scans and bright signal intensity on T2-weighted scans
   B. Dark signal intensity on T1-weighted scans and dark signal intensity on T2-weighted scans
   C. Bright signal intensity on T1-weighted scans and bright signal intensity on T2-weighted scans
   D. Bright signal intensity on T1-weighted scans and dark signal intensity on T2-weighted scans

4. Of these mass lesions of the temporomandibular joint, which is the most common?
   A. Osteochondroma
   B. Synovial chondromatosis
   C. Pigmented villonodular synovitis
   D. Chondrosarcoma
   E. Synovial sarcoma

See Supplemental Figures section for additional figures and legends for this case.

CASE 198

Synovial Chondromatosis

1. **A, B, and C.** Gout can erode and enlarge the temporomandibular joint, and pigmented villonodular synovitis is centered on the joint. Synovial chondromatosis is also correct, despite the absence of calcified matrix in this case.

2. **D.** Hemorrhagic byproducts, erosive changes of bone and cartilage, and dark signal on T2-weighted scans as a result of the presence of hemosiderin are imaging features of pigmented villonodular synovitis on MRI.

3. **A.** Early MRI findings in avascular necrosis of the condylar head are dark signal intensity on T1-weighted scans and bright signal intensity on T2-weighted scans. These findings represent edematous bone.

4. **B.** Synovial chondromatosis is the most common of the listed mass lesions of the temporomandibular joint. Chondrosarcoma may be the most common malignancy after metastases and lymphoma. Osteochondroma, pigmented villonodular synovitis, and synovial sarcoma are rare.

Comment

Diagnosing Synovial Chondromatosis

Synovial chondromatosis is not always characterized by dense loose bodies in the joint. Sometimes the lesions are noncalcified, which makes the diagnosis much more difficult, as in this case (Figures S198-1 and S198-2). In that instance, only enlargement of the joint space and remodeling of the mandibular condyle and the glenoid fossa, with possible involvement of the muscles of mastication, are visible on imaging. A more classical finding is of loose bodies that appear as multiple densities in and around the joint. The entity is more commonly monoarticular and occurs in young adults. Pain is a component of the disease. The larger joints are more commonly affected than the small ones. When the lesion is calcified, the differential diagnosis for loose bodies includes tumoral calcinosis, which produces large periarticular calcified masses, although the temporomandibular joint is much less frequently involved than the hips, elbows, and shoulders. Tumoral calcinosis occurs predominantly in young African American adults. Other entities to be considered include calcium pyrophosphate deposition disease, chronic renal failure with dystrophic calcification, dialysis-related arthropathy, and chondroosseous neoplasms.

Manifestation of Synovial Chondromatosis

The entity usually manifests with pain referred to the ear. Elsewhere in the body, it is more common in men than in women, with a mean age at onset in the fifth decade of life. However in the temporomandibular joint it affects women four times more commonly than it does men, and it is four times more common on the right side than on the left, for unknown reasons. Treatment comprises removal of the loose bodies and the affected synovium.

Reference

Koyama J, Ito J, Hayashi T, Kobayashi F. Synovial chondromatosis in the temporomandibular joint complicated by displacement and calcification of the articular disk: report of two cases. *AJNR Am J Neuroradiol.* 2001;22(6):1203-1206.

Cross-Reference

Neuroradiology: The Requisites, 3rd ed, 424-427.

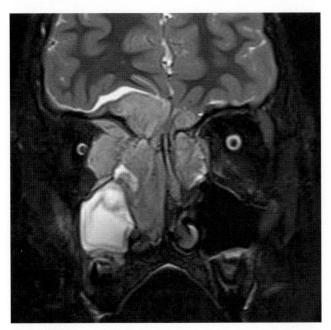

Figure 199-1

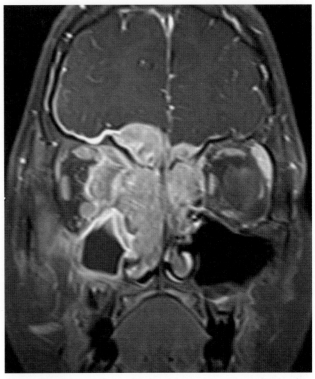

Figure 199-2

HISTORY: A teenager presents with a "stuffy nose."

1. Which of the following should be included in the differential diagnosis? (Choose all that apply.)
   A. Squamous cell carcinoma
   B. Lymphoma
   C. Rhabdomyosarcoma
   D. Esthesioneuroblastoma

2. What is the best method to distinguish inspissated secretions from tumor tissue on magnetic resonance imaging (MRI)?
   A. T1-weighted imaging
   B. T2-weighted imaging
   C. Fat-suppressed, T1-weighted, gadolinium-enhanced imaging
   D. Diffusion-weighted imaging

3. What percentage of sinonasal rhabdomyosarcomas have orbital extension?
   A. 0% to 25%
   B. 26% to 50%
   C. 51% to 75%
   D. >75%

4. What percentage of sinonasal rhabdomyosarcomas have skull base/intracranial extension?
   A. 0% to 25%
   B. 26% to 50%
   C. 51% to 75%
   D. >75%

See Supplemental Figures section for additional figures and legends for this case.

CASE 199

Sinonasal Rhabdomyosarcoma

1. **B and C.** The correct diagnosis in this case is rhabdomyosarcoma, which is expected in a child. The age and appearance of the lesion is appropriate for lymphoma as well. Squamous cell carcinoma is rare in teenagers, and esthesioneuroblastoma is rare in children. Sinonasal undifferentiated carcinoma would be included in the differential diagnosis because of the dural growth, but it is uncommon in children.

2. **C.** Fat-suppressed, T1-weighted, gadolinium-enhanced imaging is the best method for distinguishing inspissated secretions from tumor tissue on MRI. Tumors enhance and secretions do not, but T1-weighted images without gadolinium must be evaluated to make sure that secretions do not appear bright before contrast, owing to high protein content.

3. **A.** Approximately 20% of sinonasal rhabdomyosarcomas have orbital extension. Patients in whom the extension originates from the nasal cavity and maxillary sinus have the best chance of survival, and patients with ethmoid sinus malignancy have the worst rate of survival. Rhabdomyosarcomas and squamous cell carcinomas invade the orbit more than do tumors of other histologic features.

4. **B.** Close to 50% of sinonasal rhabdomyosarcomas have skull base/intracranial extension. This is why they are referred to as *parameningeal tumors.*

Comment

Rate of Survival of Sinonasal Rhabdomyosarcomas

Sinonasal rhabdomyosarcomas are considered parameningeal rhabdomyosarcomas and therefore carry a worse prognosis than do those that develop outside the parameningeal locations. Parameningeal rhabdomyosarcomas are ones that arise in the following locations: nasopharynx, nasal cavity, paranasal sinuses, middle ear, mastoid region, infratemporal fossa, and pterygopalatine fossa. Other poor prognostic factors are age older than 10, alveolar histologic features, meningeal or orbital involvement, tumor size of more than 5 cm, gross tumor residual before or after surgery, and distant metastases. In children, they are the most common malignancies of the sinonasal cavity (Figures S199-1 and S199-2). The 5-year survival rate is approximately 50%. Survival rates with botryoid and spindle cell types are better than those with the embryonal subtype, which in turn are better than those with the alveolar/undifferentiated subtype, but alveolar sinonasal rhabdomyosarcomas are more common than the embryonal subtype.

Differential Diagnosis

In children with sinonasal masses, the differential diagnosis for a sinonasal mass is broad. Polyposis is likely the most common source of a mass and is particularly frequent in children with cystic fibrosis and/or allergic syndromes. If bleeding is a component of the manifestation and the child is a boy, juvenile nasopharyngeal angiofibroma is a possible diagnosis. If the lesion shows translucency, it may be a cephalocele, whether it contains brain tissue (encephalocele) or just meninges (meningocele). Nasal gliomas are gray in color and have a solid consistency, and they may be nasal or extranasal. If hair or sebaceum is present, the lesion may be a dermoid or an epidermoid, potentially with a tract leading intracranially. If the mass is pulsatile, it should be investigated to determine whether it contains cerebrospinal fluid, inasmuch as meningoceles pulsate, but so do giant aneurysms.

Reference

Fyrmpas G, Wurm J, Athanassiadou F, Papageorgiou T, Beck JD, Iro H, et al. Management of paediatric sinonasal rhabdomyosarcoma. *J Laryngol Otol.* 2009;123(9):990-996.

Cross-Reference

Neuroradiology: The Requisites, 3rd ed, 380, 383f, 445.

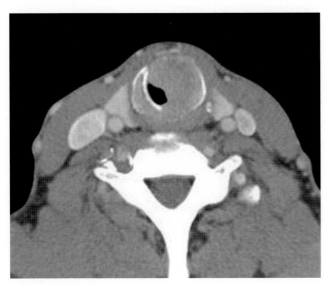

Figure 200-1

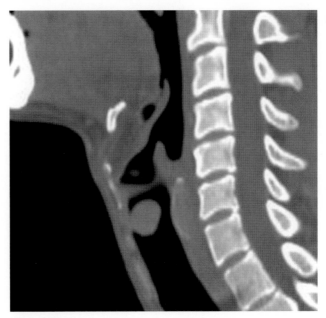

Figure 200-2

HISTORY: A man in his 30s has new onset of hoarseness.

1. Which of the following should be included in the differential diagnosis? (Choose all that apply.)
   A. Chondrosarcoma
   B. Amyloidoma
   C. Lymphoma
   D. Giant cell tumor

2. In the head and neck, what is the most common site of amyloid deposition?
   A. Orbit
   B. Larynx
   C. Nodes
   D. Hyoid bone

3. Which of the following statements is true?
   A. Giant cell tumors of the larynx most commonly affect the thyroid cartilage.
   B. Amyloidomas of the larynx most commonly affect the thyroid cartilage.
   C. Giant cell tumors of the larynx most commonly affect the cricoid cartilage.
   D. Chondrosarcomas of the larynx most commonly affect the thyroid cartilage.

4. In the head and neck, which of the following is the most common site of giant cell tumors?
   A. Mandible
   B. Hyoid bone
   C. Larynx
   D. Pharynx

See Supplemental Figures section for additional figures and legends for this case.

CASE 200

Subglottic Giant Cell Tumor

1. **A, B, C, and D.** This case's true diagnosis is giant cell tumor, which is a very rare tumor in this location. The differential diagnosis should also include chondrosarcoma, even without a calcified matrix. Amyloidoma can occur in the subglottic space. Lymphoma is possible as well, but unusual.

2. **B.** The larynx is the most common site of amyloid deposition in the head and neck. The orbit is the second most common site. Amyloid deposition may occur in nodes, but it is not common. Amyloidomas are characterized by low signal intensity on T2-weighted imaging. They rarely calcify and may simulate chondrosarcomas when they do.

3. **A.** Giant cell tumors of the larynx affect the thyroid cartilage. Amyloidomas may not affect the cartilage but may be submucosal in location. Chondrosarcomas most commonly affect the cricoid cartilage.

4. **A.** The mandible is the most common site of giant cell tumors of the head and neck. Those tumors rarely occur in the hyoid bone, larynx, and pharynx. Giant cell tumors of the salivary gland have also been reported.

Comment

Diagnosis

Giant cell tumors of the larynx are unusual. Approximately 50 have been reported in the literature. These tumors most commonly affect the thyroid cartilage and therefore manifest with hoarseness, airway obstruction, and dysphagia and have a strong predilection for men.

Imaging Findings

Imaging usually shows a submucosal mass that does not have the calcified matrix expected of a chondrosarcoma. Therefore, the differential diagnosis includes entities such as amyloidomas, which usually affect the supraglottic larynx. Amyloidomas may have stippled calcification but not dominant coarse calcification, as do chondrosarcomas. Amyloid usually appears quite dark on T2-weighted magnetic resonance imaging. Fluid levels are seen in aneurysmal bone cysts, which are associated with giant cell tumors (Figures S200-1 and S200-2).

Prognosis

The prognosis for patients with a giant cell tumor of the larynx is excellent because it is a benign condition and responds well to a variety of treatments.

Reference

Wieneke JA, Gannon FH, Heffner DK, Thompson LD. Giant cell tumor of the larynx: a clinicopathologic series of eight cases and a review of the literature. *Mod Pathol.* 2001;14(12):1209-1215.

Cross-Reference

Neuroradiology: The Requisites, 3rd ed, 467-468.

Supplemental Figures

CASE 1

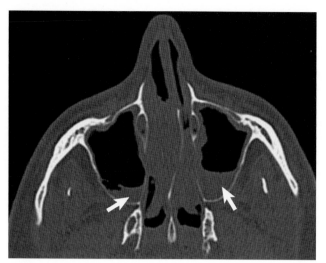

Figure S1-1. The presence of air-fluid levels signifies acute sinusitis *(arrows).*

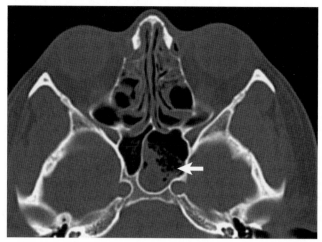

Figure S1-2. Air bubbles in the sinuses imply fluid and acute disease, even in the absence of an air-fluid level *(arrow).*

CASE 2

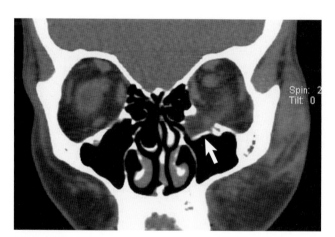

Figure S2-1. The common wall of the orbital floor and the medial orbital wall are fractured, with a depressed fragment opening like a trap door *(arrow).*

CASE 3

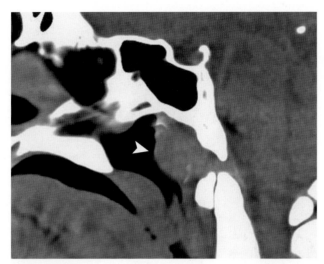

Figure S3-1. Note the fullness of the nasopharynx *(arrowhead)* on sagittal computed tomographic scan.

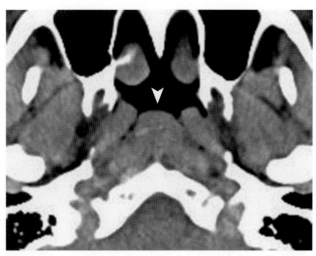

Figure S3-2. No evidence of extra-adenoidal invasion is visible *(arrowhead)* on the axial scan.

CASE 4

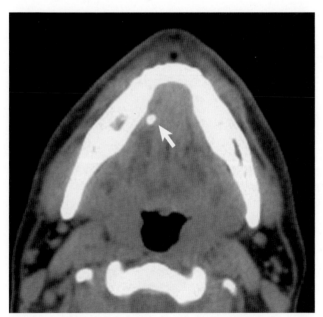

Figure S4-1. Note the small area of radiodensity *(arrow)* in the floor of the mouth on this unenhanced computed tomographic scan.

CASE 5

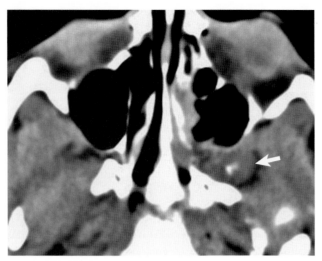

Figure S5-1. Axial computed tomographic scan shows a mass *(arrow)* in the left pterygopalatine fossa.

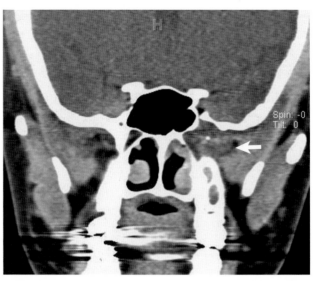

Figure S5-2. Coronal computed tomographic scan shows that mass *(arrow)* in the left pterygopalatine fossa.

CASE 6

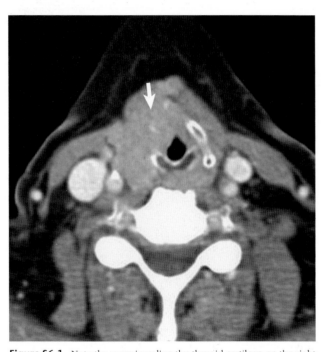

Figure S6-1. Note the mass invading the thyroid cartilage on the right *(arrow)*.

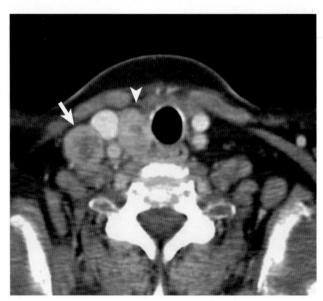

Figure S6-2. A mass in the thyroid gland *(arrowhead)* and a right-sided level IV jugular lymph node *(arrow)* are visible.

CASE 7

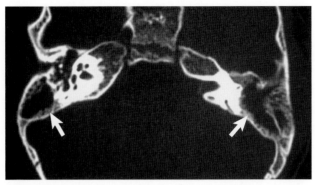

Figure S7-1. Note the destruction of mastoid septa *(arrows)* bilaterally in a young adult.

CASE 8

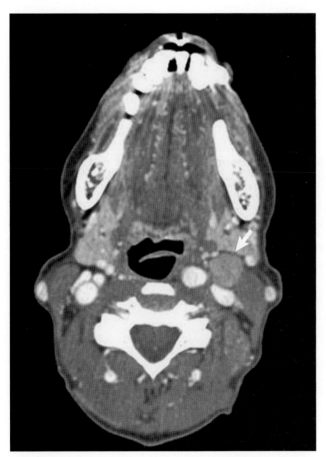

Figure S8-1. Axial computed tomographic image shows a lymph node *(arrow)* in the left jugular IIa chain.

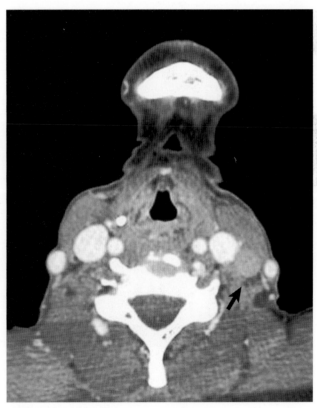

Figure S8-2. Axial computed tomographic image shows a lymph node *(arrow)* in the left jugular III chain.

CASE 9

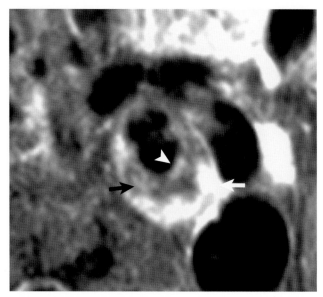

Figure S9-1. Post contrast fat-suppressed magnetic resonance image shows enhanced fibrous cap *(arrowhead)*, enhanced plaque inflammation *(white arrow)*, and fat-suppressed lipid core *(black arrow)*.

CASE 10

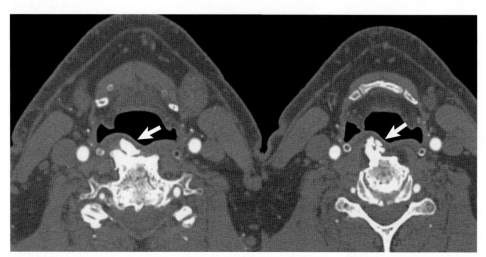

Figure S10-1. Note the large osteophytes *(arrows)* indenting the pharyngeal airway from a posterior direction.

CASE 11

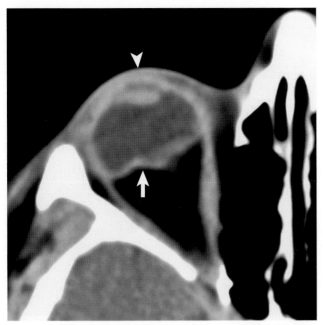

Figure S11-1. Note the decreased depth and increased density of the anterior chamber *(arrowhead)* with a disrupted malpositioned lens. The "flat tire" of the vitreous humor *(arrow)* implies rupture and low pressure.

CASE 12

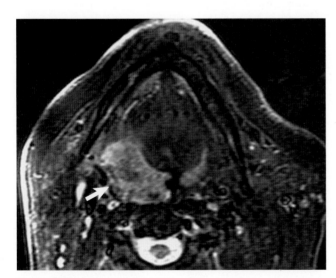

Figure S12-1. Note the bright right palatine tonsil cancer *(arrow)* on T2-weighted magnetic resonance image.

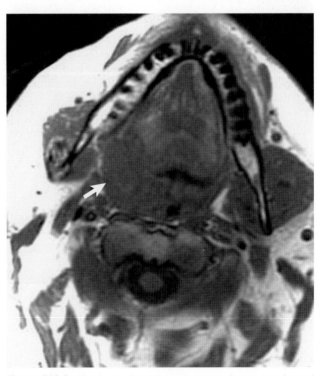

Figure S12-2. The lesion has intermediate signal intensity *(arrow)* on T1-weighted magnetic resonance image.

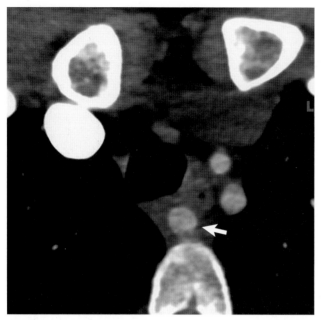

Figure S13-1. Note the enhancing vessel *(arrow)* coursing posterior to the esophagus.

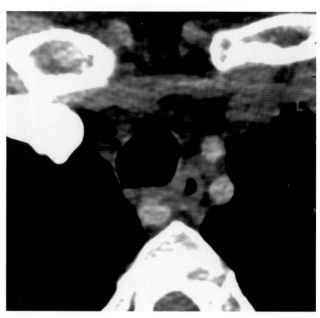

Figure S13-2. Note the enhancing vessel *(arrow)* coursing posterior to the esophagus.

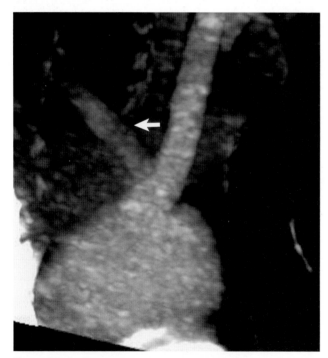

Figure S13-3. The maximum-intensity projection image of the vessel shows the left-to-right course *(arrow)*.

CASE 14

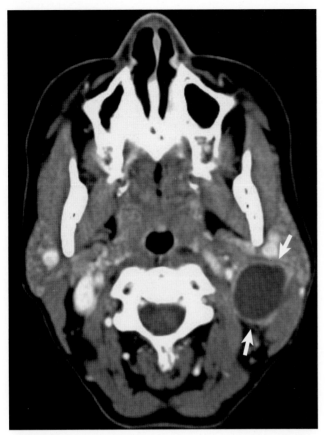

Figure S14-1. Note the large cystic structure in the lower left aspect of the neck *(arrows)*.

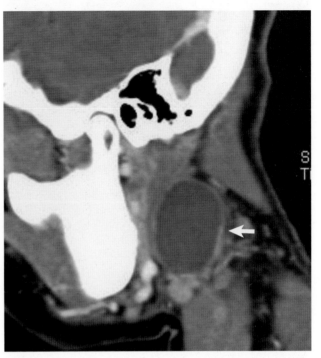

Figure S14-2. Sagittal reconstruction of the axial images shows the cyst *(arrow)* deep to the sternocleidomastoid muscle.

CASE 15

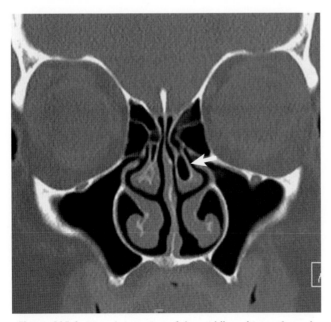

Figure S15-1. Note the aeration of the middle turbinate *(arrow)*.

CASE 16

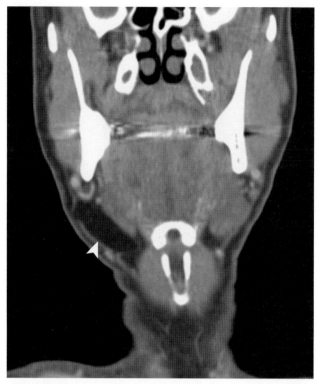

Figure S16-1. A coronal reconstruction of axial computed tomographic scans shows a low-density mass in the right side of the neck *(arrowhead)*.

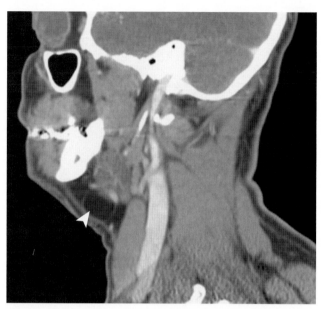

Figure S16-2. The mass *(arrowhead)* is well depicted superficial to the submandibular gland on the sagittal scan.

CASE 17

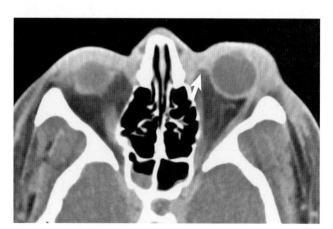

Figure S17-1. Note that the periorbital tissue anterior to the orbital septum *(arrow)* is thickened and inflamed.

CASE 18

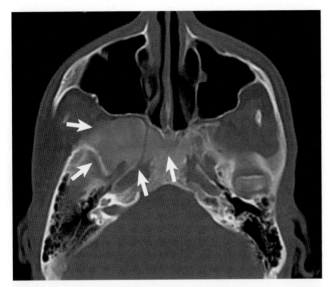

Figure S18-1. Note the ground-glass appearance *(arrows)* of the skull base around the Vidian canal.

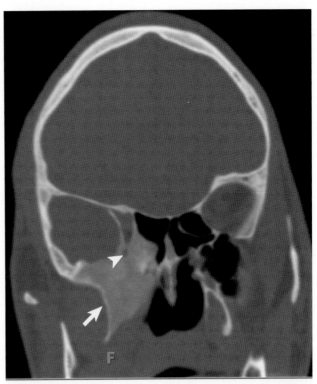

Figure S18-2. Coronal scan shows involvement of the pterygoid plates *(arrow)* and the foramen rotundum *(arrowhead)*.

CASE 19

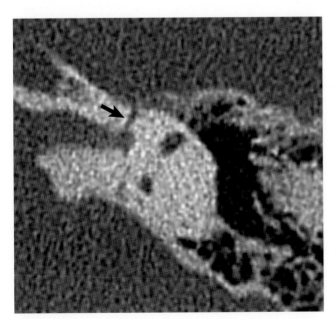

Figure S19-1. Note the lines of fracture *(arrow)* extending to inner ear structures on the axial scan.

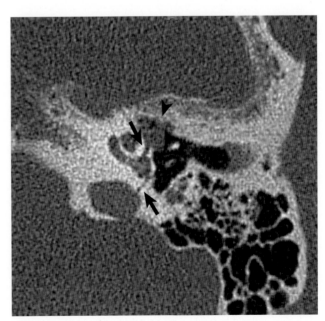

Figure S19-2. A lower section shows the involvement of the basal turn of the cochlea *(arrow)*. The *arrowhead* shows a soft tissue incidental epidermoid in the middle ear.

417

CASE 20

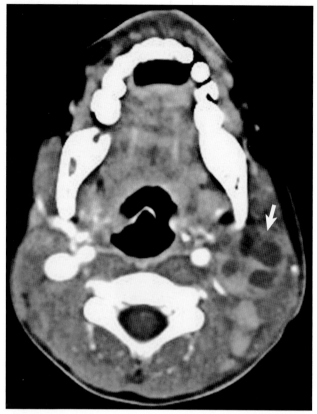

Figure S20-1. Note the necrotic multiloculated mass on the axial scan *(arrow)*. Many nonnecrotic nodes are visible posteriorly within the jugular chain on sagittal scans as well.

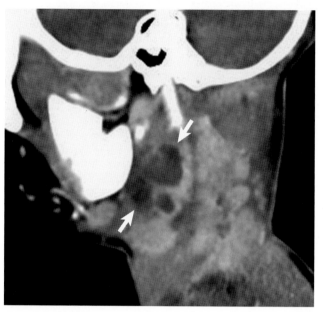

Figure S20-2. Sagittal reconstruction of the axial data shows the extensive cervical adenopathy *(arrows)*.

CASE 21

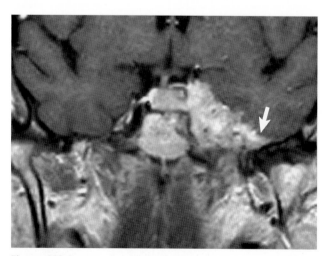

Figure S21-1. Note the dural tail along the lateral aspect of the skull base in this dura-based mass on enhanced magnetic resonance imaging (MRI).

CASE 22

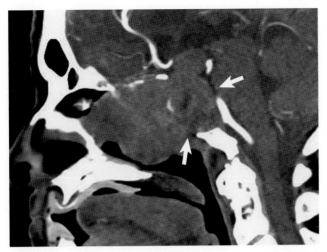

Figure S22-1. Note the aggressive nature of the mass *(arrows)*. The pituitary gland cannot be identified separately from the mass.

CASE 23

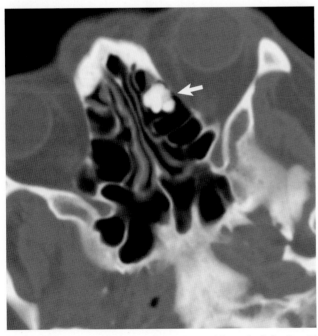

Figure S23-1. A calcified mass *(arrow)* is visible in the left ethmoid air cells.

CASE 24

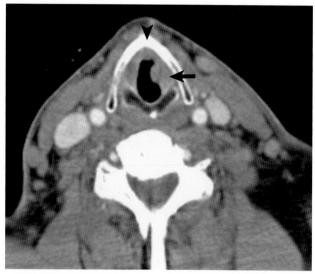

Figure S24-1. There is thickening of the true vocal cord *(arrow)*. Note that the thickness of the anterior commissure is abnormal as well *(arrowhead)*.

CASE 25

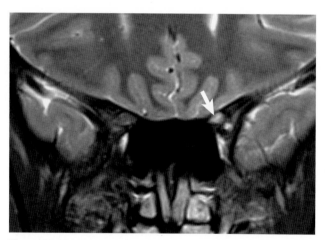

Figure S25-1. The coronal T2-weighted image shows brighter signal intensity in the swollen left optic nerve *(arrow)* than in the right optic nerve.

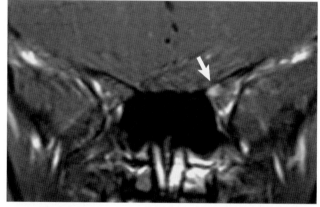

Figure S25-2. The contrast-enhanced fat-suppressed T1-weighted scan shows enhancement of the left optic nerve *(arrow)* at the orbital apex.

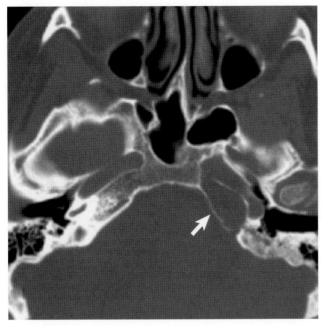

Figure S26-1. Note the opacification of the petrous apex *(arrow)* on the computed tomographic scan.

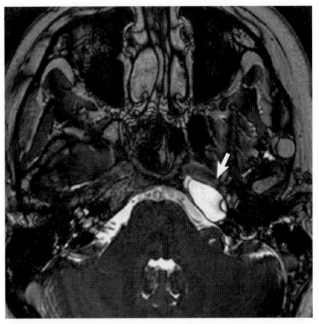

Figure S26-2. Note the bright signal of the left petrous apex collection *(arrow)* on constructive interference in steady state (CISS) imaging.

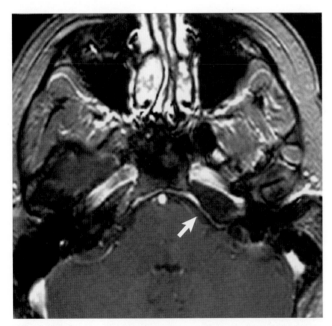

Figure S26-3. The abnormality is not enhanced *(arrow)* on post-contrast T1-weighted imaging.

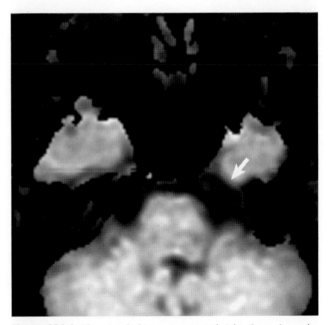

Figure S26-4. The signal does not appear bright *(arrow)* on the diffusion-weighted image; this indicates a fluid-containing lesion.

CASE 27

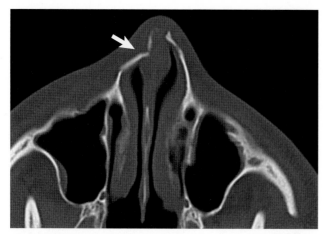

Figure S27-1. Deformity and angulation of the right nasal bone *(arrow)* are evident.

CASE 28

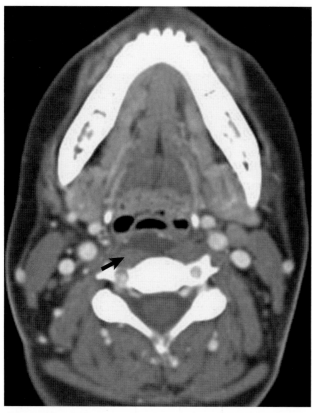

Figure S28-1. The axial image shows low density in the retropharyngeal space *(arrow)* anterior to the longus musculature but posterior to the pharyngeal musculature. No rim enhancement and no extension beyond the confines are seen. The condition resulted from radiation therapy.

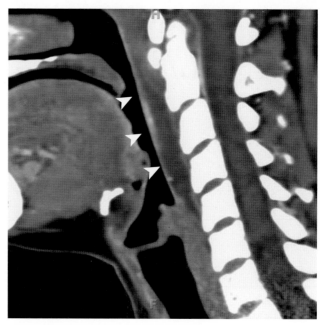

Figure S28-2. The sagittal reconstructed image shows low density in the retropharyngeal space from C1 to C5 *(arrowheads)*.

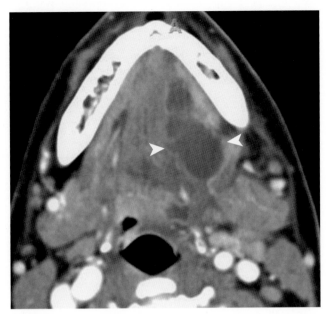

Figure S29-1. Note the low-density collection marked by the *arrowheads* in the sublingual space.

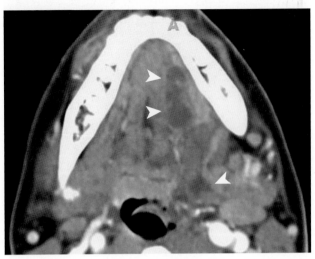

Figure S29-2. More inferiorly, an irregular low-density collection can be seen between the tongue muscles of the mylohyoid and the hyoglossus *(right-pointing arrowheads)* and genioglossus medial to that *(left-pointing arrowhead).*

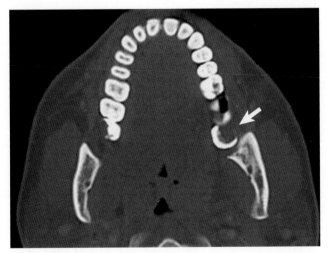

Figure S29-3. The bone window shows the low-density lytic nature in one left mandibular molar *(arrow).*

CASE 30

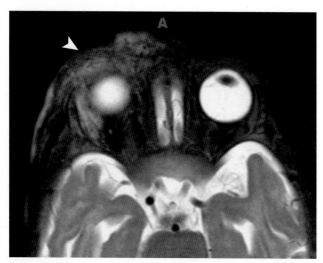

Figure S30-1. Note the irregular cutaneous and subcutaneous and orbital lesion *(arrowhead)* on the T2-weighted scan.

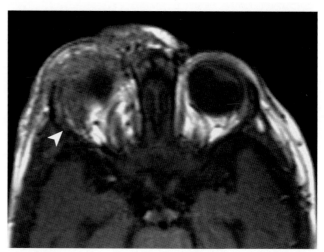

Figure S30-2. The infiltration of the extraconal fat *(arrowhead)* in the superior orbit is well seen on the T1-weighted scan.

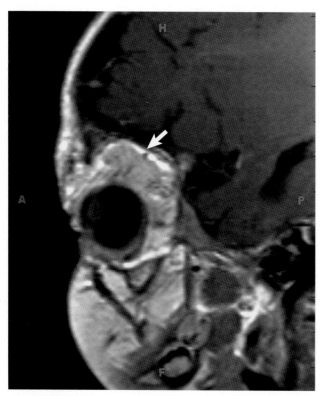

Figure S30-3. The deeper extension of the hemangioma and its intense enhancement *(arrow)* are better seen on the sagittal reconstruction.

CASE 31

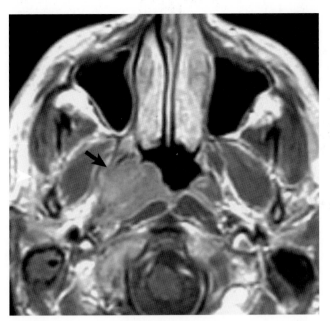

Figure S31-1. Axial scans through the nasopharynx show an infiltrative mass *(arrow)* in the right fossa of Rosenmüller. It spreads to the parapharyngeal space.

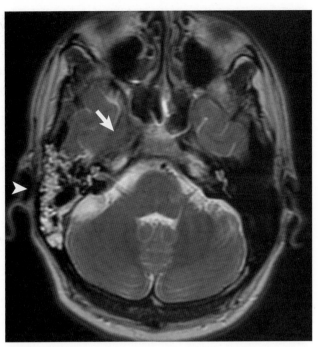

Figure S31-2. The lesion spread to the right cavernous sinus *(arrow)*, as shown on this T2-weighted image. Note also the fluid in the middle ear and mastoid *(arrowhead)*.

CASE 32

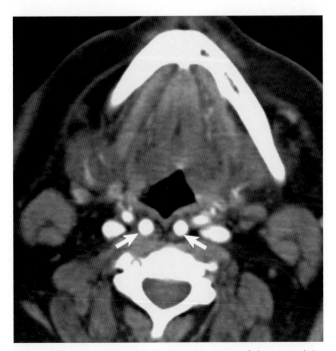

Figure S32-1. Note the retropharyngeal location of the internal (or common) carotid arteries as a normal variant *(arrows)*.

CASE 33

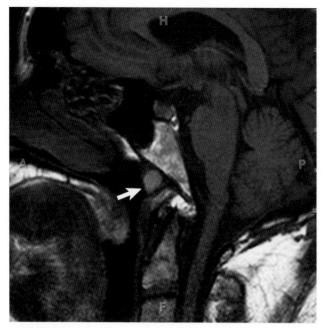

Figure S33-1. A midline nasopharyngeal lesion *(arrow)* is hyperintense on the T1-weighted image.

CASE 34

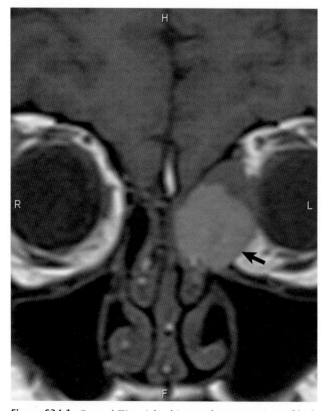

Figure S34-1. Coronal T1-weighted image shows secretions of high signal intensity within an expanded ethmoid air cell *(arrow)*. Expansion into the left orbit causes indentation of the extraocular muscles.

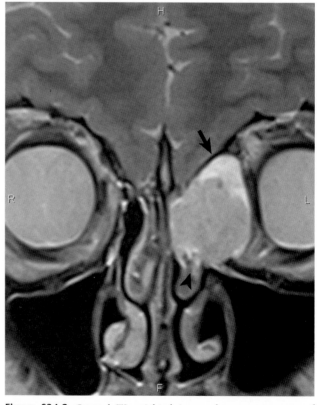

Figure S34-2. Coronal T2-weighted image shows components of both low signal intensity *(arrowhead)* and high signal intensity *(arrow)*.

CASE 35

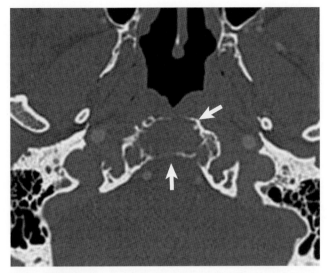

Figure S35-1. Note the lytic lesion *(arrow)* with cortical breakthrough in some areas of the clivus.

CASE 36

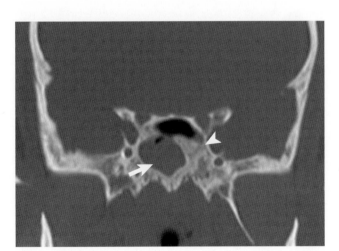

Figure S36-1. Note the opacification of the sphenoid sinus *(arrow)* and thickening of the bony walls of the sphenoid sinus *(arrowhead).*

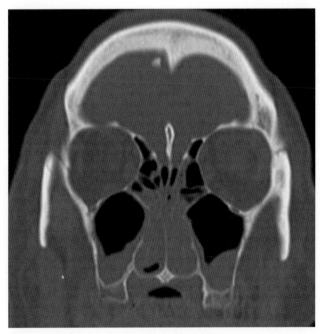

Figure S36-2. The maxillary sinus shows thick mucosa, and the nasal cavity also has congested mucosa.

CASE 37

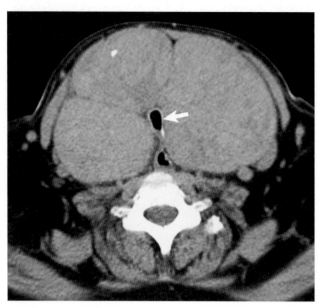

Figure S37-1. This bilateral mass shows compression of the airway in a transverse plane *(arrow)*.

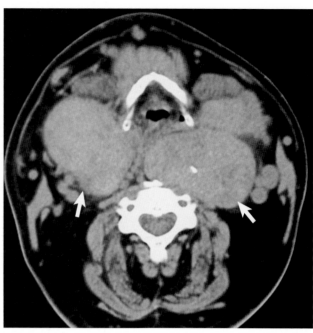

Figure S37-2. Note that the lesion ascends to at least the level of the hyoid bone bilaterally in the retropharyngeal space *(arrows)*.

CASE 38

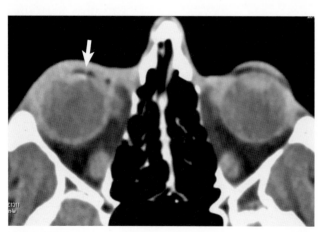

Figure S38-1. Note the tiny nonmetallic radiodensity *(arrow)* along the surface of the globe in the axial plane. This was a small piece of leaded glass.

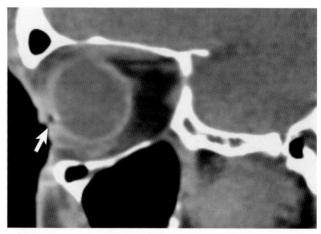

Figure S38-2. The sagittal reconstruction better shows the skin defect from the penetrating injury *(arrow)* and the tiny radiodensity on the cornea.

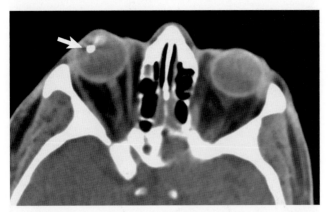

Figure S38-3. In a second case, metallic foreign body *(arrow)* from nail is visible in the axial plane. This metal fragment is in the vitreous and has gone through the corneal layer.

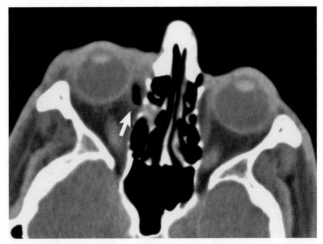

Figure S38-4. In a third case, an air density lesion is visible near the medial wall of the orbit. It was from light-weight wood penetration and, fortunately, went medial to the globe.

CASE 39

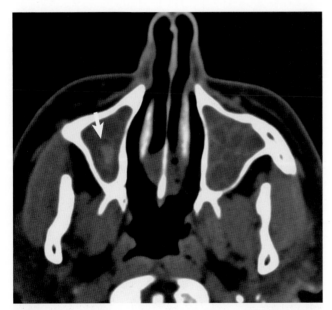

Figure S39-1. Axial computed tomographic image shows dense secretions, most apparent in the right maxillary antrum *(arrow)*.

CASE 40

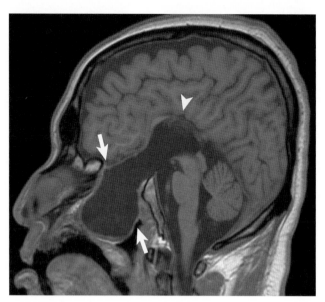

Figure S40-1. Note the protrusion of intracranial contents through the skull base *(arrows)* with an associated dysmorphic appearance of the corpus callosum *(arrowhead)*.

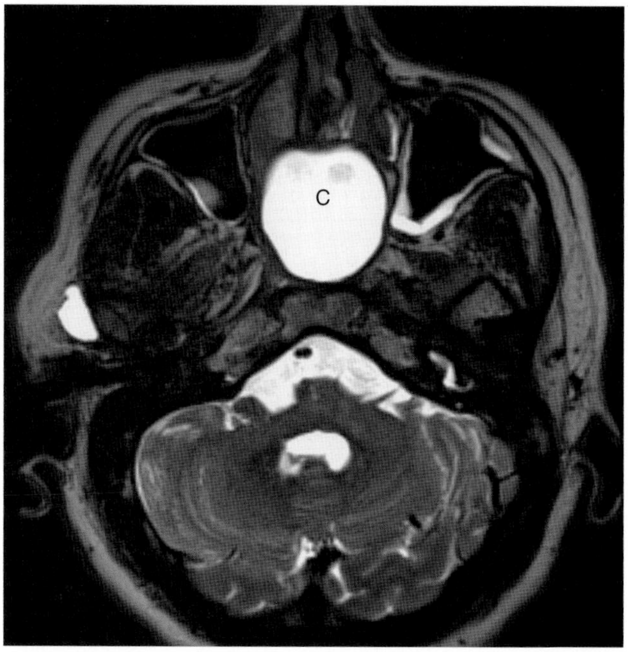

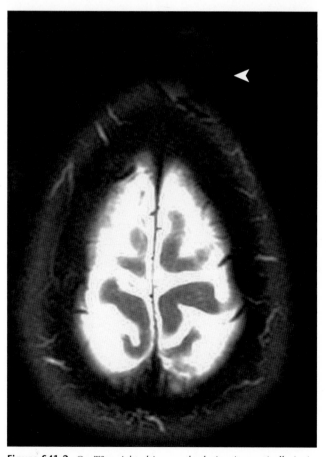

Figure S40-2. Axial T2-weighted image shows cerebrospinal fluid (C) intensity in the expected location of the sphenoid sinus. Ignore the incidental right parotid cyst.

CASE 41

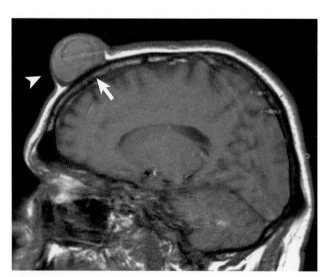

Figure S41-1. Sagittal T1-weighted image shows a scalp mass *(arrowhead)* without destruction or infiltration of the underlying bone *(arrow)*.

Figure S41-2. On T2-weighted image, the lesion is practically invisible because of low signal intensity *(arrowhead)*.

CASE 42

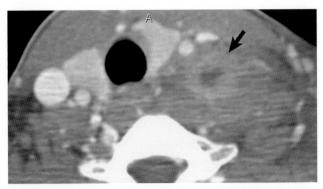

Figure S42-1. The enhanced computed tomographic scan shows a ring-enhancing, centrally necrotic mass in the left side of the neck *(arrow)*. Edema of the subcutaneous fat is present. The carotid sheath contents are displaced anteriorly. The inflammatory mass displaces the anterior scalene muscle posteriorly.

CASE 43

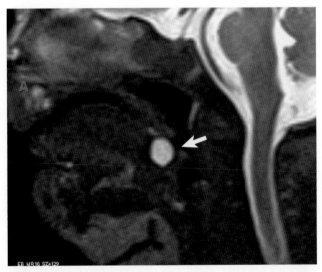

Figure S43-1. A small cyst *(arrow)* is seen in the upper part of the tongue at the junction of the oral and oropharyngeal portions of the tongue.

CASE 44

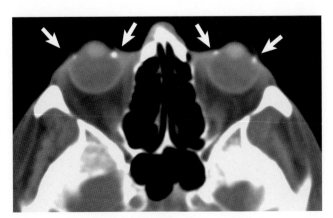

Figure S44-1. Bilateral medial and lateral punctuate calcifications of the globe *(arrows)* are visible.

CASE 45

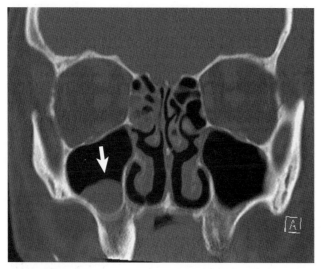

Figure S45-1. Note the smooth, unilocular lesion *(arrow)* in the inferior right maxillary antrum.

CASE 46

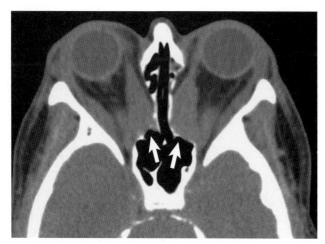

Figure S46-1. Note the enlargement of extraocular muscles *(arrows)*, sparing tendons. The infracturing of the medial orbital walls is evident.

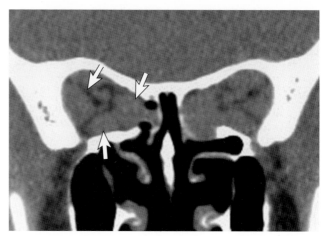

Figure S46-2. Coronal scan shows enlarged extraocular muscles *(arrows)*, but fat is still present around the optic nerves.

CASE 47

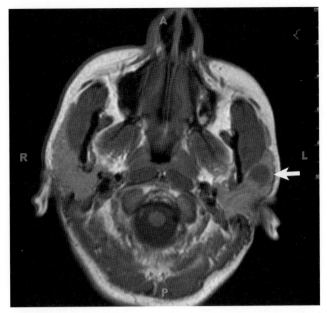

Figure S47-1. Low signal on T1-weighted images *(arrow)* is typical of these masses.

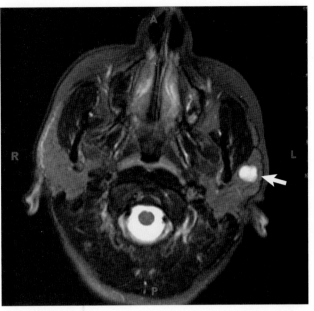

Figure S47-2. Note the mass *(arrow)* in the left parotid superficial lobe. It is very bright on the T2-weighted image.

CASE 48

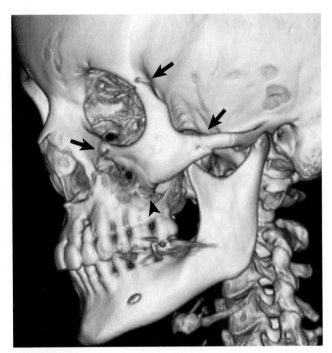

Figure S48-1. Note the locations of fractures *(arrows)* on this lateral three-dimensional view.

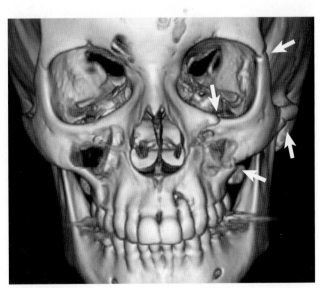

Figure S48-2. Note the locations of fractures *(arrows)* on this coronal three-dimensional view.

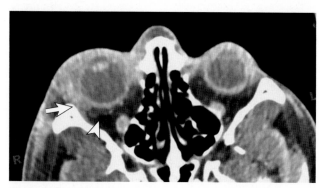

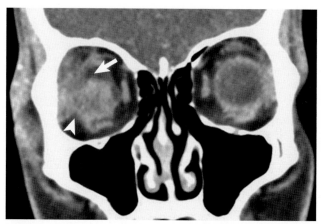

Figure S49-1. The axial scan shows edema in the retrobulbar fat *(arrowhead)* and thickening of the sclera *(arrow)*. Superficial thickening is also present. The orbital septum has been violated.

Figure S49-2. The coronal computed tomographic scan shows edema *(arrowhead)* and inflammation *(arrow)* in the extraconal fat.

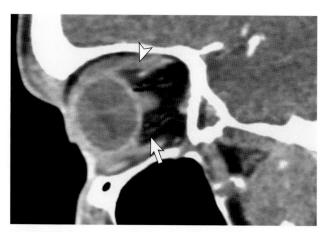

Figure S49-3. The sagittal scan shows the inflammation *(arrow, arrowhead)* extending to the superior rectus muscle.

CASE 50

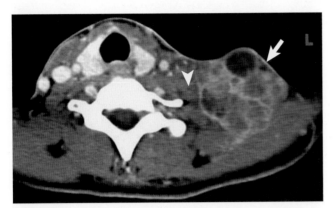

Figure S50-1. Axial computed tomographic scan shows the anterior scalene muscle *(arrowhead)* and a large nodal mass *(arrow)*.

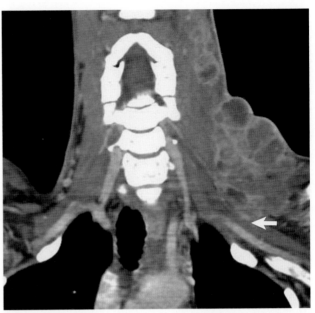

Figure S50-2. Coronal scan shows compression of the brachial plexus *(arrow)* by the necrotic nodal mass above it.

CASE 51

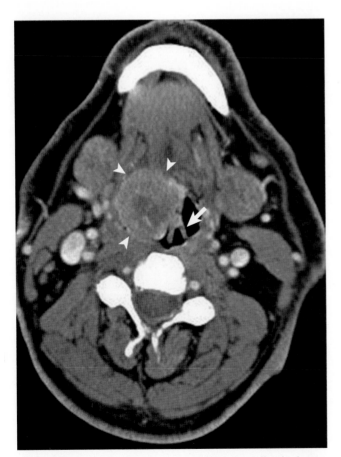

Figure S51-1. A well-defined mass is visible in the vallecula *(arrowheads)*. Epiglottis *(arrow)* is displaced to left.

CASE 52

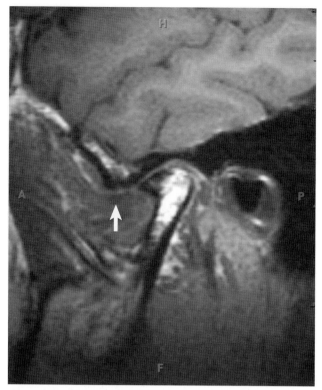

Figure S52-1. Note the anterior position of the meniscus *(arrow)* in the closed-mouth position.

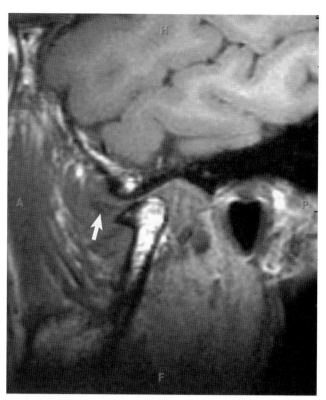

Figure S52-2. The meniscus remains anteriorly positioned in the open-mouth view. The mandibular condyle translates well, which indicates that motion is not limited.

CASE 53

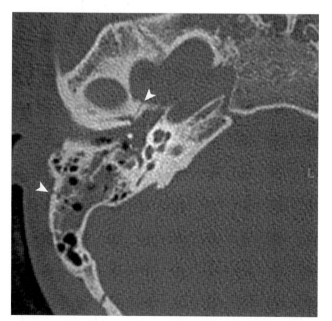

Figure S53-1. Axial computed tomography shows the opacified mastoid and middle ear cavity, as well as the fracture line across the mastoid to the anterior epitympanic margin *(arrowheads).*

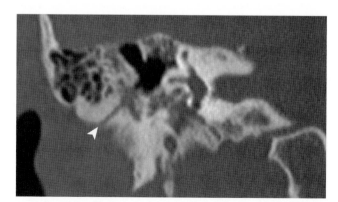

Figure S53-2. Coronal computed tomography shows the fracture *(arrowhead)* of the lateral mastoid portion of the temporal bone as well.

CASE 54

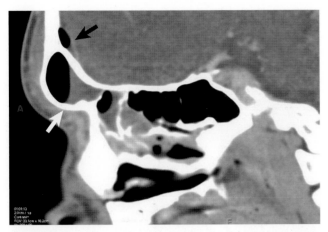

Figure S54-1. Note the air-fluid level in the frontal sinus *(white arrow)* and the epidural compartment *(black arrow)* in a patient with fever and meningismus.

CASE 55

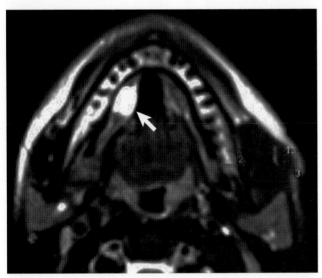

Figure S55-1. T2-weighted image shows a cystic lesion *(arrow)* in the floor of the mouth.

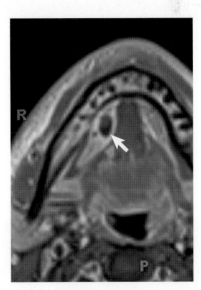

Figure S55-2. The lesion *(arrow)* does not enhance.

CASE 56

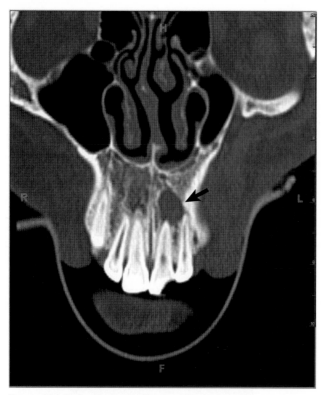

Figure S56-1. A cyst *(arrow)* is present in association with the root of the maxillary incisor.

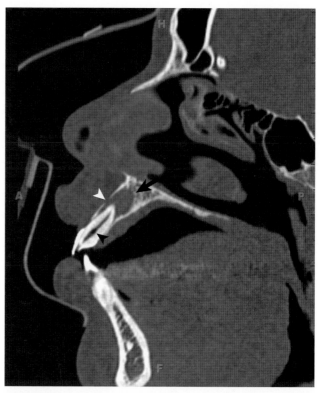

Figure S56-2. On the sagittal reconstruction, a dehiscent area at the anterior margin of the maxilla *(white arrowhead)* is associated with the cyst *(arrow)*. In addition the central root canal of the tooth is very low in density *(black arrowhead)*, which indicates that the tooth is no longer vital.

CASE 57

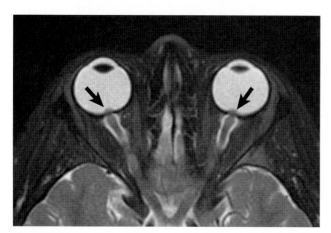

Figure S57-1. Note the enlarged optic nerve sheath complexes and the protrusion of the papilla into the posterior globes *(arrows)* on the T2-weighted image.

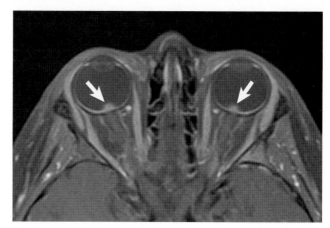

Figure S57-2. The papilla enhances *(arrows)*, which is an uncommon associated finding that may suggest papillitis and inflammation.

CASE 58

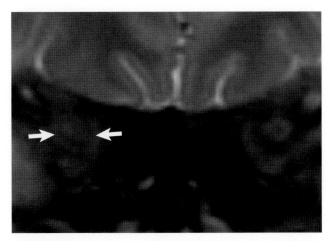

Figure S58-1. Note the expanded nerve sheath complex on the right on the T2-weighted image *(arrows)*, with obscuring of the outline of the nerve and sheath.

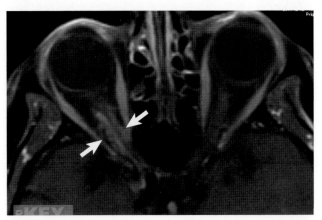

Figure S58-2. On contrast-enhanced imaging, the sheath appears prominent, although enhancement is irregular *(arrows)*, which is the tram track sign.

CASE 59

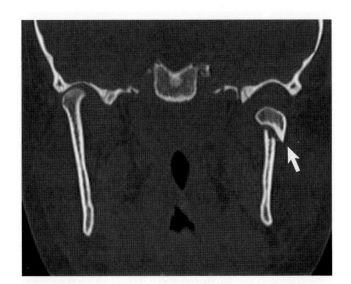

Figure S59-1. Note the abnormality *(arrow)* involving the left mandibular condyle and neck.

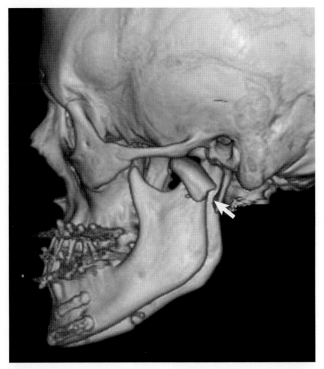

Figure S59-2. Three-dimensional reconstruction displays the angulation of the fracture fragments *(arrow)* and the fact that the patient's mouth had been previously wired for facial fractures before this latest injury.

CASE 60

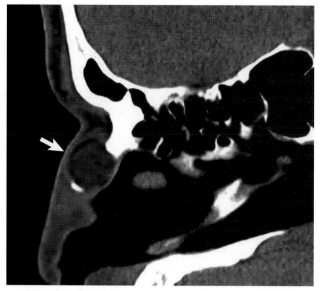

Figure S60-1. Note the low-density nasal mass *(arrow)* passing into the nasal bone.

CASE 61

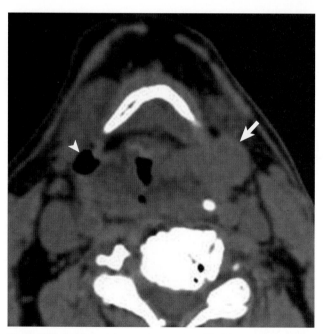

Figure S61-1. The axial scan shows an air-filled lesion *(arrowhead)* and a fluid-filled lesion *(arrow)*.

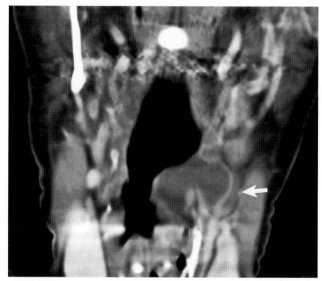

Figure S61-2. The coronal scan better demonstrates the paraglottic nature of the left-sided fluid-filled lesion *(arrow)* and the perforation across the thyrohyoid membrane.

CASE 62

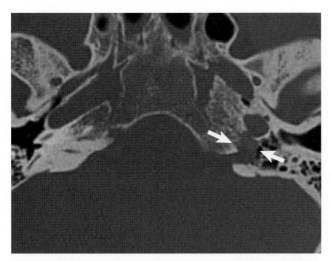

Figure S62-1. High-resolution axial computed tomography with bone algorithm reconstruction shows an erosive mass *(arrows)* posteromedial to the carotid artery on the left side and with a bone-permeative pattern.

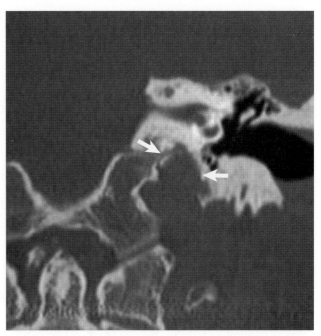

Figure S62-2. The location of the mass *(arrows)* along the superior jugular foramen is better assessed on the coronal reformatted section on the left side. The edges of the lesion are irregular.

CASE 63

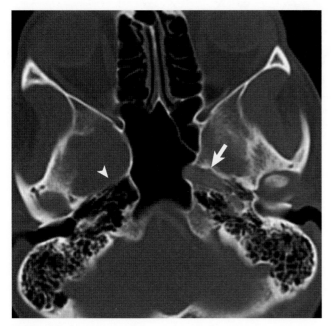

Figure S63-1. Note the absence of a petrous carotid canal on the right *(arrowhead),* in comparison with the left side *(arrow).*

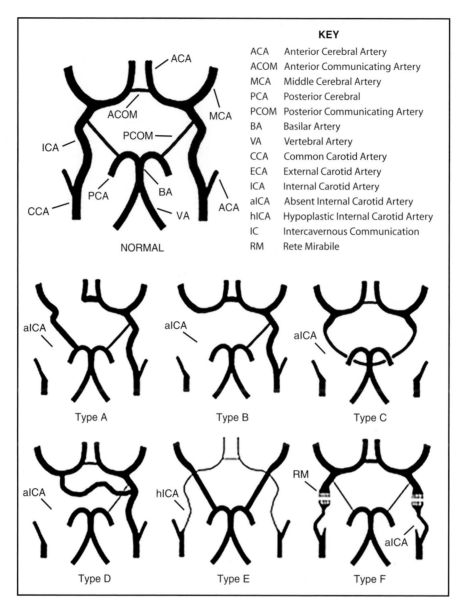

Figure S63-2. Pathways of collateral circulation in association with absence of one or both internal carotid arteries (see text for descriptions). *(From Given CA 2nd, Huang-Hellinger F, Baker MD, Chepuri NB, Morris PP. Congenital absence of the internal carotid artery: case reports and review of the collateral circulation. AJNR Am J Neuroradiol. 2001;22[10]:1953-1959.)*

CASE 64

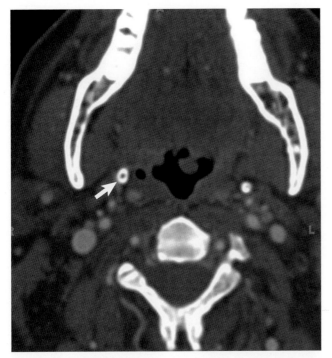

Figure S64-1. Axial computed tomography shows prominence of both stylohyoid ligaments, which are calcified *(arrow)*.

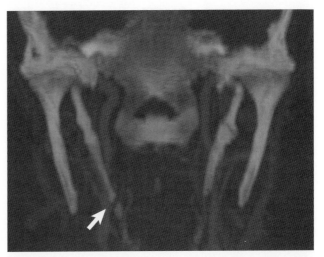

Figure S64-2. The right-sided ligament *(arrow)* runs more medial and inferior; it also appears this way on this three-dimensional reconstruction.

CASE 65

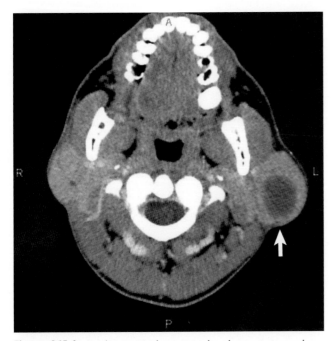

Figure S65-1. Axial computed tomography demonstrates a large midparotid cyst on the left side *(arrow)*.

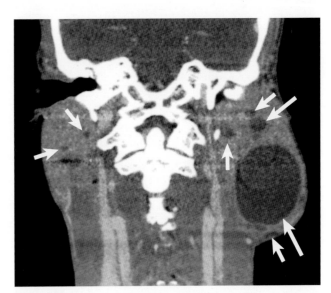

Figure S65-2. Coronal scan shows that there actually are numerous cysts *(arrows)* bilaterally in the parotid glands.

CASE 66

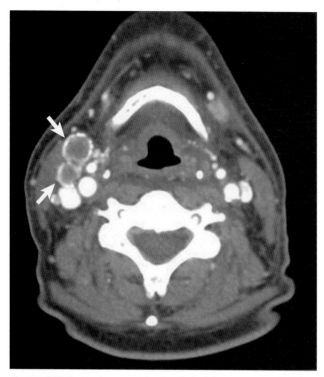

Figure S66-1. Axial scans reveal calcified lymph nodes *(arrows)* intimately associated with the jugular vein.

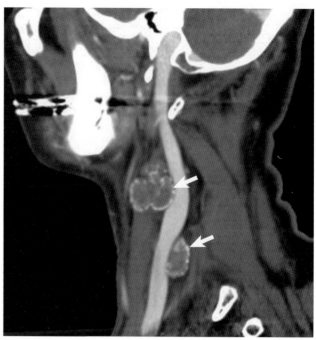

Figure S66-2. Sagittal reconstructions are often helpful in characterizing the location of nodes *(arrows)* with regard to the hyoid bone and cricoid cartilage.

CASE 67

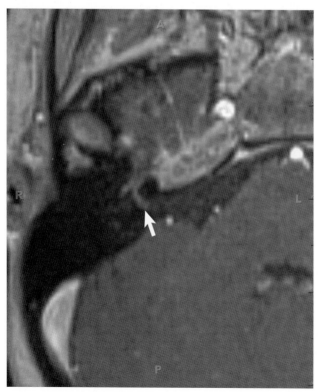

Figure S67-1. Note the enhancement of the labyrinthine portion *(arrow)* of the facial nerve.

CASE 68

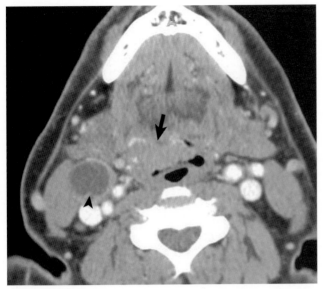

Figure S68-1. In addition to the cystic and solid left jugular lymph node *(arrowhead)*, there is a mass in the base of the tongue *(arrow)*.

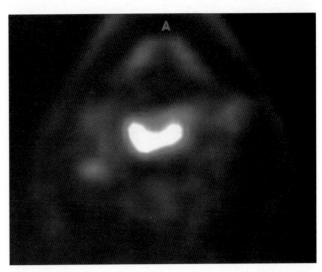

Figure S68-2. Note the high avidity on the positron emission tomographic (PET) scan.

CASE 69

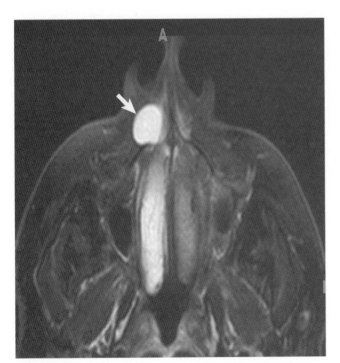

Figure S69-1. T2-weighted image shows a cyst *(arrow)* anterior to the right maxillary spine, displacing the right naris/nasal aperture anteriorly.

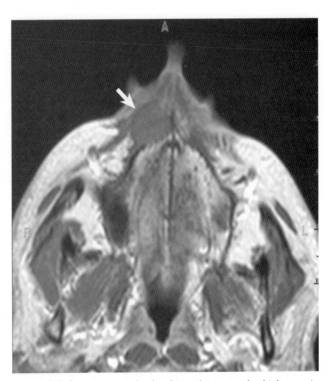

Figure S69-2. On T1-weighted enhanced images, the high protein content in the cyst *(arrow)* leads to intermediate signal intensity but does not enhance.

CASE 70

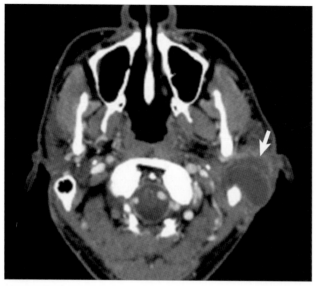

Figure S70-1. Note the large, irregularly shaped cyst *(arrow)* in the left parotid gland. This curvilinear shape is typical of the diagnosis.

CASE 71

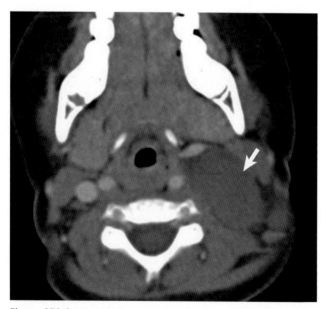

Figure S71-1. Note the large cystic structure in the lower left aspect of the neck *(arrow)*.

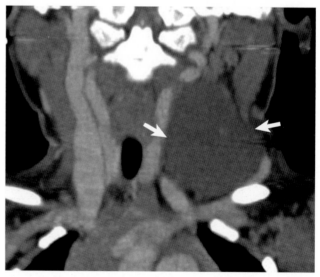

Figure S71-2. Coronal reconstruction provides a better view of the size and location of the node *(arrows)*.

CASE 72

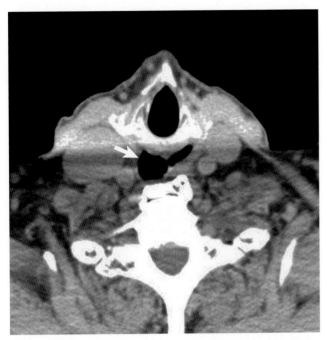

Figure S72-1. A right-sided eccentric air collection *(arrow)* is associated with the esophagus on this axial unenhanced computed tomographic scan.

CASE 73

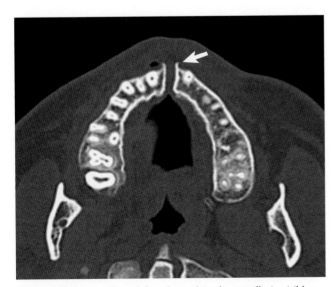

Figure S73-1. A midline defect *(arrow)* in the maxilla is visible on the axial CT scan.

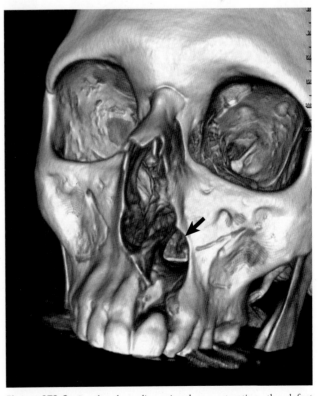

Figure S73-2. On the three-dimensional reconstruction, the defect *(arrow)* in the hard palate is better depicted; the deformity was more extensive than expected.

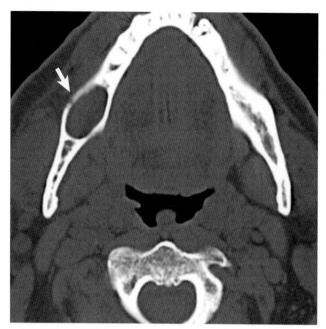

Figure S74-1. Axial scan with bone algorithm reconstruction shows an ovoid lesion in the right mandible with benign expansion of the medullary cavity *(arrow).*

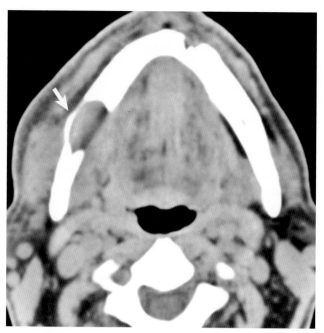

Figure S74-2. The soft tissue window shows preservation of the buccal bony margin *(arrow),* but the lingual side is dehiscent. The lesion has low density.

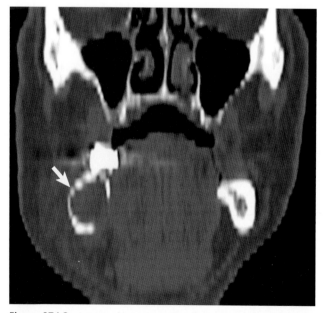

Figure S74-3. A coronal reconstruction shows no relationship of the lesion *(arrow)* with a tooth root and confirms the absence of bone along the medial lingual surface.

CASE 75

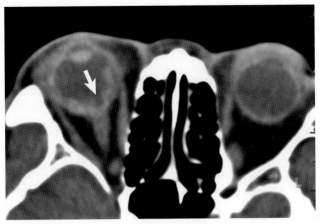

Figure S75-1. The axial computed tomographic image demonstrates collections of hyperdense material in the right globe, which converges on the optic nerve insertion to the globe *(arrow)*.

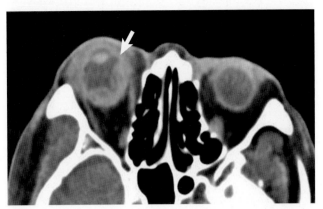

Figure S75-2. The medial collection terminates shy of the ciliary apparatus, at a point referred to as the *ora serrata (arrow)*.

CASE 76

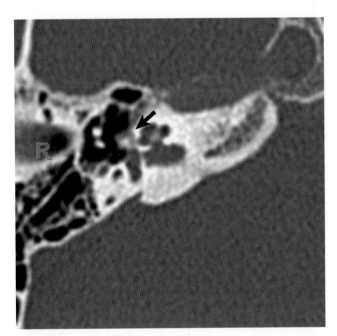

Figure S76-1. Note the new bone growth *(arrow)* just anterior to the oval window.

CASE 77

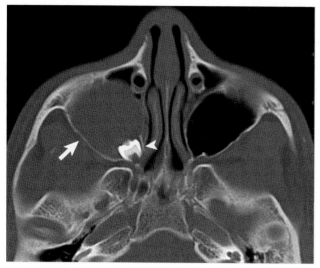

Figure S77-1. Note the unerupted tooth *(arrowhead)* associated with the cyst *(arrow)* in the maxillary antrum.

CASE 78

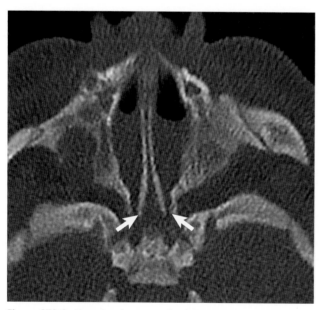

Figure S78-1. Note the obstruction by soft tissue of the nasal cavities bilaterally *(arrows)*.

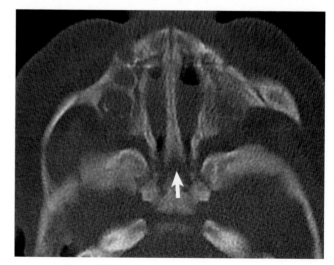

Figure S78-2. The vomer is widened *(arrow)*.

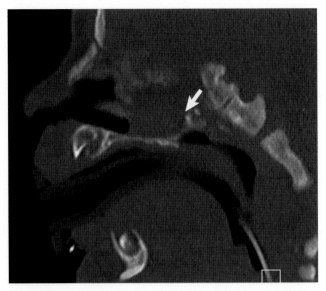

Figure S78-3. Sagittal scan best depicts the obstructing secretions or membranous soft tissue mass *(arrow)*.

CASE 79

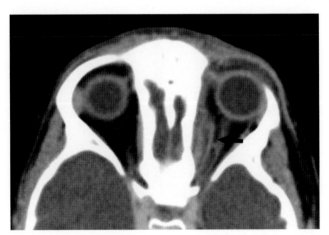

Figure S79-1. Axial scans show a low-density collection *(arrow)* along the medial aspect of the left eye.

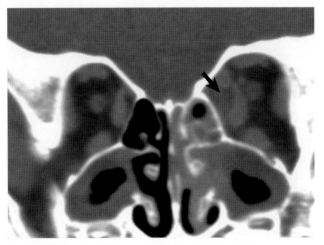

Figure S79-2. The collection *(arrow)* is also seen in the superomedial compartment on the coronal study.

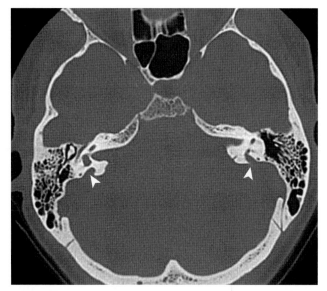

Figure S80-1. Computed tomography demonstrates the enlargement of the bony structure *(arrowheads).*

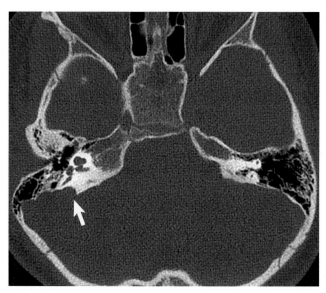

Figure S80-2. Another scan shows the appearance of incomplete turns of the cochlea on the right side, with a large right vestibular aqueduct *(arrow).*

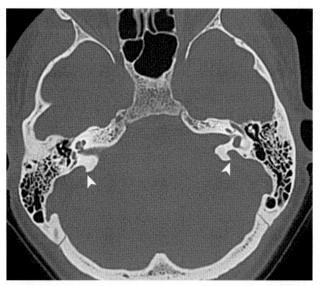

Figure S80-3. A third view demonstrates bilateral enlargement of the vestibular aqueducts *(arrowheads).*

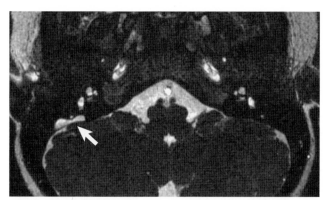

Figure S80-4. On T2-weighted magnetic resonance imaging, the intensity of the cerebrospinal fluid *(arrow)* running parallel to the temporal bone represents the enlarged endolymphatic sac.

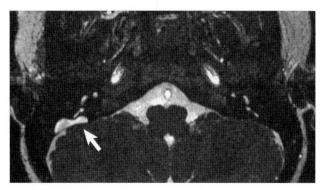

Figure S80-5. The endolymphatic sac *(arrow)* is too large. Normally it is nearly invisible.

CASE 81

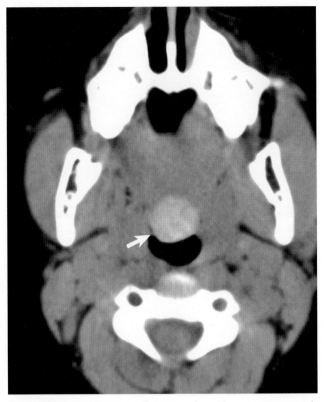

Figure S81-1. Axial computed tomography without contrast reveals a markedly hyperdense mass *(arrow)* in the midline of the base of the tongue.

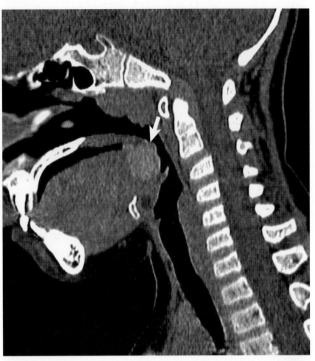

Figure S81-2. Sagittal reconstruction of the axial scans shows the expected location of the hyperdense mass at the foramen cecum of the tongue, representing the junction of the base of the tongue and the oral portion of the tongue.

CASE 82

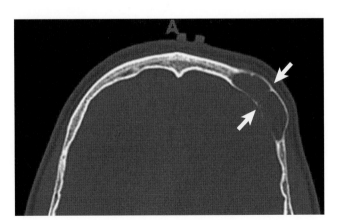

Figure S82-1. Bone window shows thinned inner and outer margins of the left frontal bone lesion *(arrow).*

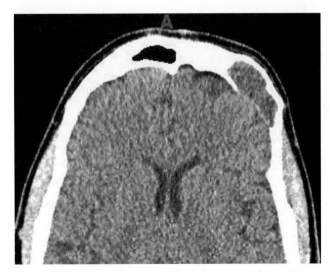

Figure S82-2. The soft tissue windowing shows a lower density lesion.

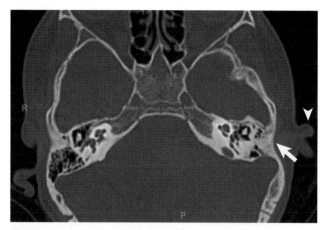

Figure S83-1. The external auditory canal is blocked by bone *(arrow),* and the external ear is small *(arrowhead).*

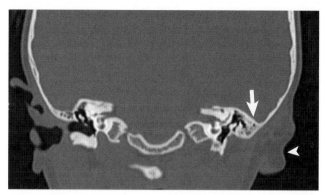

Figure S83-2. Coronal computed tomography shows the malformed pinna of the ear *(arrowhead)* and absence of the external auditory canal *(arrow).*

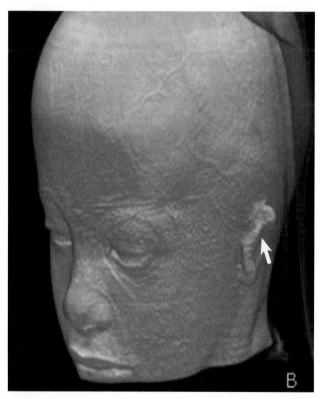

Figure S83-3. Surface reconstruction of the scans shows the congenital deformity of the left ear *(arrow).*

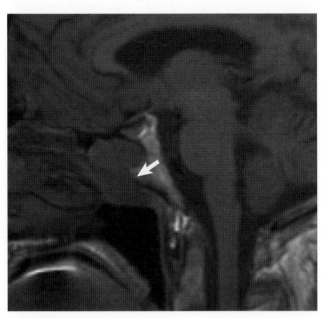

Figure S84-1. The origin of this lesion is actually along the left lateral edge of the nasopharynx *(arrow)* with growth into the nasal cavity and sphenoid sinus.

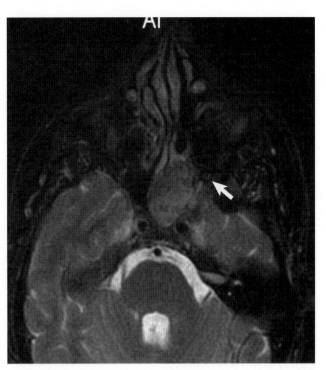

Figure S84-2. The mass does not appear bright *(arrow)* on a T2-weighted image, and thus it is less likely to be an inflammatory lesion.

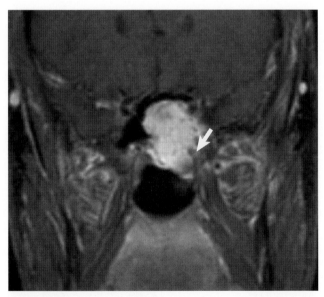

Figure S84-3. On coronal scan, the enhancement is marked, and the attachment to the lateral wall of the left side of the nasopharynx is better seen *(arrow)*.

CASE 85

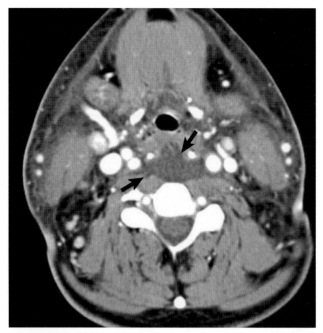

Figure S85-1. Note the low-density collection *(arrows)* seen anterior to the longus colli muscles.

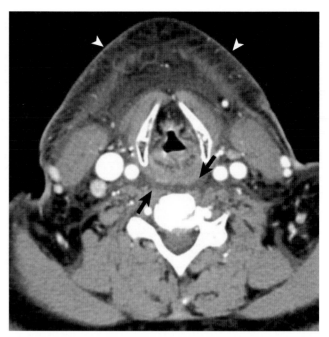

Figure S85-2. The inflammatory nature of the collection *(arrows)* is supported by the evidence of subcutaneous fat stranding *(arrowheads)*.

CASE 86

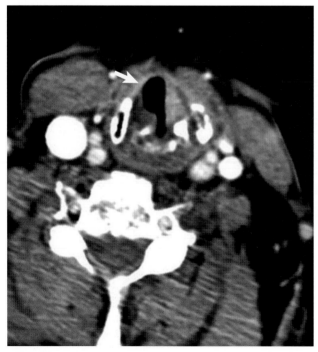

Figure S86-1. Note the medialization and atrophy of the true vocal cord on the right side *(arrow)*.

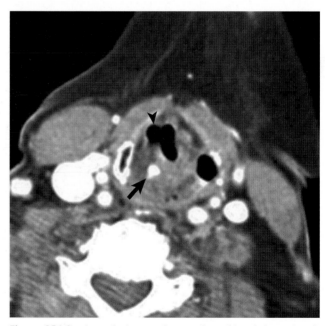

Figure S86-2. The right laryngeal ventricle is dilated *(arrowhead)*, and the arytenoid cartilage is in a medial position *(arrow)*.

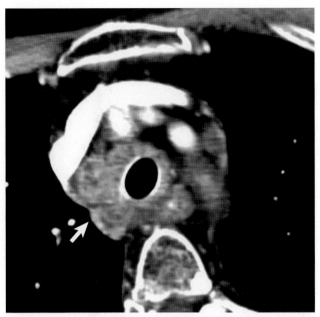

Figure S86-3. A mass along the tracheoesophageal groove in the upper chest is visible *(arrow)*.

CASE 87

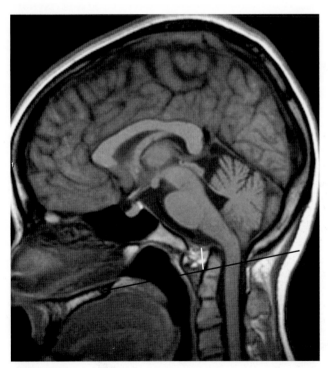

Figure S87-1. In this case, the odontoid process projects 9 mm above the Chamberlain line.

CASE 88

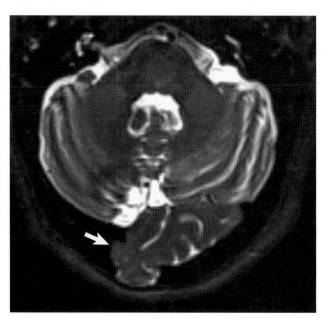

Figure S88-1. Note the herniated tissue *(arrow)* outside the skull on the axial scan.

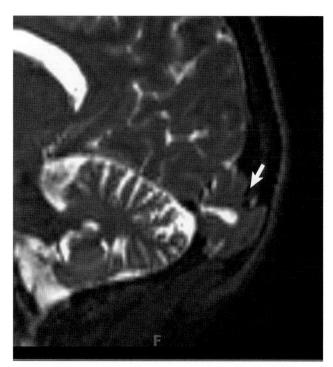

Figure S88-2. The relationship to the native occipital lobe and the herniated tissue *(arrow)* can be seen on the sagittal T2-weighted scan. The herniated tissue is not cerebellar tissue.

CASE 89

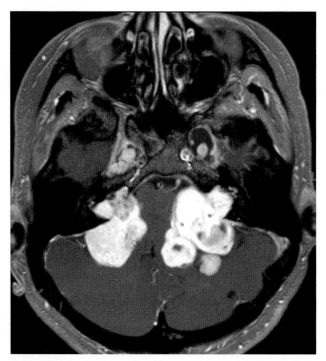

Figure S89-1. Note the bilateral cerebellopontine angle and intra-canalicular masses.

CASE 90

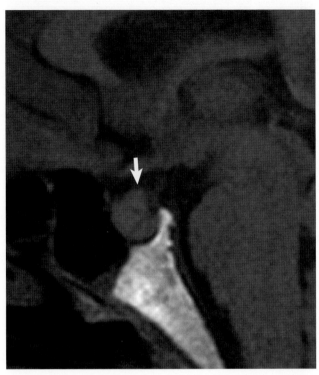

Figure S90-1. The sagittal T1-weighted image shows a mass *(arrow)* just above the normal pituitary gland.

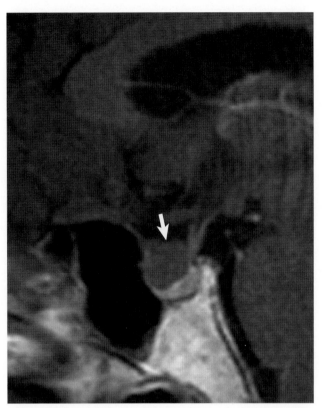

Figure S90-2. On the sagittal image obtained after gadolinium administration, note the absence of cyst enhancement *(arrow)* above the enhanced pituitary gland.

CASE 91

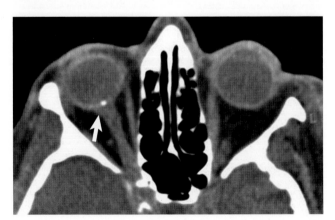

Figure S91-1. Note the calcification *(arrow)* at the optic nerve head insertion to the globe.

CASE 92

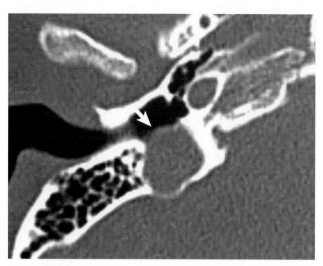

Figure S92-1. Note the lack of bone overlying the superior and anterior wall of the jugular bulb *(arrow)* in the right temporal bone.

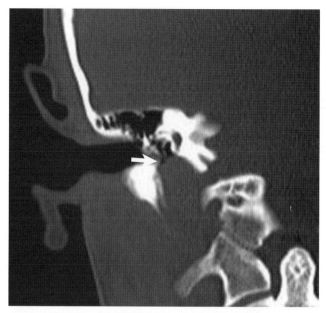

Figure S92-2. The lack of overlying bone *(arrow)* is also well seen on the coronal scan.

CASE 93

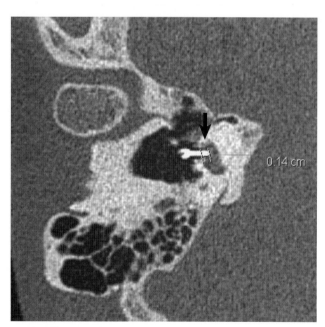

Figure S93-1. The stapes prosthesis *(arrow)* is 1.4 mm deep into the vestibule, as shown on this axial scan.

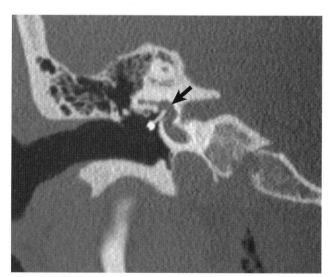

Figure S93-2. Note the depth of penetration of the implant *(arrow)* into the oval window of the vestibule.

CASE 94

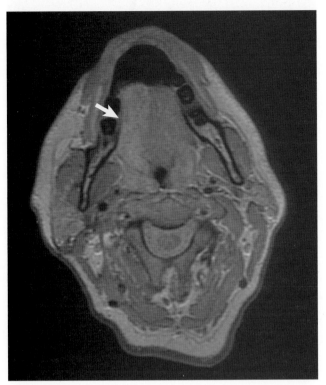

Figure S94-1. The right side of the tongue *(arrow)* has high signal.

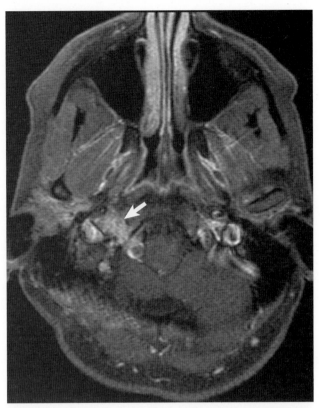

Figure S94-2. There is a mass *(arrow)* in the right hypoglossal canal.

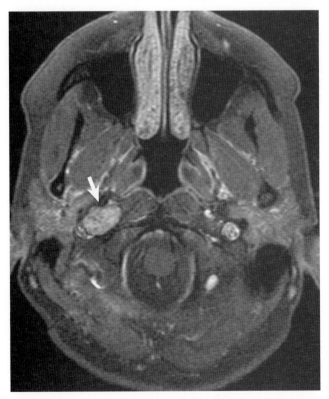

Figure S94-3. The mass *(arrow)* extends inferiorly into the upper carotid space.

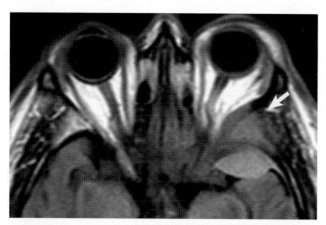

Figure S95-1. T1-weighted image shows a mass *(arrow)* infiltrating the greater wing of the left sphenoid bone. This causes the proptosis.

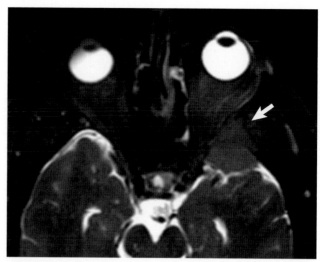

Figure S95-2. Note the low signal intensity *(arrow)* on the T2-weighted image.

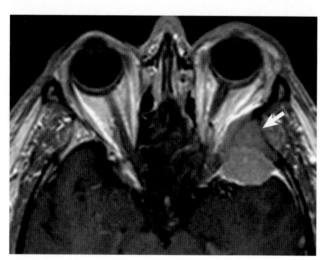

Figure S95-3. Enhancement of the lesion *(arrow)* and both an intra-orbital component and an intracranial component are visible.

CASE 96

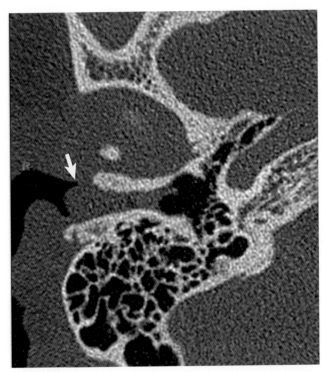

Figure S96-1. Note the soft tissue mass with a convex bulge laterally *(arrow)* that projects in the right external auditory canal on the axial scan.

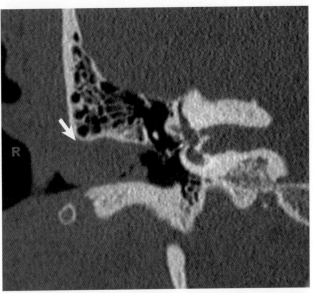

Figure S96-2. The lesion's attachment to the superior wall of the external auditory canal *(arrow)* is well depicted on the coronal scan.

CASE 97

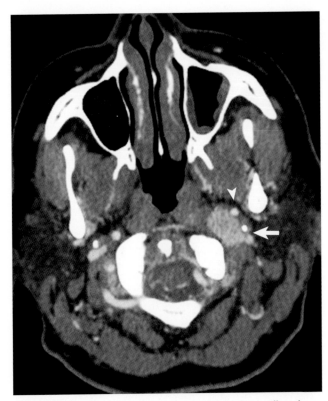

Figure S97-1. Axial computed tomography shows an avidly enhancing mass *(arrow)* in the carotid space in the upper portion of the neck. The internal carotid artery is marked by the *arrowhead.*

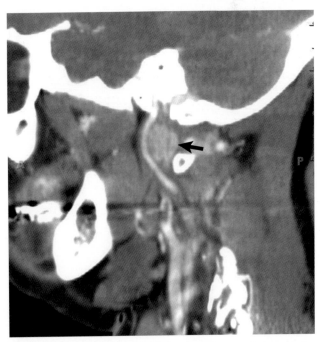

Figure S97-2. Reconstruction of the sagittal scan shows anterior displacement of the carotid artery by the mass *(arrow).*

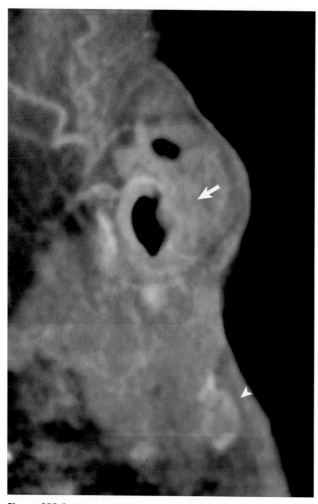

Figure S98-1. Note the thickening of the external ear that causes the pinna to encroach on the external auditory canal cartilage *(arrow)* and the node *(arrowhead)*.

CASE 99

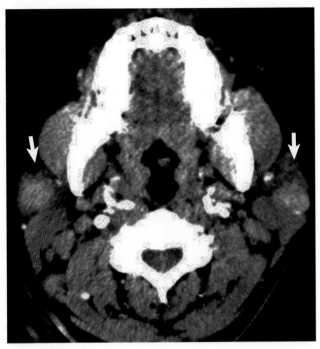

Figure S99-1. Note the bilateral soft tissue masses *(arrows)* in the parotid glands.

CASE 100

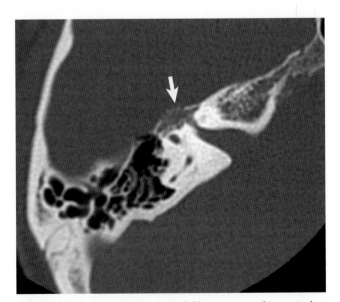

Figure S100-1. Note the honeycomb-like matrix in this geniculate ganglion region mass *(arrow)*.

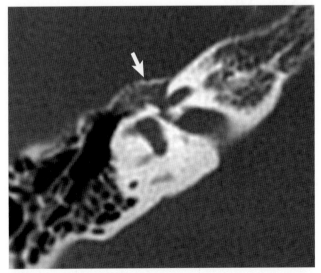

Figure S100-2. The position along the anterior aspect of the petrous temporal bone *(arrow)*, where the geniculate ganglion is located, is stereotypical of this lesion.

CASE 101

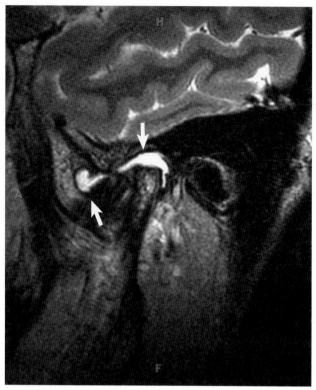

Figure S101-1. Note the large amount of fluid *(arrows)* visible on this T2-weighted image.

CASE 102

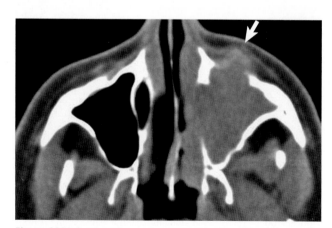

Figure S102-1. The CT scan shows opacification of the left maxillary antrum and breakthrough of the maxillary sinus anterior wall *(arrow)*.

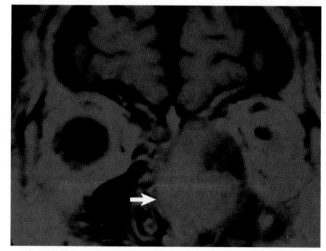

Figure S102-2. Note the bright signal *(arrow)* in the mass on this T1-weighted image without contrast.

CASE 103

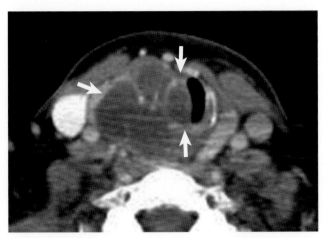

Figure S103-1. Note involvement of the cricoid cartilage *(arrows)* by a mass that appears to arise from an extramucosal location.

CASE 104

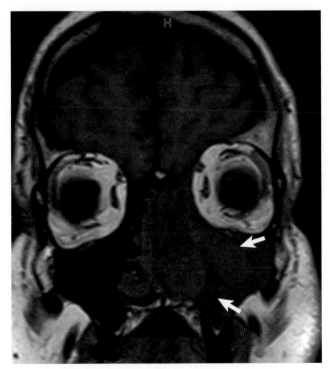

Figure S104-1. Opacification of the maxillary sinus *(arrows)* and ethmoid sinus is visible on T1-weighted image. Tissue discrimination is poor.

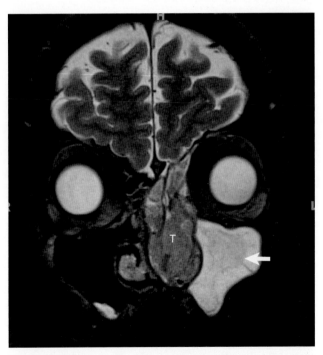

Figure S104-2. On T2-weighted image, the obstructed secretions in the antrum *(arrow)* can be distinguished from the nasal cavity tumor (T).

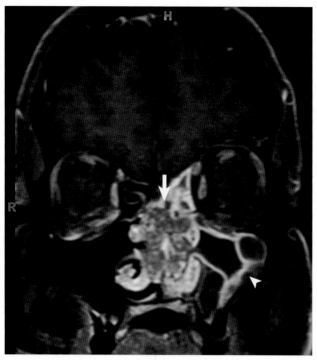

Figure S104-3. Note the difference in enhancement between the mass *(arrow)* and the sinus secretions *(arrowhead)*.

CASE 105

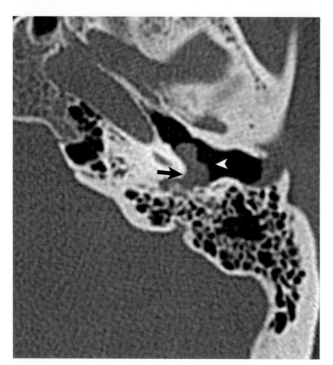

Figure S105-1. A mass *(arrowhead)* is seen lateral to the cochlear promontory *(arrow)*.

CASE 106

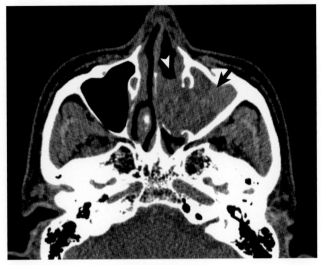

Figure S106-1. Note that this mass extends from the left maxillary sinus *(arrow)* to the nasal cavity *(arrowhead)*.

CASE 107

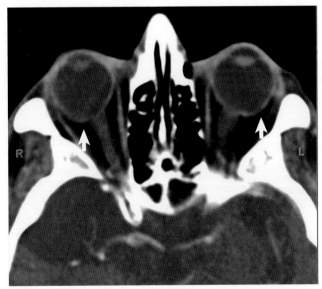

Figure S107-1. Note the scleral thinning *(arrows)* of the globes.

CASE 108

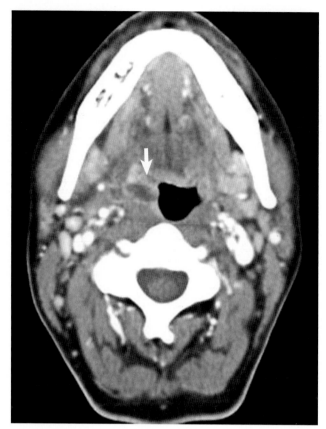

Figure S108-1. Note the ring-enhancing lesion *(arrow)* in the right peritonsillar zone.

CASE 109

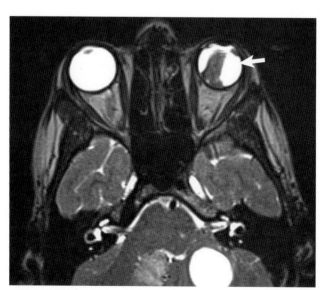

Figure S109-1. Note the lesion in the globe on the T2-weighted scan *(arrow)*. Findings in the posterior fossa may help establish the final diagnosis.

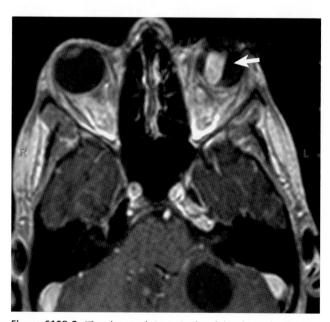

Figure S109-2. The abnormal tissue in the globe *(arrow)* enhances.

CASE 110

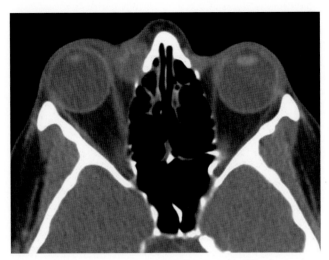

Figure S110-1. The axial scan shows enlargement of the lacrimal sac on the right, in comparison with the left.

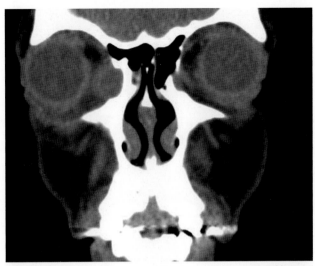

Figure S110-2. The coronal scan is useful in the right-left comparison showing the right lacrimal sac abnormality.

CASE 111

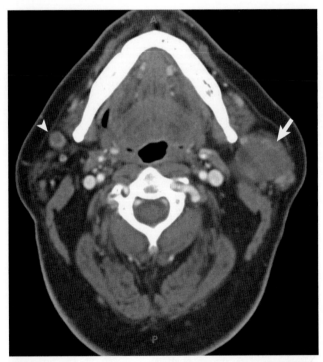

Figure S111-1. A septated cyst is seen in the left parotid gland *(arrow)*. A second smaller lesion is seen on the right parotid gland *(arrowhead)*.

CASE 112

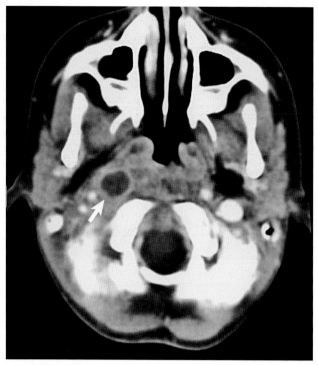

Figure S112-1. Note the low-density, peripherally enhancing lesion *(arrow)* in the retropharyngeal space.

CASE 113

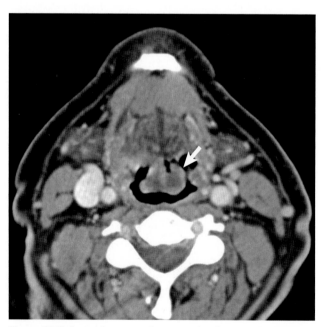

Figure S113-1. Axial computed tomography shows marked thickening of the epiglottis *(arrow)*.

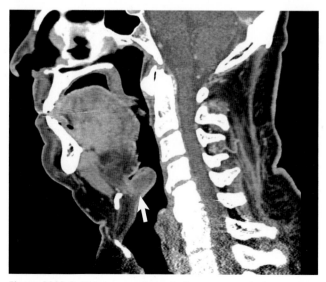

Figure S113-2. This is more dramatically seen on sagittal reconstruction, in which the whole epiglottis appears swollen *(arrow)* and yet the pharyngeal tissues are normal.

CASE 114

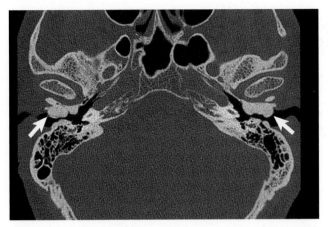

Figure S114-1. Axial scan shows bilateral bony lesions *(arrows)* with smooth narrowing in the external auditory canals.

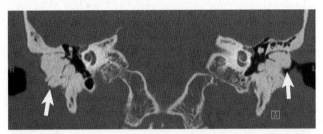

Figure S114-2. The coronal image suggests high-grade stenosis on the left side, which is simulating atresia of the external auditory canal. Bilateral bony overgrowths are present *(arrows)*.

CASE 115

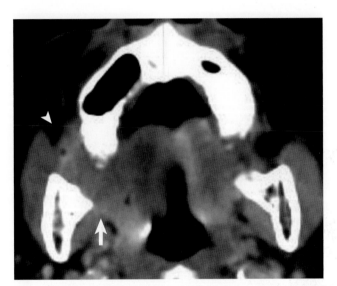

Figure S115-1. Note the mass outlined by the *arrow* and *arrowhead* in the retromolar trigone.

CASE 116

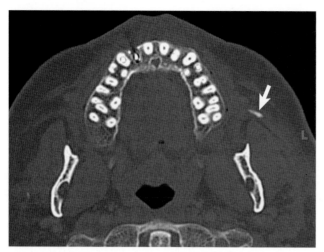

Figure S116-1. There is a hyperdensity *(arrow)* in the left cheek tracking along Stensen duct.

CASE 117

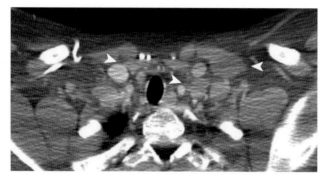

Figure S117-1. Computed tomography shows multiple nodules *(arrowheads)* in the lower neck bilaterally.

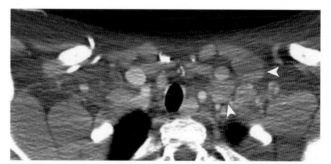

Figure S117-2. This image shows additional nodules *(arrowheads)* more on the left side than the right.

CASE 118

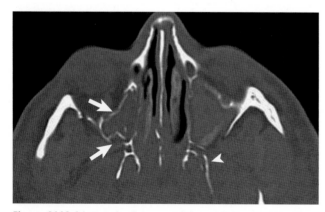

Figure S118-1. Note the fractures of the medial and lateral orbital walls *(arrows)* and the pterygoid plate *(arrowhead)*.

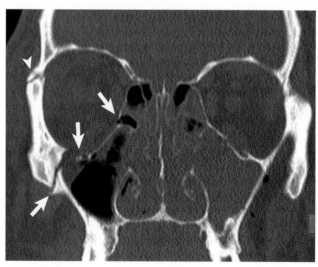

Figure S118-2. The orbital floors and medial orbital walls are fractured *(arrows)*, and the right lateral orbital wall also appears abnormal *(arrowhead)*.

CASE 119

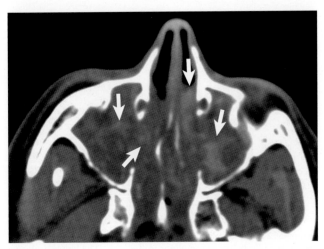

Figure S119-1. Note the marked thickening of the mucosa, the hyperdense sinus and nasal cavity *(arrows)* centrally, and the eroded medial maxillary sinus wall.

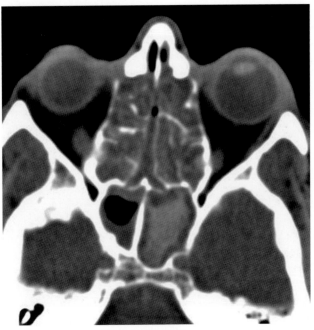

Figure S119-2. Further superiorly, high-density contents in ethmoid and left sphenoid sinuses are visible, without aggressive wall destruction.

CASE 120

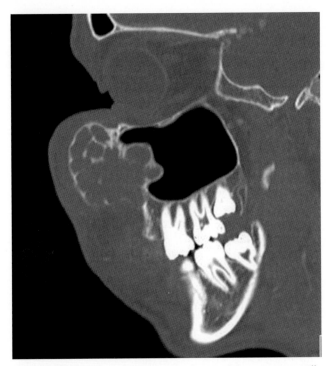

Figure S120-1. Note the bubbly bone lesion of the anterior maxilla on this sagittal reconstruction from axial raw data.

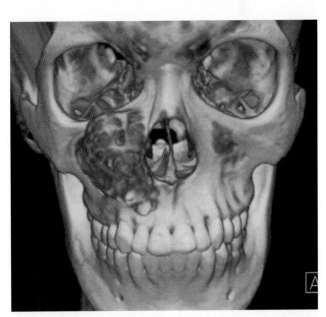

Figure S120-2. The honeycomb-like appearance of the right maxilla lesion is well portrayed on this three-dimensional reconstruction.

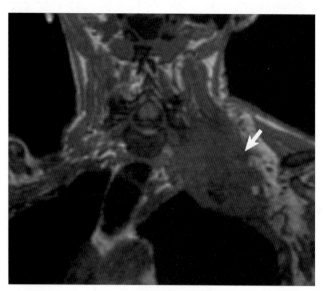

Figure S121-1. Note the infiltrative mass *(arrow)* stemming from the chest and infiltrating the brachial plexus region.

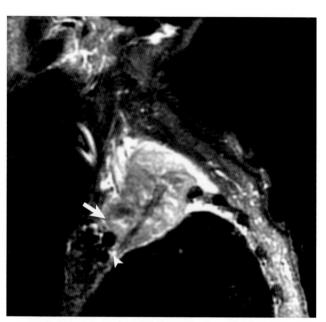

Figure S121-2. The subclavian vein and artery *(arrowhead)* on the sagittal scan lie below and anterior to the mass. The brachial plexus, which lies just superior and posterior to the subclavian artery, is infiltrated *(arrow)*.

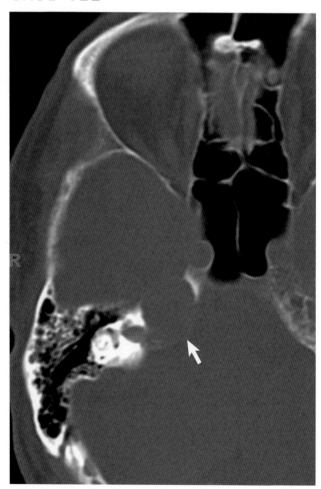

Figure S122-1. Note the lytic expansile lesion *(arrow)* in the right petrous apex on axial computed tomography.

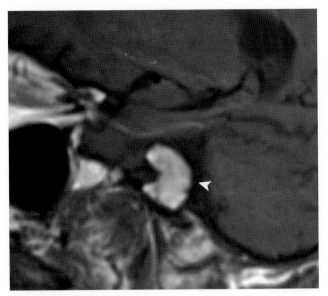

Figure S122-2. This lesion *(arrowhead)* shows high signal on the T1-weighted sagittal scan.

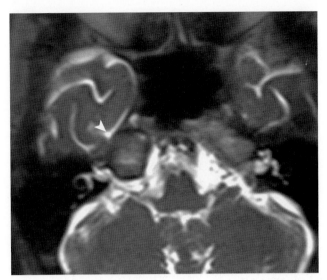

Figure S122-3. The axial T2-weighted scan shows mixed signal in the petrous apex with expansion *(arrowhead)*.

CASE 123

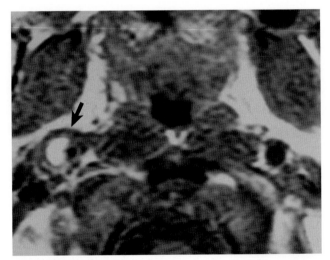

Figure S123-1. Note the narrowed lumen and high signal *(arrow)* in the wall of the right internal carotid artery.

CASE 124

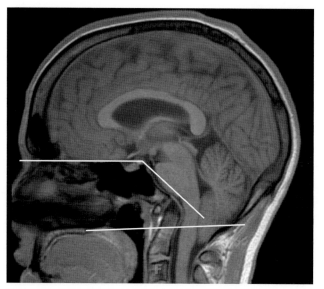

Figure S124-1. Note the unusual appearance of the skull base with abnormal position of the tonsils in the foramen magnum, the position of the odontoid process with McGregor's line, and the angulation of the clivus in relation to the anterior cranial fossa *(lines)*.

CASE 125

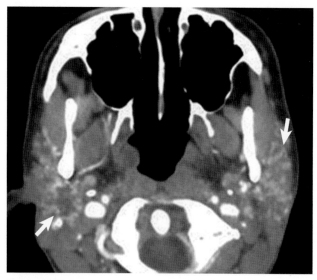

Figure S125-1. Note the enhancing and enlarged glands bilaterally *(arrows)*.

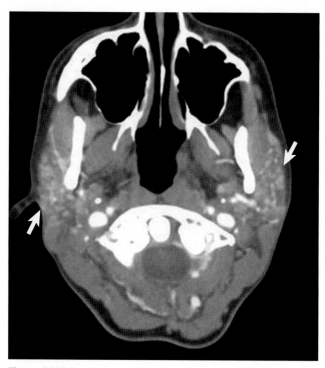

Figure S125-2. Overlying subcutaneous edema *(arrows)* adjacent to the parotid gland indicates an inflammatory process.

CASE 126

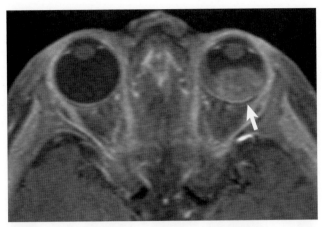

Figure S126-1. Fat-suppressed enhanced T1-weighted scan in the axial plane shows a left ocular mass *(arrow)* in an infant.

CASE 127

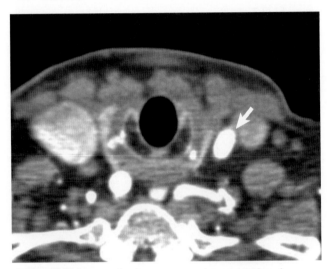

Figure S127-1. Arterial phase computed tomography shows an avidly enhancing nodule posteriorly *(arrow)*. (Note no enhancement of the left jugular vein.)

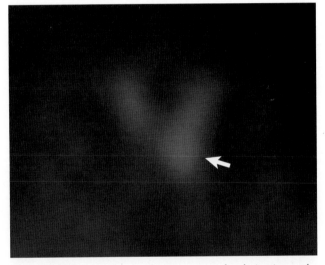

Figure S127-2. Frontal sestamibi imaging reveals a lesion just to the left of midline *(arrow)*.

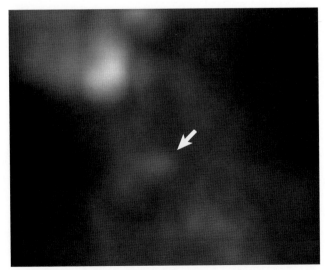

Figure S127-3. Note that the lesion *(arrow)* is posteriorly located in the neck on sestamibi scan.

479

CASE 128

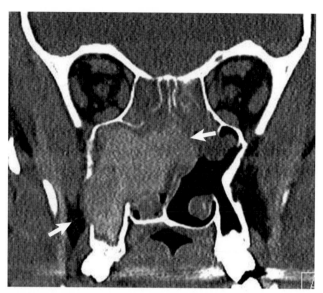

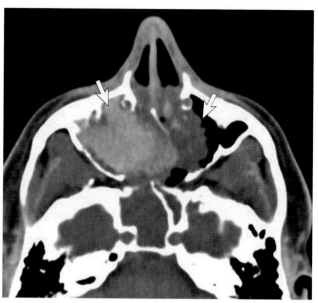

Figure S128-1. Coronal scans show hyperdense material *(arrows)* in the right maxillary antrum with mass effect on the medial sinus wall and erosion of the lateral sinus wall but not in an aggressive manner. Polypoid change on the left side is also visible.

Figure S128-2. On the axial scan, the polypoid changes are visible bilaterally *(arrows)*. The hyperdensity of the sinus contents is well depicted on the patient's right side.

CASE 129

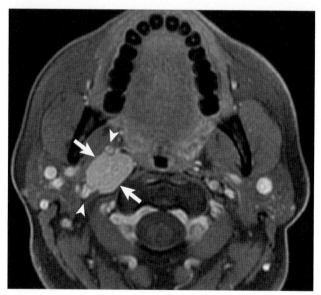

Figure S129-1. Note the avidly enhancing mass *(arrows)* located between the internal and external carotid arteries *(arrowheads)* on this contrast-enhanced, fat-suppressed T1-weighted image.

CASE 130

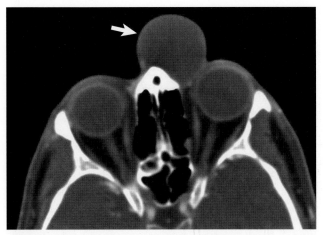

Figure S130-1. Cystic lesion is seen to the left of midline at the tip of the nose *(arrow)*. No intracranial extension was identified.

CASE 131

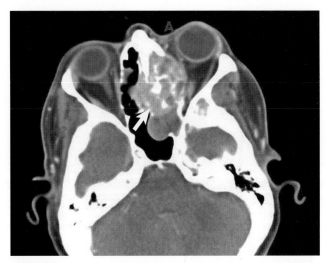

Figure S131-1. Axial computed tomographic image shows a mass *(arrow)* centered in the left ethmoid sinus.

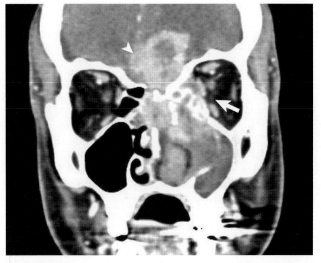

Figure S131-2. Extension of the mass is intracranial *(arrowhead)* and intraorbital *(arrow)*.

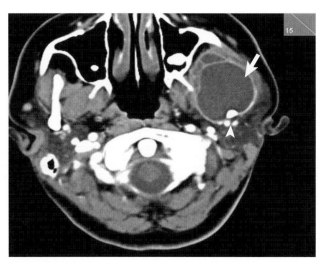

Figure S132-1. Axial image showing a predominately cystic mass affecting the left mandible *(arrow)*, which expands the bone. Note the tooth associated with the mass *(arrowhead)*.

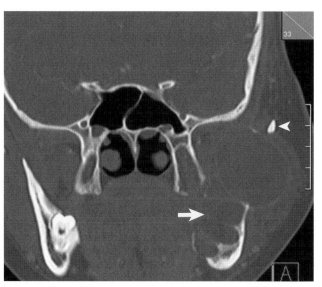

Figure S132-2. Extension into the extraosseous soft tissue is best depicted on the coronal image with dental residual *(arrowhead)* and expansion of the left mandible *(arrow)*.

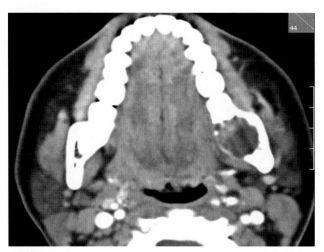

Figure S132-3. The extension to the angle of the mandible is evident on this axial scan with soft tissue algorithm reconstruction.

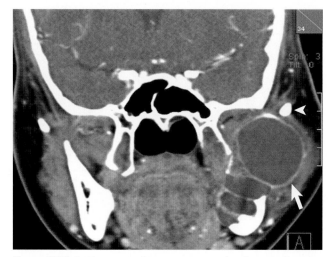

Figure S132-4. The image of Figure S132-2 with soft tissue algorithm reconstruction better depicts the extent of the extra-osseous growth of this mass *(arrow)* and the dental residual *(arrowhead)*.

CASE 133

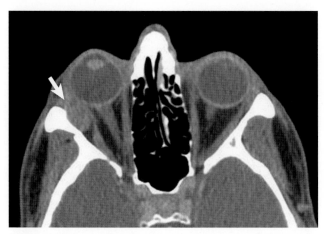

Figure S133-1. A well-defined mass *(arrow)* is enlarging the right lacrimal gland.

CASE 134

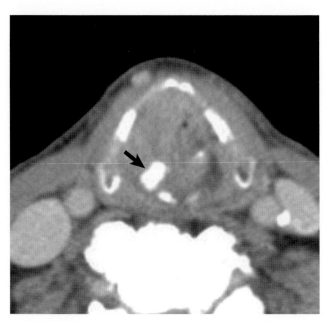

Figure S134-1. Note the marked sclerosis of the arytenoid cartilage *(arrow)* and the thickening of the true vocal cord and paraglottic soft tissues on the right side.

CASE 135

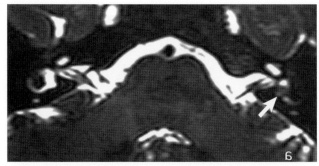

Figure S135-1. Note the low signal intensity of the tissue in the left vestibule *(arrow)* on high-resolution T2-weighted (constructive interference in steady state [CISS]) images.

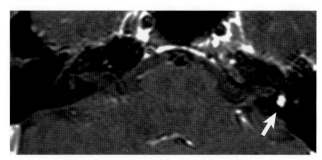

Figure S135-2. This mass enhances *(arrow).*

483

CASE 136

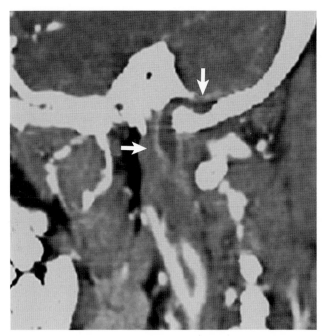

Figure S136-1. Note the low-density material *(arrows)* that follows the vascular structures, descending from intracranially into the jugular vein.

CASE 137

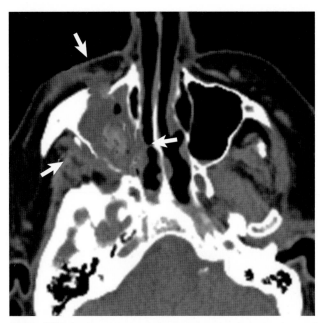

Figure S137-1. Note the areas of aggressive growth *(arrows)* out of the maxillary sinus along the anterior, medial, and posterior walls of the antrum, with edema of perisinus fat.

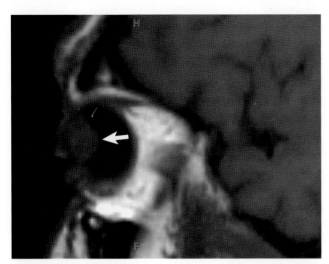

Figure S138-1. Note the mass associated with the left lateral ciliary apparatus of the globe, which is slightly hyperintense *(arrow)* on sagittal T1-weighted images without contrast.

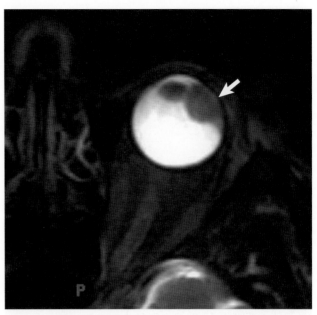

Figure S138-2. The intermediate signal intensity *(arrow)* on T2-weighted image is a typical histologic feature of this lesion.

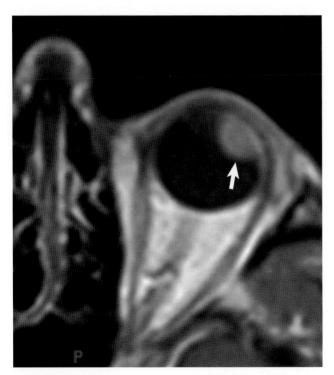

Figure S138-3. Enhancement suggests that the lesion *(arrow)* is a tumor that is closely associated with the uveal tract.

CASE 139

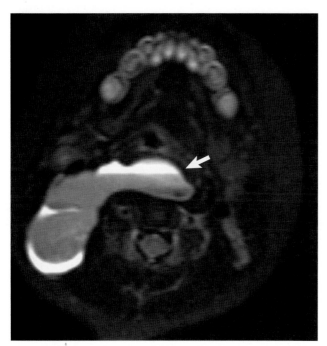

Figure S139-1. Note the blood-fluid levels in this multicompartmental, multiloculated lesion *(arrow)* in the neck on the T2-weighted image.

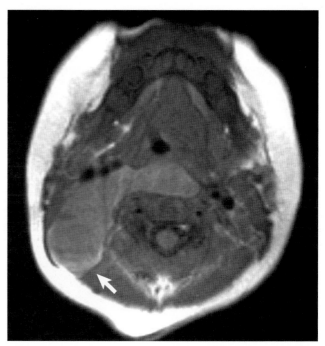

Figure S139-2. On the T1-weighted scan, the lesion has a bright signal, and its contents are therefore not pure fluid in intensity. A blood-fluid level is seen *(arrow)*.

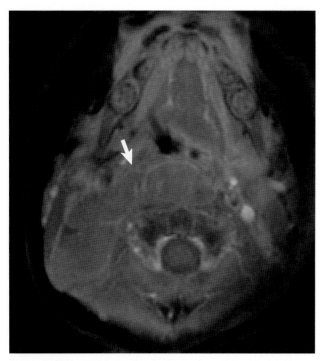

Figure S139-3. On T1-weighted scans with contrast, the abnormality does not show enhancement *(arrow)*.

CASE 140

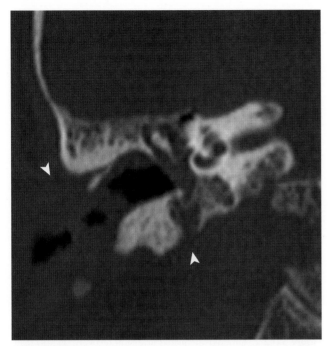

Figure S140-1. Note the soft tissue *(arrowheads)* in the cartilaginous and bony portion of the external auditory canal. The *lower arrowhead* shows erosion of the inferior wall of the external auditory canal leading to the skull base. *(Image courtesy Carolina Paulazo, MD.)*

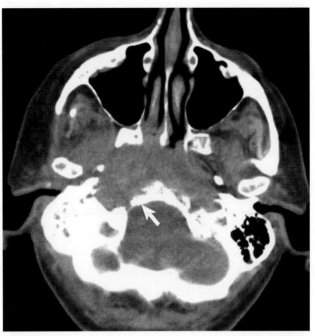

Figure S140-2. The image of the skull base shows erosion at the lower right clivus *(arrow)* with soft tissue infiltrating the parapharyngeal soft tissues. *(Image courtesy Carolina Paulazo, MD.)*

CASE 141

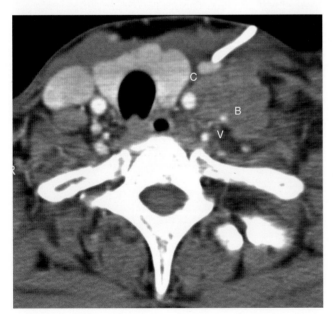

Figure S141-1. The mass is depicted involving 180 degrees of the carotid artery (C), not encroaching on the vertebral artery (V), but encircling the branch vessel (B).

CASE 142

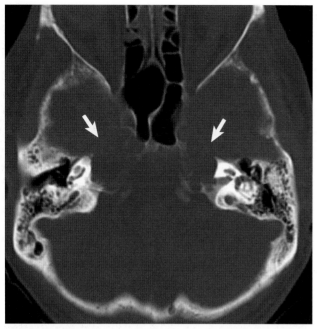

Figure S142-1. Note the expansile bilateral lesion on computed tomogram of the petrous apex *(arrows)*.

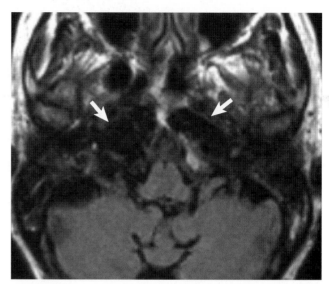

Figure S142-2. On fluid-attenuated inversion recovery (FLAIR) magnetic resonance imaging, the signal intensity is that of cerebrospinal fluid *(arrows)*.

CASE 143

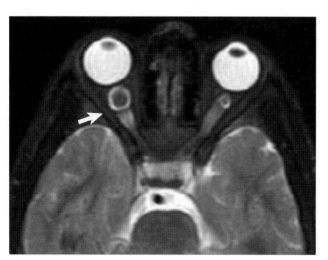

Figure S143-1. Note the enlarged right optic nerve and sheath *(arrow)* on this T2-weighted scan at the level of the optic canal.

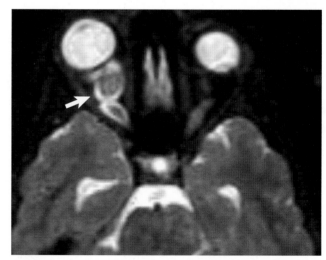

Figure S143-2. The enlargement of the right optic nerve *(arrow)* and its redundancy appears slightly worse on this section.

CASE 144

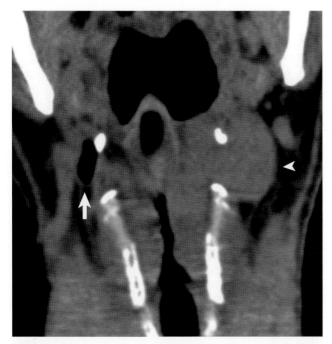

Figure S144-1. Note the fluid-filled left-sided lesion *(arrowhead)* and the air-filled right-sided structure *(arrow)* on a coronal reconstruction of the axial scans.

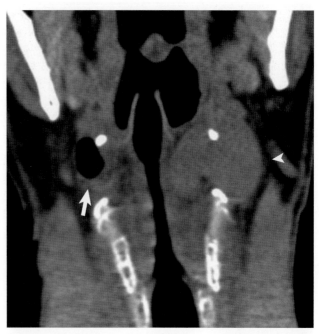

Figure S144-2. The communication of the left-sided lesion *(arrowhead)* with the paraglottic space is best seen on a more posterior coronal section, which also shows the right-sided lesion *(arrow)*.

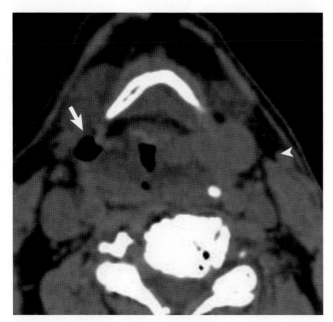

Figure S144-3. The positions of the air-filled lesion *(arrow)* and fluid-filled lesion *(arrowhead)* with regard to the thyrohyoid membrane are better depicted on an axial scan.

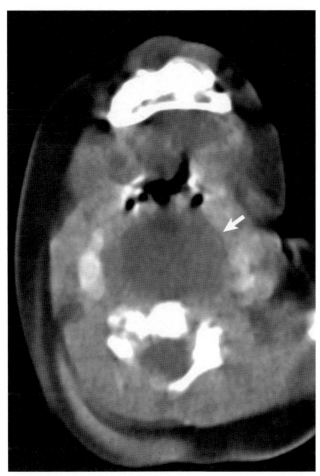

Figure S145-1. Axial scan at the level of the mandible shows a large, low-density mass *(arrow)* anterior to the longus musculature and pushing the airway anteriorly.

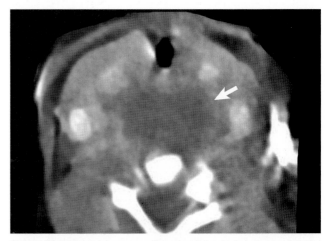

Figure S145-2. Axial scan at the cricoid level also shows that the lesion *(arrow)* is large and compressive.

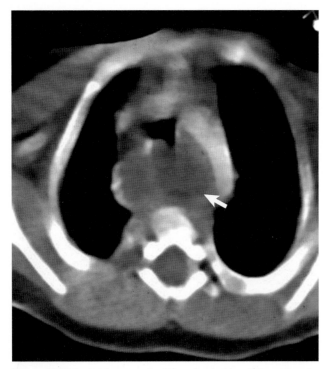

Figure S145-3. Axial scan at the T6 mediastinal level shows that the trachea is pushed forward by the mass *(arrow)*.

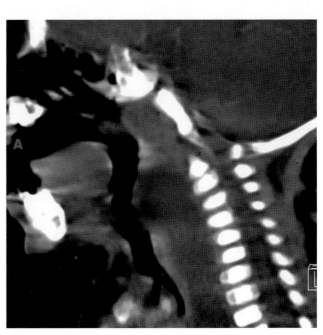

Figure S145-4. The sagittal reconstruction shows how the lesion extends from superiorly at the clivus level all the way into the thoracic level.

CASE 146

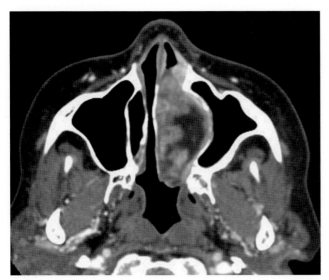

Figure S146-1. Note the mass centered in the left nasal cavity.

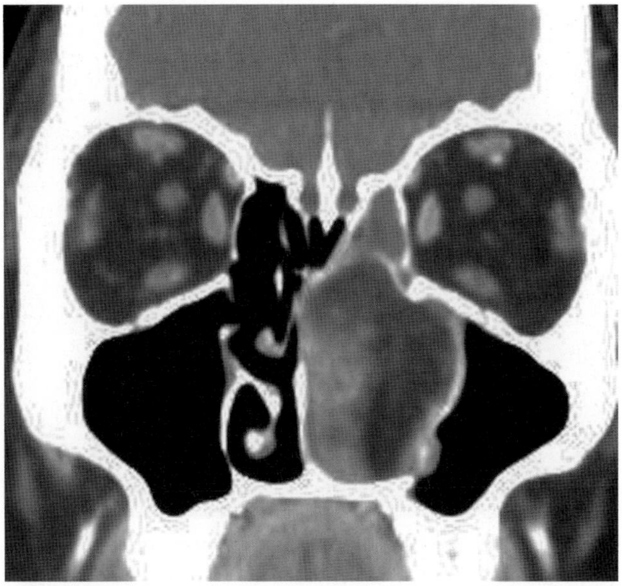

Figure S146-2. The coronal reconstruction shows the heterogeneous density to this mass and the obstructed left ethmoid air cell. The architecture of the left nasal cavity is grossly distorted.

CASE 147

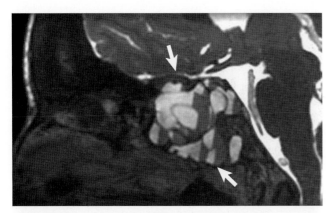

Figure S147-1. Note the fluid-fluid levels *(arrows)* in this paranasal sinus lesion on sagittal T2-weighted image.

CASE 148

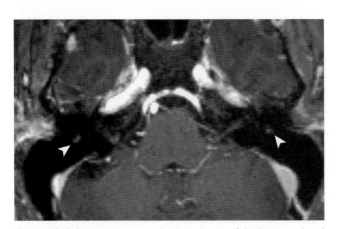

Figure S148-1. Note the normal enhancement of the horizontal and descending portions of the facial nerve *(arrowheads)*.

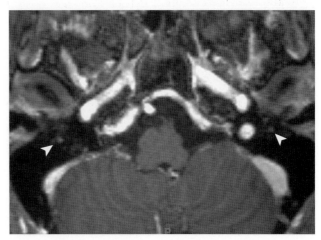

Figure S148-2. Asymmetry in enhancement *(arrowheads)* is more common than not.

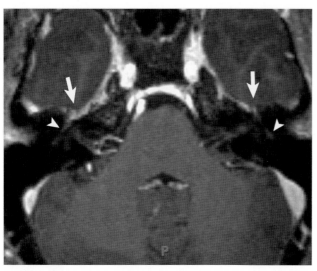

Figure S148-3. The geniculate ganglia enhances *(arrows)*, in addition to the tympanic portion of the facial nerve *(arrowheads)*.

CASE 149

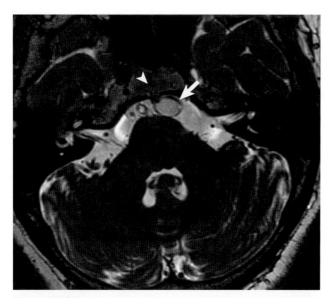

Figure S149-1. Note the exophytic lesion *(arrow)* arising from the clivus *(arrowhead)* extending into the prepontine cistern. *(Image courtesy Gul Moonis, MD.)*

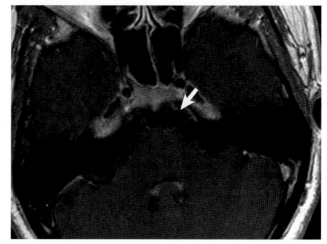

Figure S149-2. The abnormality *(arrow)* does not enhance. *(Image courtesy Gul Moonis, MD.)*

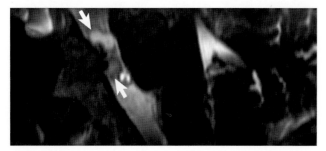

Figure S149-3. Note the relationship of the lesion (between *arrows*) to the skull base. *(Image courtesy Gul Moonis, MD.)*

CASE 150

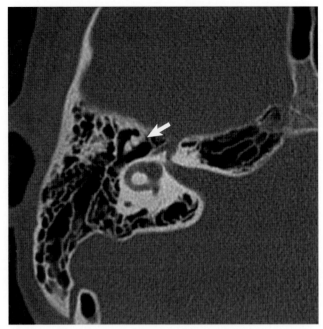

Figure S150-1. Note the calcified connection *(arrow)* of the malleus to the tympanic wall. *(Image courtesy Gul Moonis, MD.)*

CASE 151

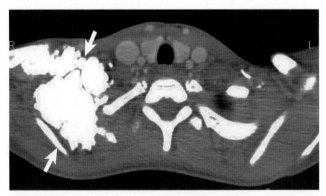

Figure S151-1. Note the dense matrix in the soft tissues (between the *arrows*) that is probably impacting the brachial plexus.

CASE 152

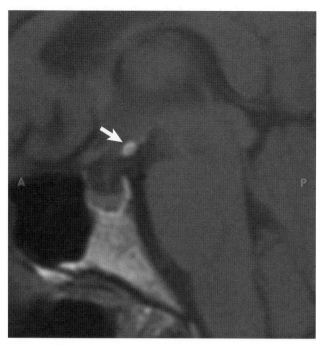

Figure S152-1. Sagittal T1-weighted image shows the hyperintense tissue *(arrow)* at the base of the hypothalamus.

CASE 153

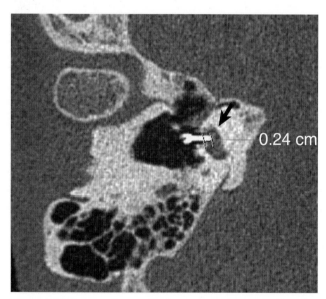

Figure S153-1. Note the metallic device *(arrow)* and its relationship to the ossicles and the labyrinthine structures, particularly the vestibule.

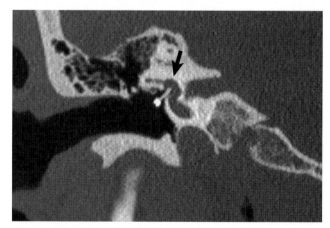

Figure S153-2. The coronal view shows the deep penetration of the stapes implant *(arrow)* into the vestibule.

0.24 cm

CASE 154

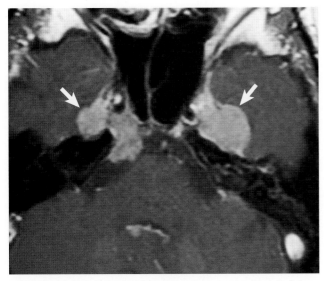

Figure S154-1. Note dura-based masses *(arrows)* at the skull base and cavernous sinus–Meckel cave junction.

CASE 155

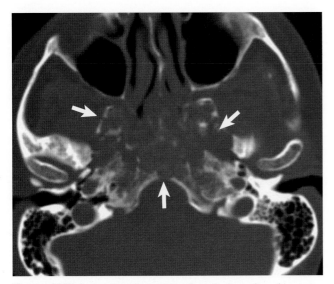

Figure S155-1. Computed tomography depicts the destructive process eroding the clivus and pterygoid plates *(arrows)*.

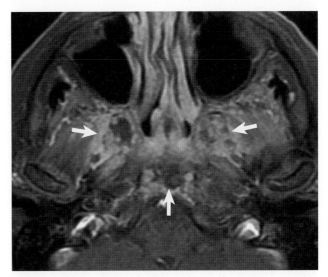

Figure S155-2. The lesion shows contrast enhancement and necrosis *(arrows)* on the axial post-contrast image.

CASE 156

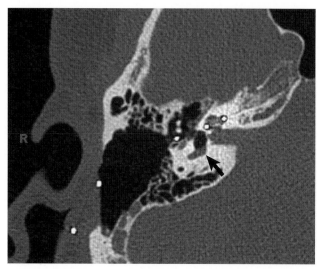

Figure S156-1. Note the air *(black arrow)* in the vestibule in this postoperative case.

CASE 157

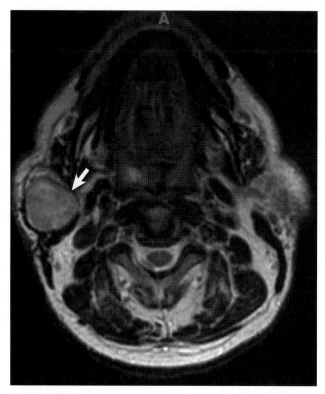

Figure S157-1. Note the mass *(arrow)* in the tail of the right parotid gland.

CASE 158

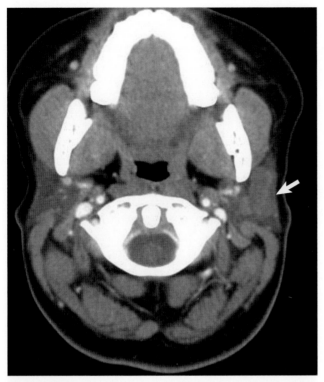

Figure S158-1. Note the two irregularly shaped masses in the left parotid gland *(arrow)*.

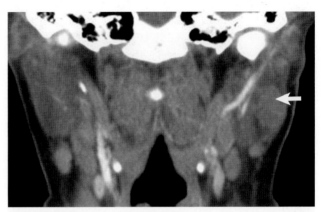

Figure S158-2. The lesion *(arrow)* is confined to the left parotid gland with no extracapsular extension.

CASE 159

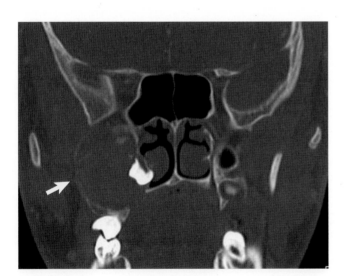

Figure S159-1. Coronal computed tomography shows the expansile nature of the mass with benign bony remodeling laterally *(arrow)*.

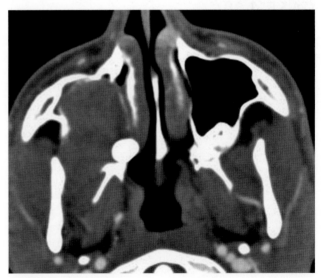

Figure S159-2. Note that on soft tissue imaging windows, the lesion appears solid, not cystic.

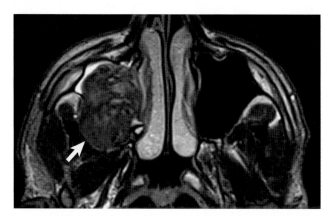

Figure S159-3. The lesion *(arrow)* appears dark on T2-weighted magnetic resonance imaging.

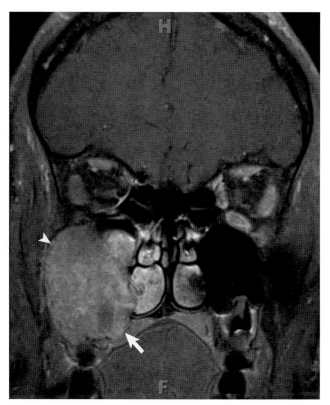

Figure S159-4. The lesion *(arrow and arrowhead)* enhances homogeneously and avidly on coronal contrast-enhanced, fat-suppressed, T1-weighted magnetic resonance imaging.

CASE 160

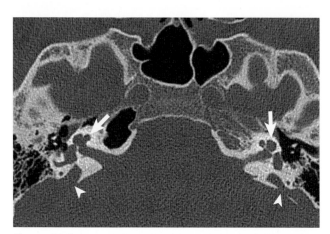

Figure S160-1. Note the incomplete rotations of the cochlea bilaterally *(arrows)*, as well as the enlarged vestibular aqueducts *(arrowheads)*.

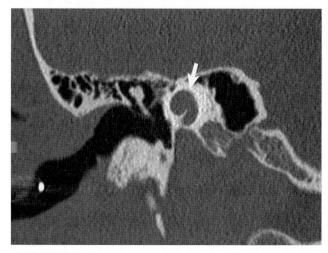

Figure S160-2. Coronal scan best depicts the incomplete development of the cochlear modiolus *(arrow)*.

CASE 161

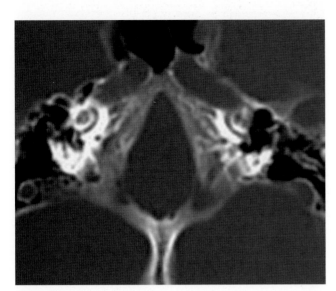

Figure S161-1. Note the small size of the foramen magnum in this patient.

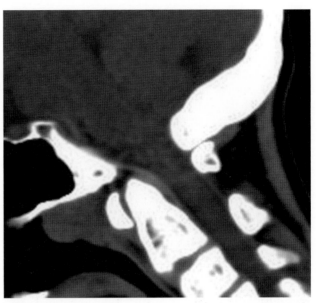

Figure S161-2. The sagittal scan shows the narrowing and its potential effect on the cervicomedullary junction.

CASE 162

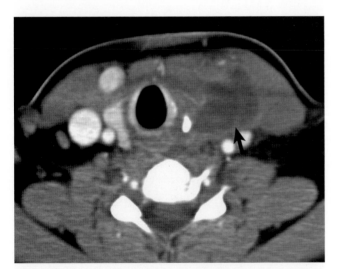

Figure S162-1. Note the cystic mass *(black arrow),* on the lower left side of the neck, displacing the carotid sheath vessels posteriorly. The thyroid gland on the left side is not showing enhancement, which may indicate concomitant thyroiditis.

CASE 163

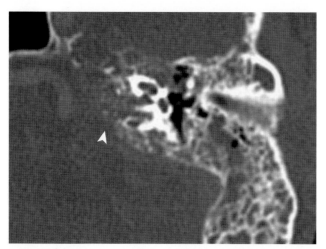

Figure S163-1. Computed tomography shows a destructive mass in the left petrous portion *(arrowhead)* of the temporal bone extending towards the mastoid portion.

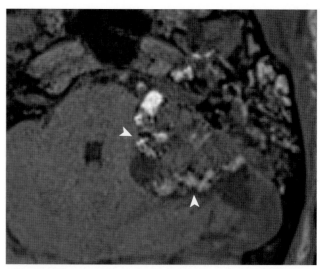

Figure S163-2. The lesion *(arrowheads)* has areas of high signal on the unenhanced T1-weighted image.

CASE 164

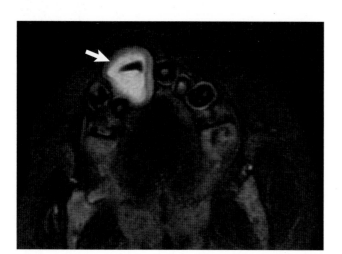

Figure S164-1. T2-weighted image demonstrates a cystic lesion between the medial incisor and the canine tooth on the right *(arrow)*.

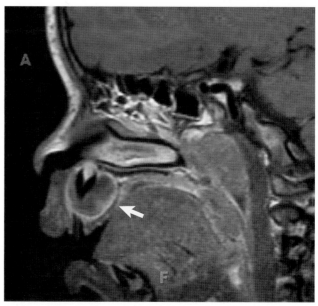

Figure S164-2. Axial magnetic resonance study with contrast shows only rim enhancement *(arrow)*. This implies that the lesion is not a tumor.

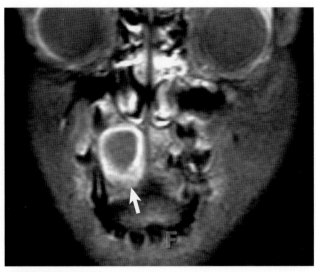

Figure S164-3. Coronal magnetic resonance image with contrast confirms absence of solid enhancement *(arrow)*.

CASE 165

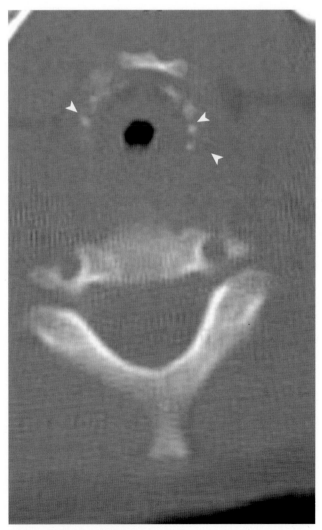

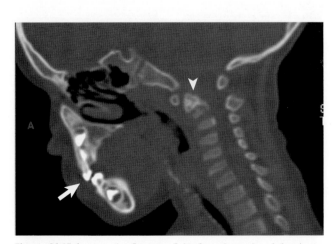

Figure S165-1. Note the flatness of the face *(arrow)* and dysplastic, clefted C1-C2 junction *(arrowhead)* on this sagittal reconstruction.

Figure S165-2. The thyroid cartilage has a stippled appearance on imaging *(arrowheads)*.

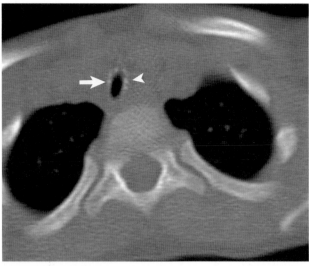

Figure S165-3. The tracheal cartilage also has a stippled appearance on imaging *(arrow and arrowhead)*, and the transverse diameter is narrowed (tracheal stenosis).

CASE 166

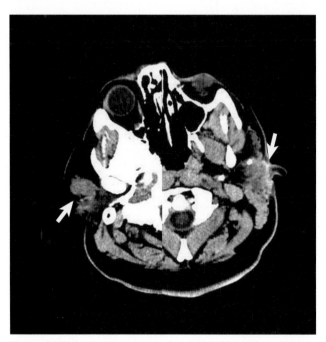

Figure S166-1. The first patient has bilateral irregular infiltrative masses in the superficial portion of the parotid glands *(arrows)*.

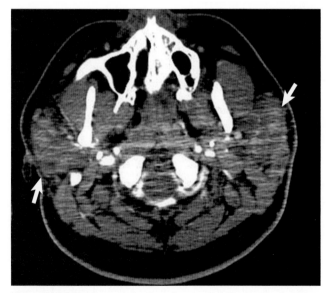

Figure S166-2. The second patient has more diffuse parotid enlargement *(arrows)*, with lymphonodular infiltrates in the glands.

CASE 167

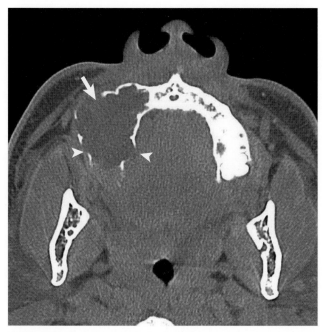

Figure S167-1. Axial computed tomography reveals a lytic expansile mass *(arrow and arrowheads)* of the maxilla.

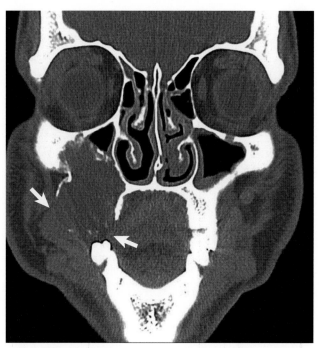

Figure S167-2. The expanded walls without aggressive erosion *(arrows)* are well seen on the coronal computed tomographic reformatted scan.

CASE 168

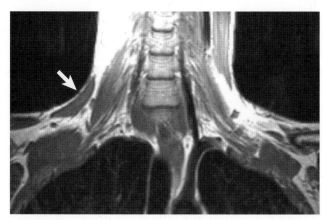

Figure S168-1. Coronal T1-weighted imaging shows a structure with the intensity of muscle along the right side of the neck *(arrow)*.

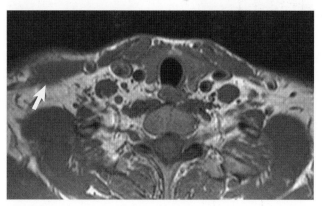

Figure S168-2. Axial T1-weighted imaging confirms the presence of soft tissue in the anterior right portion of the neck *(arrow)*.

CASE 169

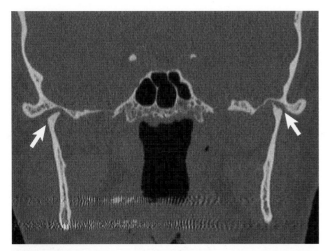

Figure S169-1. Coronal reconstruction of axial computed tomographic data shows bilateral deformation of the mandibular condyles *(arrows)*.

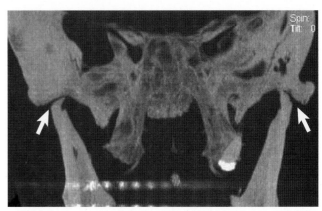

Figure S169-2. Note the pointy nature and increased density of the condyles *(arrows)* on this three-dimensional reconstruction.

CASE 170

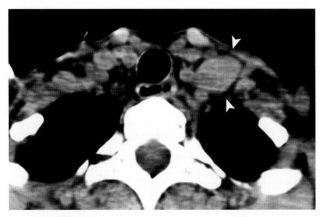

Figure S170-1. An ovoid stricture *(arrowheads)* is visible in the lower left aspect of the neck, lateral to the carotid sheath. Ultrasonography demonstrated that it was cystic.

CASE 171

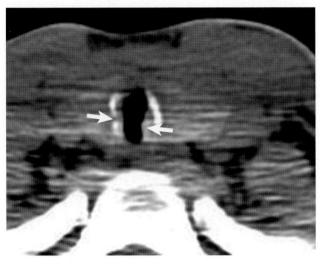

Figure S171-1. Axial scan shows narrowing of the airway's transverse diameter *(arrows)* in an irregular contour at the level of the trachea.

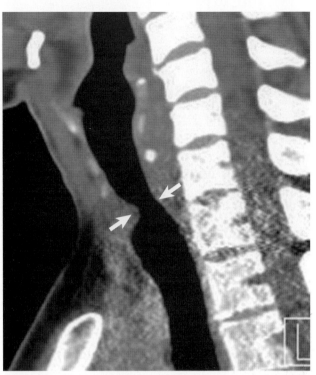

Figure S171-2. The sagittal image confirms the narrowing *(arrows)* below the cricoid cartilage.

CASE 172

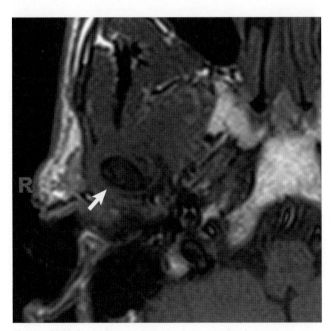

Figure S172-1. On the unenhanced T1-weighted magnetic resonance image, the marrow signal of the mandibular condyle *(arrow)* is abnormal.

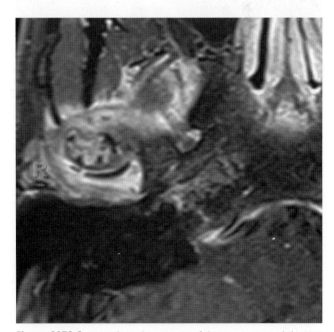

Figure S172-2. Note the enhancement of the tissues around the TMJ and the abnormal signal of the condylar marrow on post-contrast scan.

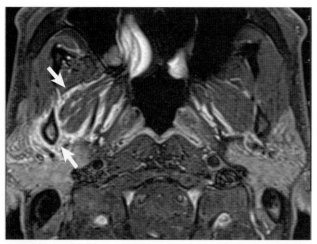

Figure S172-3. Enhancement of the muscles of mastication *(arrows)* indicates inflammation.

CASE 173

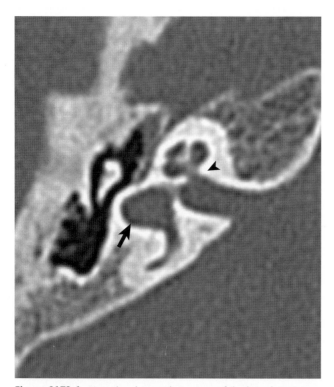

Figure S173-1. Note the abnormal structure of the lateral semicircular canal *(arrow)* and the bone seen within the canal. In this case, the cochlear aperture is also narrowed *(arrowhead).*

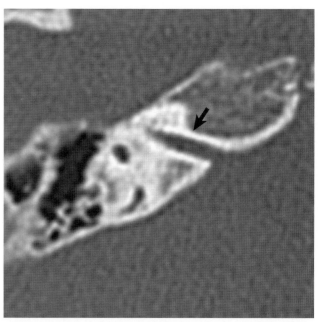

Figure S173-2. A second patient has narrowing of the internal auditory canal *(arrow)* on the right side. These imaging findings are indicative of a particular diagnosis.

CASE 174

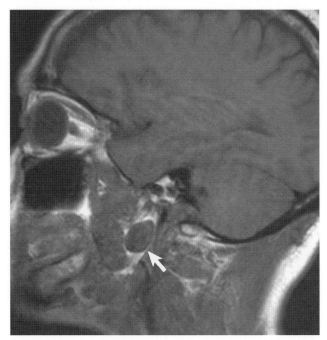

Figure S174-1. T1-weighted scout view of the brain shows a mass *(arrow)* in the parapharyngeal space, surrounded by the intrinsic fat of the space.

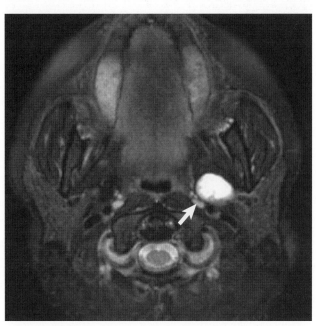

Figure S174-2. Note the high signal intensity of the mass *(arrow)* on the axial fat-suppressed T2-weighted image.

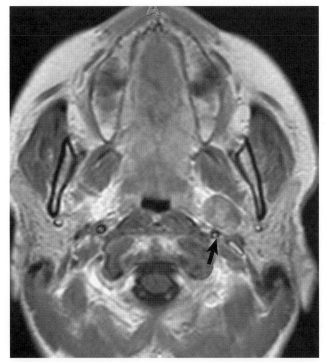

Figure S174-3. With gadolinium enhancement (but without fat suppression), the mass *(arrow)* appears less conspicuous as parts become nearly isointense to the fat in the parapharyngeal space.

CASE 175

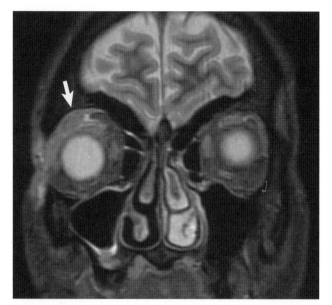

Figure S175-1. The coronal T2-weighted image shows infiltration of the right lacrimal gland *(arrow)*.

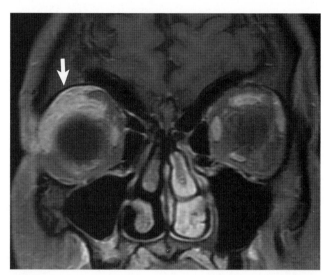

Figure S175-2. On T1-weighted imaging with contrast and fat suppression, the right lacrimal gland *(arrow)* is enlarged and enhances uniformly.

CASE 176

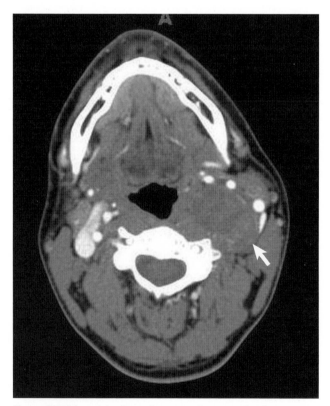

Figure S176-1. Axial enhanced computed tomography shows a mass *(arrow)* causing the carotid artery and jugular vein to splay apart.

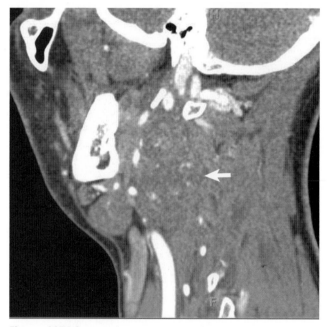

Figure S176-2. Sagittal reconstruction shows speckled areas of enhancement *(arrow)*.

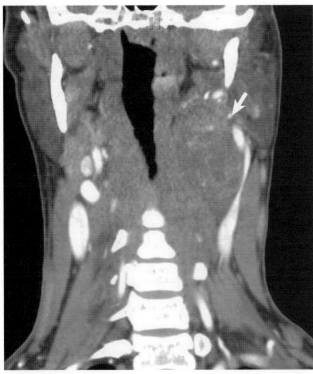

Figure S176-3. The internal architecture of the mass *(arrow)* on coronal reformatted image, although heterogeneous, is predominantly not enhancing.

CASE 177

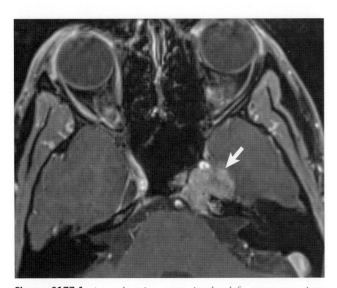

Figure S177-1. An enhancing mass in the left cavernous sinus *(arrow)* is visible.

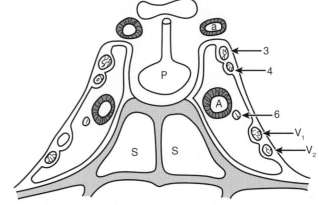

Figure S177-2. This schematic shows the location of cranial nerves in the cavernous sinus. The oculomotor, trochlear, and abducens nerves are represented by "3," "4," and "6," respectively. V₁ and V₂ represent the ophthalmic and maxillary branches, respectively, of the trigeminal nerve. *A,* Cavernous carotid artery; *a,* supraclinoid internal carotid artery; *P,* pituitary gland; *S,* sphenoid sinus.

CASE 178

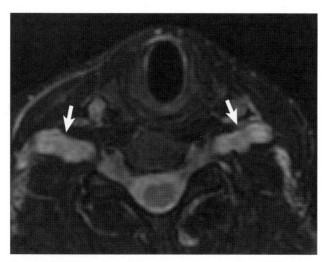

Figure S178-1. Marked bilateral enlargement of brachial plexus nerves is visible on the T2-weighted image *(arrows)*.

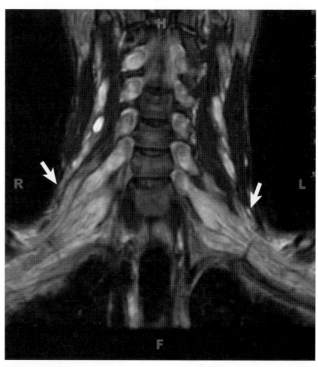

Figure S178-2. Coronal scan shows the diffuse bilateral nature of the process *(arrows)*.

CASE 179

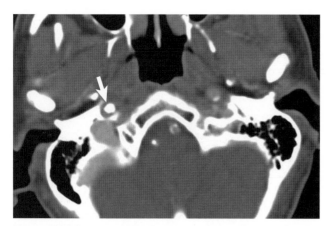

Figure S179-1. Note the calcified outpouching *(arrow)* of the right internal carotid artery on the axial scan.

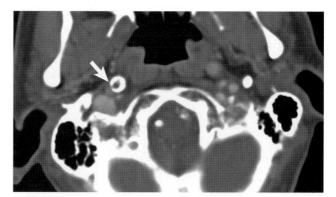

Figure S179-2. The calcified wall and the patent lumen that projects posterolaterally *(arrow)* is visible farther superiorly on the axial scan with contrast.

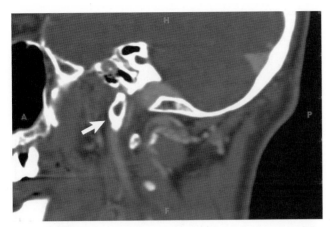

Figure S179-3. The sagittal reconstruction shows the location of the calcified vessel wall *(arrow)* just below the skull base.

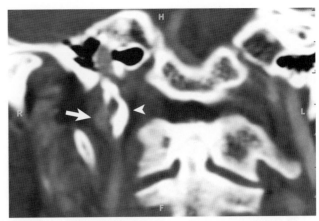

Figure S179-4. The coronal scan best shows the patent lumen of the carotid artery *(arrow)* and the calcified pseudoaneurysm projecting medially *(arrowhead)*.

CASE 180

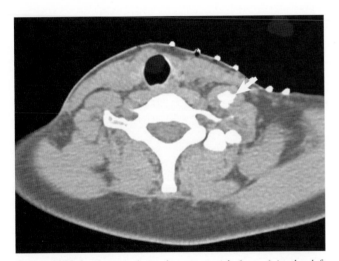

Figure S180-1. There is hyperdense material *(arrow)* in the left anterior scalene muscle.

CASE 181

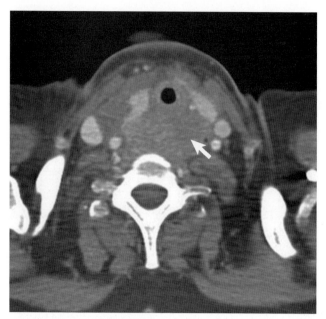

Figure S181-1. A large mass *(arrow)* that originated in the hypopharynx is now also invading the upper esophagus.

CASE 182

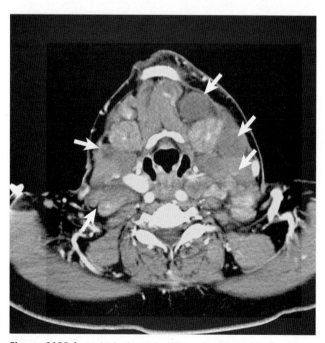

Figure S182-1. Multiple large lymph nodes *(arrows)* are present bilaterally in the neck.

CASE 183

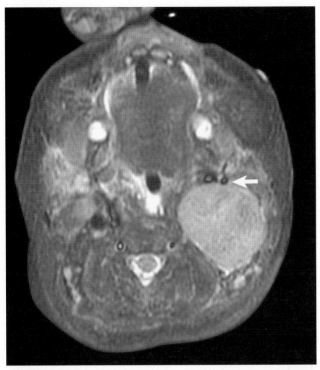

Figure S183-1. Note the mass *(arrow)* in the left side of the neck on axial imaging with short tau inversion recovery (STIR). It is intimately associated with the left carotid artery, which is displaced by the large mass.

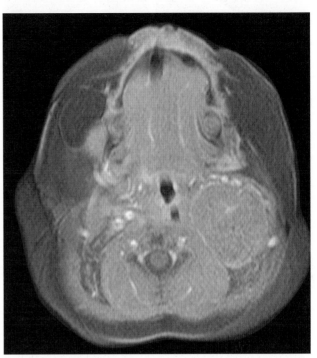

Figure S183-2. The enhancement of the mass is minimal.

CASE 184

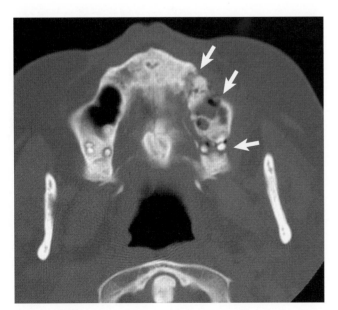

Figure S184-1. The axial computed tomographic image shows erosion of the maxilla *(arrows)* in a moth-eaten pattern with the suggestion of floating teeth. The bone has increased density and erosions.

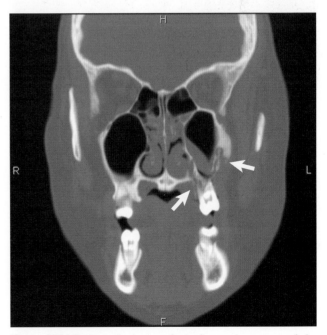

Figure S184-2. Coronal view confirms the erosive nature of the lesion in the base of the maxilla *(arrows)*.

CASE 185

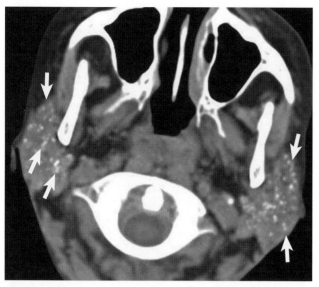

Figure S185-1. Computed tomography shows bilateral tiny calculi *(arrows)* in the parotid glands.

CASE 186

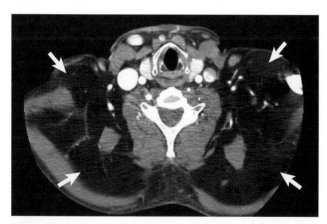

Figure S186-1. Axial computed tomography shows bilateral symmetric enlargement of the fat of the neck, manifested by bulky supraclavicular and posterior fat deposits *(arrows)*.

CASE 187

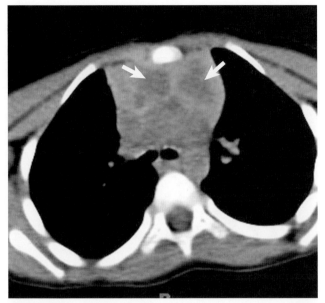

Figure S187-1. Note the low-density cystic areas *(arrows)* within the mediastinal tissue in front of the great vessels.

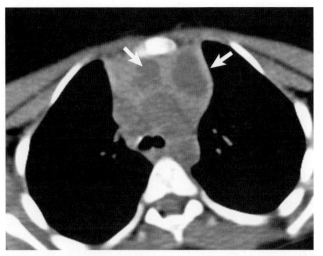

Figure S187-2. Lower section of scan shows similar infiltration of the mediastinum *(arrows)*.

CASE 188

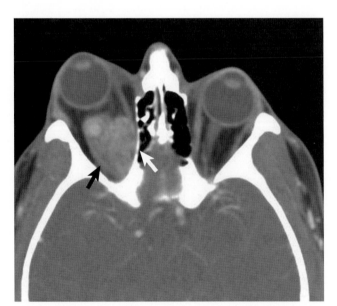

Figure S188-1. Axial scan with contrast shows a mass *(black arrow)* in the intraconal space that is causing proptosis and stretching of the medial rectus muscle. Note the bone remodeling *(white arrow)*.

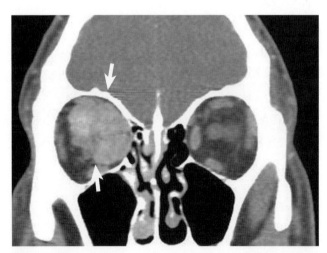

Figure S188-2. On the coronal image, bone remodeling of the orbital roof is present with infiltration around the optic nerve. The enhancement in the mass *(arrows)* is more heterogeneous than would be expected for a hemangioma or venous vascular malformation.

CASE 189

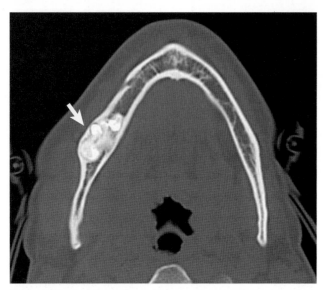

Figure S189-1. A hyperdense mass is causing the right side of the mandible to expand *(arrow)*.

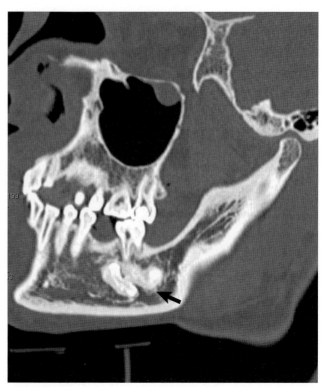

Figure S189-2. The sagittal reconstruction shows that the lesion is made of primordial teeth and is not associated with a cyst or supernumerary teeth *(arrow)*.

CASE 190

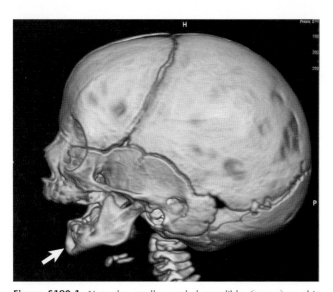

Figure S190-1. Note the small, receded mandible *(arrow)* on this three-dimensional reconstruction of a facial computed tomographic scan.

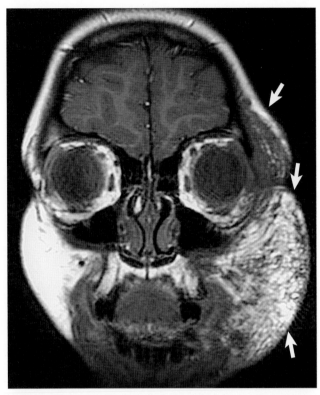

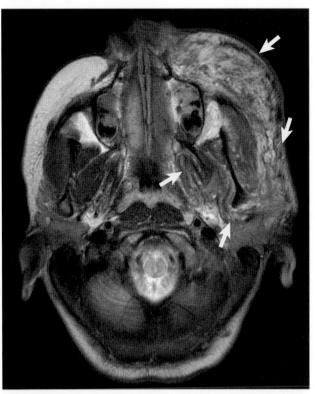

Figure S191-1. Coronal T1-weighted image shows diffuse enlargement of the soft tissues of the face *(arrows)*. Some areas have fatty intensity, and others show soft tissue intensity.

Figure S191-2. On axial T2-weighted image, it is evident that this is not merely swelling from trauma but an infiltrative mass *(arrows)* that also affects the muscles of mastication.

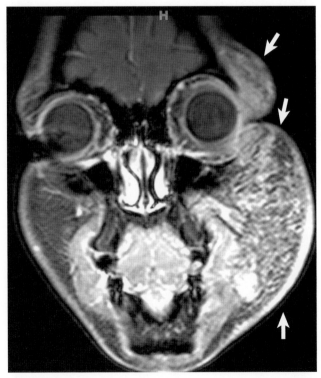

Figure S191-3. On fat-suppressed scanning with contrast, diffuse enhancement is present. Note the effect on the orbicularis oris muscle on the patient's left.

CASE 192

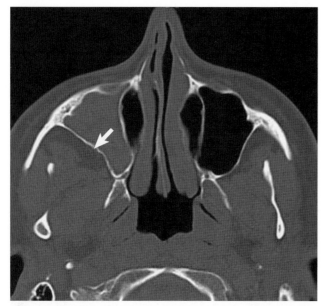

Figure S192-1. Note the increased perimaxillary fat *(arrow)* and the small retracted maxillary sinus.

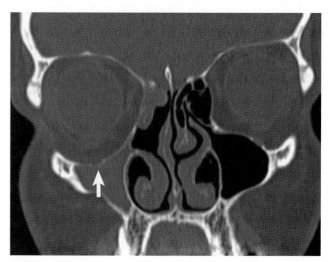

Figure S192-2. On the coronal scan, the orbital floor appears depressed *(arrow)*.

CASE 193

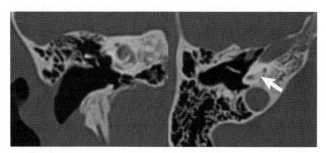

Figure S193-1. There is high density *(arrow)* in the otic capsule. *Left,* Coronal image; *right,* axial image.

CASE 194

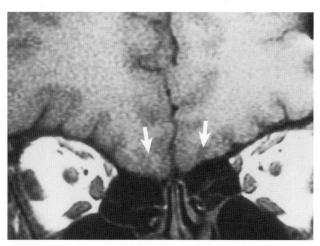

Figure S194-1. The olfactory bulbs and tracts are absent bilaterally, and the olfactory sulci are blunted *(arrows)*.

CASE 195

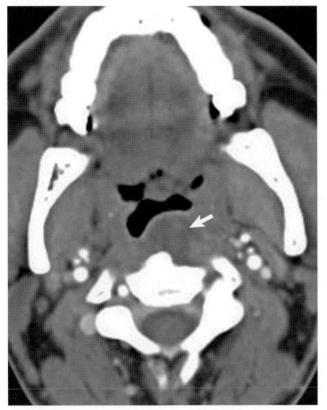

Figure S195-1. Note the low-density mass *(arrow)*, causing a submucosal impression on the aerodigestive system at the level of the palatine tonsils.

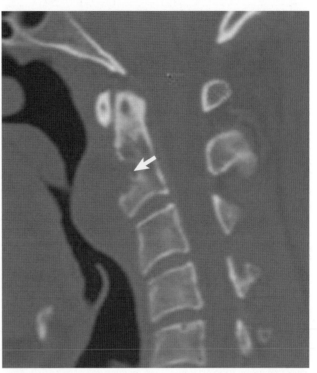

Figure S195-2. Associated changes in the anterior aspect of the C2 vertebra *(arrow)* are better shown on the sagittal scan. The bony derivation may be subtle on imaging.

CASE 196

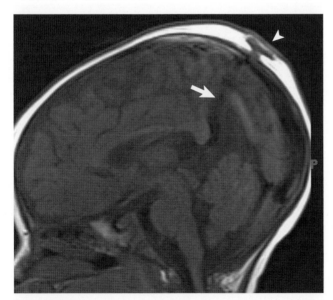

Figure S196-1. Note the vertically oriented vascular structure *(arrow)* that leads to an extracranial nubbin of soft tissue *(arrowhead)*.

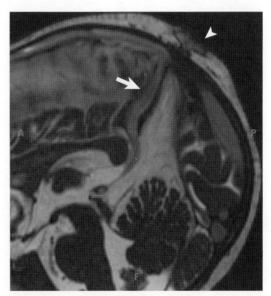

Figure S196-2. The T2-weighted image shows the straight sinus *(arrow)*, the normal-appearing corpus callosum, and the brain tissue tented to the encephalocele *(arrowhead)*.

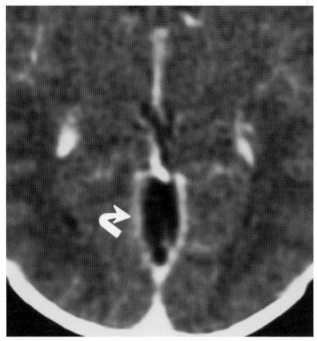

Figure S196-3. Axial contrast-enhanced computed tomographic scan shows the typical "spinning-top" configuration of the tentorial incisura *(arrow)* that results from the prominent superior cerebellar cistern in association with the high position of the tentorium. *(From Patterson RJ, Egelhoff JC, Crone KR, Ball WS Jr. Atretic parietal cephaloceles revisited: an enlarging clinical and imaging spectrum?* AJNR Am J Neuroradiol. *1998;19[4]:791-795.)*

CASE 197

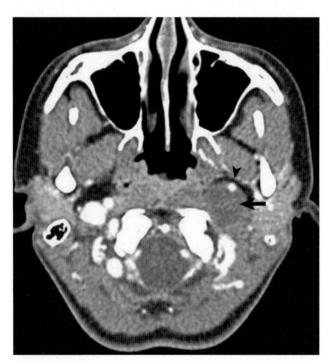

Figure S197-1. Soft tissue windows show a nonenhancing mass *(arrow)* in the carotid sheath that displaces the carotid artery *(arrowhead)* anteriorly.

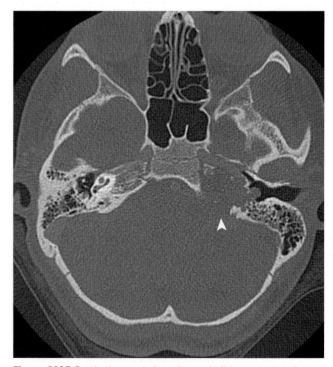

Figure S197-2. The bone window shows skull base erosion *(arrowhead)* of the petrous portion of the left temporal bone.

CASE 198

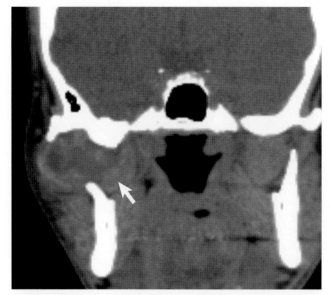

Figure S198-1. Computed tomographic image in soft tissue algorithm shows marked widening of the temporomandibular joint with a mass of mixed attenuation *(arrow)*.

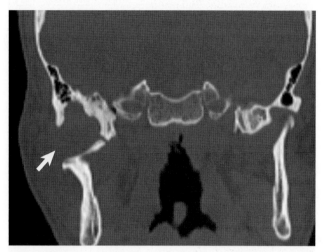

Figure S198-2. Computed tomographic image in bone algorithm shows remodeling of the mandibular condyle *(arrow)* and glenoid fossa.

CASE 199

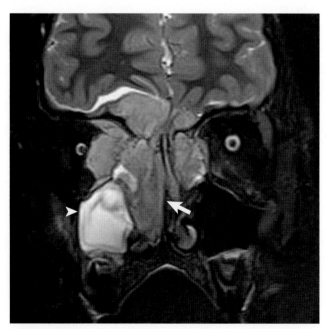

Figure S199-1. Note the low signal intensity on T2-weighted scan of the mass *(arrow)*, as opposed to the bright obstructed secretions in the maxillary sinus *(arrowhead)*.

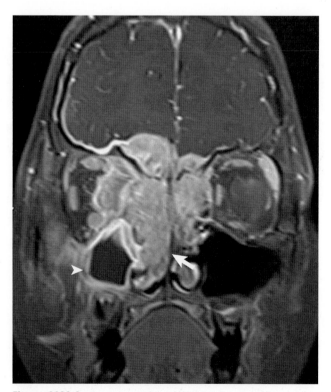

Figure S199-2. On scans with gadolinium, the mass *(arrow)* has solid enhancement, whereas the secretions *(arrowhead)* show the typical linear peripheral enhancement. The intracranial spread along the dura is extensive. Fortunately, the brain is not invaded.

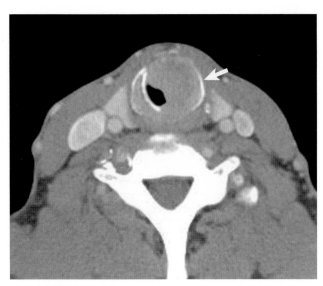

Figure S200-1. Note the submucosal mass *(arrow)* in the subglottic region without tumoral matrix.

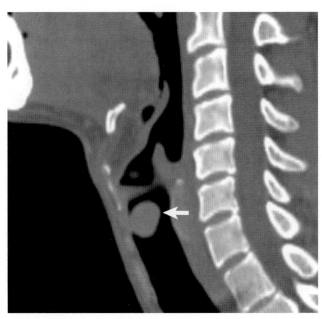

Figure S200-2. The subglottic location of the mass *(arrow)* is well depicted on the sagittal reconstruction of the axial computed tomographic slices.

Page numbers followed by "f" indicate figures.